PEDIATRIC MASSAGE THERAPY

2nd EDITION

D1341668

PEDIATRIC MASSAGE THERAPY

2nd EDITION

MARYBETTS SINCLAIR, LMT

Corvallis, Oregon

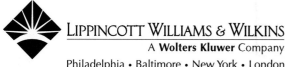

LIPPINCOTT WILLIAMS & WILKINS
A **Wolters Kluwer** Company

Philadelphia • Baltimore • New York • London
Buenos Aires • Hong Kong • Sydney • Tokyo

Senior Acquisitions Editor: Peter J. Darcy
Associate Development Editor: David Payne
Senior Marketing Manager: Christen DeMarco
Project Editor: Caroline Define
Indexer: Angie Wiley

Designer: Doug Smock
Art Direction: Jonathan Dimes
Artwork: David Rini and Kim Battista
Typesetter: Lippincott Williams & Wilkins
Printer: Quebecor

The publisher is not responsible (as a matter of product liability, negligence or otherwise) for any injury resulting from any material contained herein. This publication contains information relating to general principles of medical care which should not be construed as specific instructions for individual patients.

Printed in the United States of America

Library of Congress Cataloging-in-Publication Data

Sinclair, Marybetts.
    Pediatric massage therapy / Marybetts Sinclair.—2nd ed.
       p. ; cm.
    Rev. ed. of: Massage for healthier children, 1992.
    Includes bibliographical references and index.
    ISBN 0-7817-4219-6
       1. Massage for children. I. Sinclair, Marybetts. Massage for healthier children. II. Title.
    [DNLM: 1. Massage—methods—Child. WB 537 S616p 2005]
RJ53.M35S56 2005
615.8'22'083—dc22

                                                              2003069525

The publishers have made every effort to trace the copyright holders for borrowed material. If they have inadvertently overlooked any, they will be pleased to make the necessary arrangements at the first opportunity.

To purchase additional copies of this book, call our customer service department at **(800) 638-3030** or fax orders to **(301) 824-7390**. For other book services, including chapter reprints and large quantity sales, ask for the Special Sales department.

For all other calls originating outside of the United States, please call **(301)714-2324**.

Visit Lippincott Williams & Wilkins on the Internet: http://www.lww.com. Lippincott Williams & Wilkins customer service representatives are available from 8:30 am to 6:00 pm, EST, Monday through Friday, for telephone access.

05 06 07 08 09

1 2 3 4 5 6 7 8 9 1

This book is dedicated to two groups of people.

First, those giants upon whose shoulders this work stands:
Judith Bluestone, Moshe Feldenkrais, Tiffany Field, Karen Olness,
Meir Schneider, Agatha Thrash, and Janet Travell.

and

Second, my children, Rachel and Daniel. I love you with all my heart.

FOREWORD

Perhaps the last place in the world one would think of looking to find evidence for the powerful effects of human touch and human contact on physical health would be in the social isolation of a soundproofed Pavlovian Chamber. Yet it was precisely there, in 1962, at the Johns Hopkins Medical School, where I first witnessed the remarkable ways that human touch could alter heart rate, blood pressure, and coronary blood flow in dogs. It was there too that I first had the privilege of meeting my graduate school professor, W. Horsley Gantt, M.D. (a physician who had studied with Ivan P. Pavlov for 7 years and translated his research into English), and come to learn of his research studies on what he called "The Effect of Person." He would have easily recognized Marybetts Sinclair's text, *Pediatric Massage Therapy*, as an elementary component of his "Effect of Person," and he would have been delighted to see it emerge as an integral part of pediatric care.

Ironically, 1962 was part of an era in which mechanistic medicine had reached its high water mark. Dr. Christian Barnard electrified the world when he performed the first heart transplant operation in South Africa in 1969, helping to solidify the impression that the human heart was nothing more and nothing less than a mere pump. A few years earlier, the genetic code had been cracked, and the double helix was unraveled, helping to reinforce the perception that all disease could be unraveled and controlled within a few years. In that era, it was difficult to generate much excitement in the scientific community about research findings demonstrating that petting a dog could elicit an immediate 50% reduction in heart rate or blood pressure or that human contact could elicit greater increases in coronary blood flow than vigorous exercise. There seemed to be little room within the protein molecules of the double helix or within air compressors helping to keep mechanical hearts beating to fully appreciate the vital importance of human touch or human contact on our physical health. It was an era in which Marybetts' text on pediatric massage would have had a difficult time finding a receptive audience.

Fortunately, over the past 40 years, much has changed. A large number of studies have shown that even the most elementary forms of human touch can have dramatic effects on the heart rate, heart rhythm, and blood pressure of patients in coronary care and shock trauma units. In the intervening years, an ever-burgeoning literature has shown that social isolation, lack of social support, and human loneliness are major contributors to sharply increased risks of disease and premature death. We have also come to understand that dialogue, both verbal and nonverbal, has highly significant effects on the human cardiovascular system and exerts a vital role in physical health. Our understanding also has come full circle in this regard. Now it is well recognized that not only can human beings elicit major changes in a dog's heart rate and blood pressure, but also that the simple act of petting a dog can have a reciprocal and equally profound influence on human cardiovascular health. We have come to recognize that dialogue is the elixir of life.

The most elementary component of dialogue begins at birth and involves tactile contact. Fortunately, few health professionals would argue any longer that pediatric massage does not have important, indeed vital, consequences for the health of infants and children. Marybetts Sinclair's revised and beautifully illustrated text, *Pediatric Massage Therapy*, is a gift to all health professionals. It is a source of great satisfaction to recognize that her book has found an enduring home within the health community. It is especially gratifying to recognize that legions of infants and children, not yet able to read her book, will be the primary beneficiaries.

James J. Lynch, Ph.D.
Baltimore, Maryland
Professor Emeritus, Johns Hopkins Medical School
Author of: (1) The Broken Heart:
The Medical Consequences of Loneliness;
(2) The Language of the Heart:
The Body's Response to Human Dialogue;
(3) A Cry Unheard: New Insights into the Medical
Consequences of Loneliness

PREFACE

PURPOSE

Because of an increased acceptance of massage by the general public and greatly increased educational requirements for massage practitioners, the field of professional massage therapy has expanded significantly in the last few decades. In addition to normal healthy people, many special populations who can especially benefit from massage have been identified, such as athletes, the elderly, and abuse victims. However, almost all of the emphasis has been on massage for adults. Little information has been available about why and how to apply the hands-on therapist's knowledge of massage to children. *Pediatric Massage Therapy* has been written to fill this gap in information. It provides students and the practitioners of massage with the information and tools they need to apply it to children. It contains information on using massage to: (1) enhance both the development and the quality of life of normal children, (2) treat a wide variety of pediatric aches and pains and injuries, and (3) improve the lives of children with disabilities in many ways.

APPROACH

Pediatric Massage Therapy is based upon my 30 years of experience of giving massages to infants, children, and adults in a variety of settings including health spas, private homes, counseling centers, infant massage classes, low-income medical clinics, nursing homes, chiropractic offices, and third-world medical clinics. During that time, I learned that massage could help relieve suffering caused by many types of injuries, many types of stress, and many chronic conditions. However, my close observation of adults and children also gave rise to many difficult questions, such as:

- How do children develop chronic tension in various places in their bodies at such young ages?
- How do children develop areas of hypersensitivity and deep tension, of which they can be completely unaware?

- How does emotional stress manifest itself in so many different places in their bodies at different times, and in such very different ways?
- Why do so many adults have deeply ingrained patterns of muscle tension whose effects can be alleviated with massage but never really go away?

These unanswered questions spurred me to study the process of normal child development, to investigate research on touch and massage, and to learn about many specific fields of knowledge that, in some way, touch upon massage and bodywork; these include psychology, the history of medicine, biology, medical and physical anthropology, and naturopathic medicine. I found classic case studies detailing the use of massage for various pediatric problems. I listened carefully to the experiences of a great variety of healthcare professionals who work with children and to the experiences of the parents, who know their children the best. Their stories were often inspiring and offered insight into the various effects of massage and caring touch, and into the questions mentioned above. Their well-documented anecdotes did not offer hard and fast rules, but instead, they provided an idea of the possibilities of massage with children and the importance of working with children while their open minds, hearts, and bodies can allow change.

Furthermore, because there are currently no sufficient large-scale, rigorous scientific studies that can document the effects of massage on children, the use of such information from healthcare professionals probably gives the best picture of the possibilities of massage therapy with children. Of course, not every positive effect seen by these professionals will be replicated by every other trained practitioner, but this should not stop us from considering the possibility of massage therapy being beneficial for a host of different conditions. As long as no unfounded claims are made and contraindications are observed, massage with children is safe; at the very least, children will be given the opportunity to experience safe and nurturing touch. Quite possibly, they will benefit from massage in many other ways.

Thus, I incorporate in this book the results of investigations and case studies from my own practice. I have also included clinical reports from as long as two generations ago, which clearly demonstrate that healthy touch during childhood has been a concern for a long time.

ORGANIZATION AND FEATURES

As mentioned above, it is the goal of this book to guide the reader on how to use massage with healthy children, children experiencing common discomforts or injuries, and children with disabilities. Thus, the first three chapters of the book, "The Benefits of Massage for Children," "Not a Miniature Adult: The Unique Dynamics of Pediatric Massage," and "Pediatric Massage and Hydrotherapy Techniques," cover general principles and techniques of pediatric massage that are useful for working with all children. Chapter 4, "Massage and Hydrotherapy for Pediatric Injuries," and Chapter 5, "Massage and Hydrotherapy for the Common Discomforts of Childhood," cover the treatment of common pediatric injuries and discomforts. Chapter 6, "Massage and Hydrotherapy for Children with Disabilities," covers a number of common pediatric disabilities and diseases, and how to use massage and hydrotherapy to treat the children who have them. Finally, Appendix A provides guidelines on how to instruct parents in using massage with their children.

The following features are included in the book as learning aids:

- Key Points at the beginning of each chapter provide critical learning objectives for students.
- Point of Interest Boxes highlight interesting facts and concepts related to the content.
- Case Studies put concepts presented in the text into a real-life context.
- Checklist Boxes summarize specific massage protocols in quick-reference lists.
- Review Questions at the end of each chapter allow students to self-review the information they've just read.

A NOTE ON GENDER LANGUAGE

Every effort has been made to keep the language in this book gender-neutral, except in portions of the book that relate exclusively to boys or to girls. However, in the instruction sections, when a child is pictured, the gender of that child is used.

A NOTE ON THERAPIES NOT SUBSTANTIATED BY SCIENTIFIC EVIDENCE

Hands-on therapies such as craniosacral therapy, acupressure, and Polarity therapy, are not accepted as valid by the scientific community at this time. However, because so many experienced, long-time practitioners and their patients have found that these therapies have important benefits, I have included information about them. Hopefully in the future, as research is done on these therapies and as our understanding of the human mind and body becomes more sophisticated, we will understand the mechanisms by which they work. (It is even possible that the explanations now given for their therapeutic effects may be shown to be invalid).

FINAL NOTE

It is important to understand that because children are so dependent upon adults for support, the quality of the environment in which they live has even more influence upon them than it does upon adults. For children to flourish, their immediate families, the societies in which they live, the type of schools they attend, the state of the environment in their communities, and the political situation in their countries must be healthy. Let us all work toward improving this "big picture" to support the physical and emotional health of our children.

Marybetts Sinclair, LMT

ACKNOWLEDGMENTS

A book such as this is never only the work of one person, and the author has many people to thank. First of all, thanks to Lippincott Williams & Wilkins for recognizing the desire of many massage therapists for a book like this and for helping me so much in bringing it to completion. A special thanks to my hard-working and dedicated editor David Payne. Developmental editor Laura Bonazzoli, the queen of turning straw into gold, deserves huge thanks for her excellent feedback, which was based on her wide experience in medical writing, great organizational and editorial skills, and her compassionate nature. This book owes its present improved form more to her help than to anyone's. Ruth Werner provided me with insightful, informed, right-on-the money criticism—thanks Ruth! Also, many thanks to my good friend Robert Baldwin for a heroic editing job and for those handouts from your high school writing class; I'm pretty sure I should have taken your class more than once!

Many thanks to all those who consented to be interviewed for the special needs chapter: Brian Athorp, Diane Keene, Mary Polk, Eugenio Bruni, Lyse Lussier, Pamela Marshalla, Kathy Knowles, Pamela Yeaton, Meir Schneider, Diane Charmley, Renee Weaver, Helen Campbell, Marty Folin, Larry Burns-Vidlak, Deborah Bowes, Ann Perrault, and Kathleen Weber. A special thanks to longtime myotherapist Bonnie Prudden for consenting to share her years of expertise.

The reference librarians at the Corvallis Public Library carried on their tradition of being resourceful, cheerful, and efficient throughout the writing of this book; they have been a huge help to me in all the writing I have done and to our family during our homeschooling years. Good Samaritan Hospital librarians Dorothy O'Brien and Anna Mihok came through for me at the last minute a number of times with obscure articles. Thanks to "Dear Diedrich" Dasenbrock for the wonderful photographs that served as the source of the drawings, and thanks to all my charming models and their parents. Additional photographs were kindly taken by Michael McWilliams. David Rini and Kim Battista have enriched the book immeasurably with their artistic skill in turning the photographs and other illustrations into gorgeous drawings.

My personal Corvallis community has given me great emotional support during some critical times, including my Poplar Place neighbors (Darrylann and Bill Peterson, Margaret and Joaquim Kummerow, Rolland Roberts, Lea Lutz, and Mauren Beezhold), Ann Huster, Karan Fairchild, Judi and Peter, my dear Mary Orr, Sharon Rose, Scott Gentry, Diana Artemis, Mark Giblin, the lovely Rolfettes, and the ever-supportive mom's group. A special thanks to Dean and Lila McQueen, whose support has been both gracious and kind and who gave me the tools to use my brain to more of its full potential. I am also deeply indebted to Michael McWilliams, whose support for my work has come in many forms and without whom *Pediatric Massage Therapy* would never have been written. I thank my wonderful children, Rachel and Daniel, who have been teaching me about being a parent and what it means to love a child since the day they were born. Surely they have taught me more about the growth and development of children than all the textbooks in the world. May their own children enrich their lives in as many ways as they have mine. And finally, thank you, Mom—I appreciate you more all the time.

Marybetts Sinclair, LMT

REVIEWERS

Diane Charmley, RN, LMT
Portland, OR

Terry Graham, PT
Performance Physical Therapy
Seattle, WA

Kimberlee Hoover, CMT
SPARTA, Inc.
Orlando, FL

Dawn Tierno, LMT
New Milford, CT

Ruth Werner, LMT, NCTMB
Myotherapy College of Utah
Layton, UT

CONTENTS

APPENDIX

TEACHING MASSAGE TO PARENTS   201

THE BENEFITS OF MASSAGE FOR CHILDREN

After completing this chapter, the student will be able to:

1. Explain the physiologic effects of massage with children.
2. Explain the emotional benefits of massage with children.
3. Explain the importance of touch in the emotional development of children.
4. Identify the major stressors in the lives of modern children.
5. Describe the signs of stress in modern children.
6. Describe the fight-or-flight reaction in children.
7. Explain how children may react when confronted with overwhelming levels of stress.
8. Describe the long-term effects of local physical stress and pain on children.
9. Describe mind-body approaches to stress-related health problems of children.
10. Explain how the individual's body image develops.
11. Explain how touch and massage help develop a healthy body image in children.

Every massage therapist has had the sad experience of treating adults who have come in for hands-on treatment, yet are afraid of being touched. As children, these fearful adults might have grown up in nontouching families or suffered physical trauma, painful medical treatment, or even physical or sexual abuse. With these experiences, children often learn to avoid and deny their need for touch. As a result, as adults, they may be touch deprived, socially isolated, and have difficulty forming and maintaining intimate relationships. Because receiving health care—especially massage therapy—almost always involves touch, it may be difficult for them to accept. In contrast, those who are exposed to sensitive, caring massage when they are children learn to have a healthy adult attitude toward touch. Giving and receiving massage is a normal part of their lives—a tool that helps them relax, helps injuries heal, and enhances their health.

Massage therapy can be equally important as a way to improve the quality of a child's life. This chapter will demonstrate that massage has proven physiologic benefits, reduces stress, and provides perceptual feedback that is vital to help children form a strong and positive body image. Chapter 4 will demonstrate how massage can treat common pediatric injuries, Chapter 5 will explore the many ways that massage can relieve common pediatric discomforts, and, in Chapter 6, the reader will learn that children with disabilities and chronic musculoskeletal problems can benefit tremendously from regular massage. From helping to heal birth trauma to soothing a stressed-out teenager, massage can dramatically help children. Many adults with long-term physical pain and dysfunction that began with a severe childhood injury or trauma could have escaped long-term effects if they had received massage therapy at the time of injury (see Figure 1–1).

PHYSIOLOGIC BENEFITS OF MASSAGE

Although comparatively little research has been done on the effects of massage on children, research has

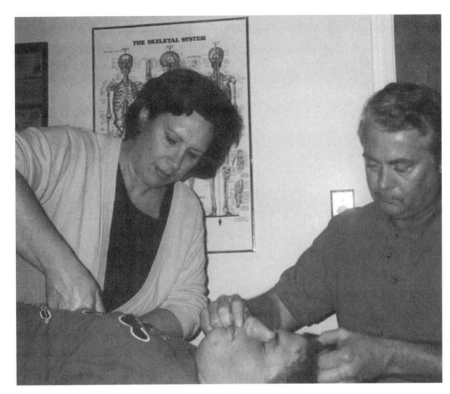

FIGURE 1–1 ■ Massage therapists Dianne and Rich Keene use massage to help their son Tim. Photo courtesy of Theresa George, Warren, MI.

confirmed that massage with adults has the following effects:

- prevents chronic musculoskeletal problems through early treatment of fascial restriction and myofascial trigger points
- relaxes muscles
- stretches muscle and connective tissue
- increases venous blood and lymph flow
- relieves pain
- reduces heart rate and blood pressure (temporarily)
- promotes deep relaxation
- changes production of certain hormones
- promotes deeper breathing
- stimulates the flow of cerebrospinal fluid
- improves immune function
- reduces anxiety, insomnia, and depression[1-4]

This is a current discussion of the physiologic effects of massage with children; however, it is hoped that as more research is completed in the near future, far more information will be available. With little or no documentation that is specific to children available, firsthand observations can help us understand the effects of massage.

Before we begin, please note that splitting the experience of touch into different "effects" is an oversimplification of a truly complex process. As infants, all mammals, including humans, depend on the physical contact of their mother for both warmth and food; they will die without her contact. Our mammalian craving for touch is originally a matter of pure survival; our reaction to touch is primal, and the effects that touch has on us are profound. When one human being touches another, we respond with our whole being. In reality, physiologic effects cannot be separated from the emotional effects. Physiologic effects, emotional effects, and even spiritual effects all happen at once. Our knowledge about the effects of human contact is still rather primitive and will certainly change as we learn more. The study described in Point of Interest Box 1-1 demonstrates that only four decades ago, science thought that the effects of touch could be separated from the effects of one person on another. While this study may seem laughably primitive to today's reader, our present understanding about touch and its effects may soon be just as outdated.

PREVENTION OF CHRONIC MUSCULOSKELETAL PROBLEMS

Note: for more information on fascial shortening and trigger points in children, see Chapter 2, page 39.

Myofascial release techniques have been successful in releasing fascial restriction and changing posture in children (see Figure 1–2). Fascial restriction may occur in utero and be present at birth. For example, autopsies of infants who died at birth have disclosed fascial shortness along large functional areas, such as the

(text continues on page 4)

POINT OF INTEREST BOX 1–1
The Problem of Isolating the Effects of Touch

In a now-classic study, Temerlin et al. tried to separate the effects of "mothering" from that of tactile stimulation. Thirty-two institutionalized, developmentally disabled boys received special mothering for 10 minutes a day, 5 days a week, for 8 weeks. Group 1 received hugging, cuddling, and rocking, during which time the "mothers" continually rubbed the boys' skin. Group 2 received the same treatment except that the mothers wore long-sleeved plastic raincoats and surgical gloves. Group 3 received passive mothering; the mothers were sitting completely still with their arms at their sides, looking straight ahead and saying nothing. Group 4 also received passive mothering, except that the mothers not only sat motionless, they wore plastic raincoats and surgical gloves.

The boys who received active mothering with actual skin-to-skin contact made significantly higher weight gains than any other group during the period of the experiment. Two boys who had been mute began saying "ma-ma" to their "mother." The most striking finding of this study is that the children did respond physiologically and emotionally to what was only a small fraction of the normal loving interaction between mother and child. Today, we know that it is not possible to separate the effects of touch from the interaction between the person touching and the person being touched, and this study appears ridiculous in its attempt to do so. Because our understanding of touch and its effects is still evolving, however, our present knowledge may look just as primitive in the future. This study was also clearly unethical, subjecting the boys to probable emotional trauma, and would never be allowed to take place today.[5]

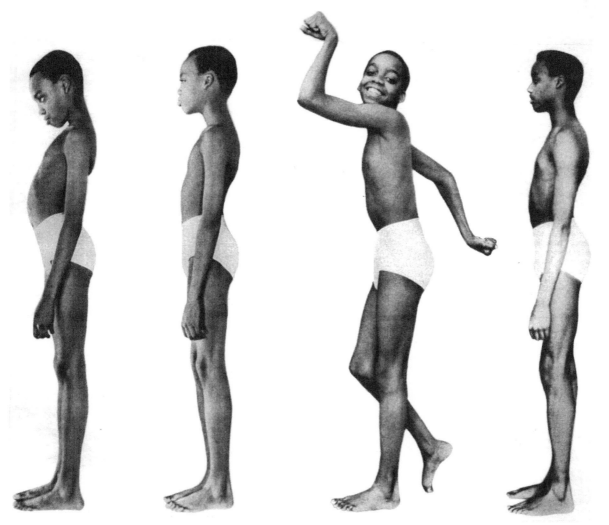

FIGURE 1–2 ■ Eleven-year-old boy, before and after ten rolfing sessions. Rolfing has greatly improved this boy's alignment. Reprinted with permission from: Toporek R: *The Promise of Rolfing Children* (monograph). Philadelphia, PA: Transformation Network, 1981.

lower back or the outside of the thigh, and muscle ad-herence to fascial wrappings. These fascial restrictions are probably caused by the child's position in utero.[6] Although children may appear to outgrow some de-formities as they become increasingly mobile, fascial shortening may remain for life and have profound ef-fects on movement and posture. For example, fibrous shortening of the sternocleidomastoid, acquired by a twisted neck in utero, may not only remain, it may cause discomfort and pain and affect the child's head posture, cervical spine mobility, and even the growth of the cranial bones (see Torticollis, page 147).

Myofascial trigger points are common in children (see Figure 1–3). They have been treated successfully

(text continues on page 7)

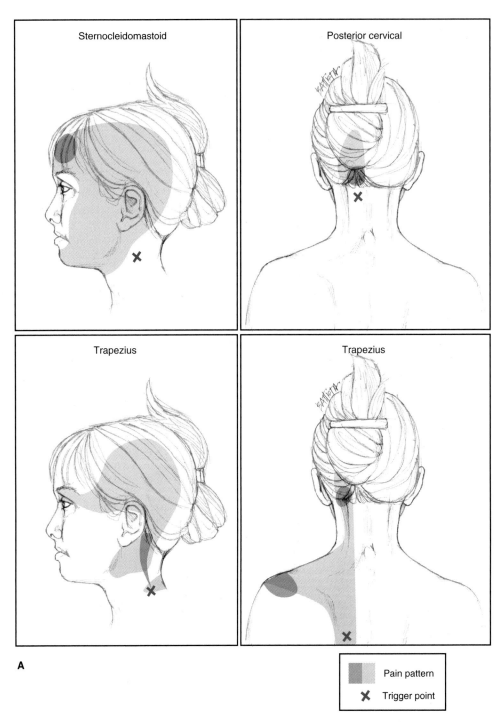

Sternocleidomastoid

Posterior cervical

Trapezius

Trapezius

A

Pain pattern

✖ Trigger point

FIGURE 1–3 ■ Trigger points in children. Trigger points can be initiated by many factors, including physical trauma or injury, sustained contrac-tion of a muscle, and prolonged poor posture.

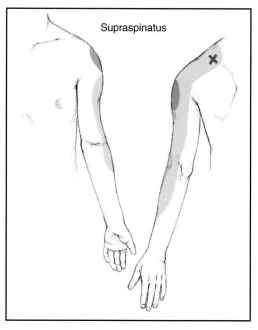

Supraspinatus

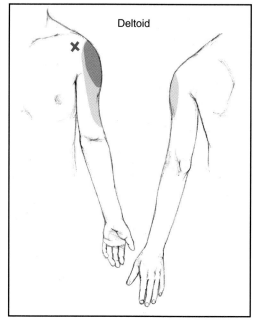

Deltoid

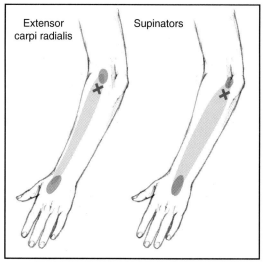

Extensor carpi radialis Supinators

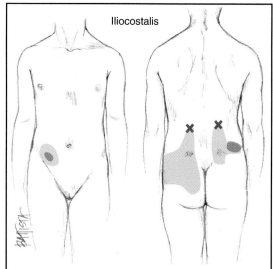

Iliocostalis

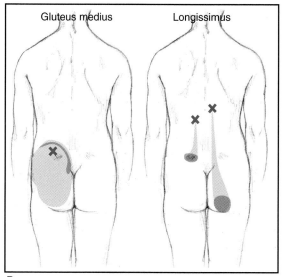

Gluteus medius Longissimus

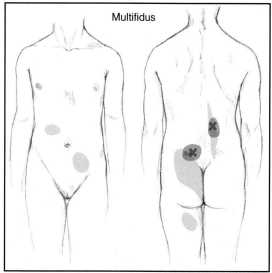

Multifidus

B

Gluteus minimus

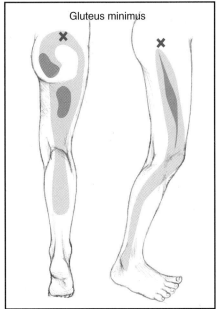

Abductor longus

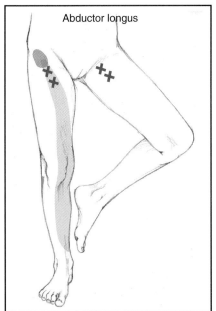

Vastus
medialis

Vastus
lateralis

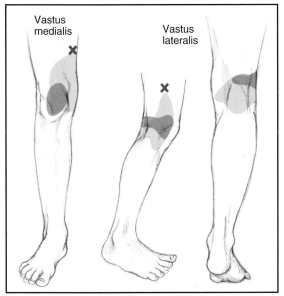

Biceps
femoris

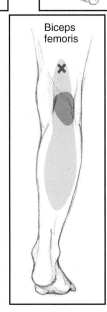

Soleus   Gastrocnemius

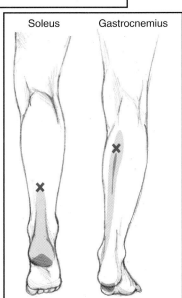

Tibialis
anterior

Long
extensors

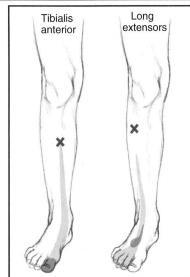

Short
extensors

Peroneus
longus

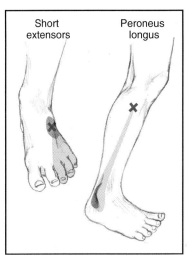

Abductor hallucis

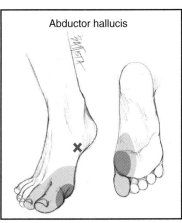

c

with ischemic compression and deep friction, as well as with injection and coolant spray.[4,7-10] Trigger points can be caused by the position of the fetus in utero; the normal birth process; and by birth trauma, such as extreme pressure on the head, traction on the head, or a forceps delivery.

Trigger points in children may be also be initiated by upper respiratory and other infections and injuries.[7] Unless treated, these trigger points may cause problems during childhood and on into adulthood; for example, trigger points in the temporalis, occipitalis, and posterior cervicals, all of which may be caused by birth trauma, are known to induce migraine headaches in adults.[4]

MUSCLE RELAXATION

Hernandez-Reif et al. found that Swedish massage reduced spasticity and improved muscular flexibility in infants with cerebral palsy.[11] The authors noted decreased muscle tension in children with cerebral palsy and spinal cord injuries after massage. (Because both conditions originate from damage to the central nervous system, and this damage is not directly impacted by massage, massage must be frequent and regular to maintain improvement.) Normal children also have decreased muscle tension after massage. The therapist can see this decrease after a massage session—when the tense muscles of a certain area are more relaxed after massage, that area will lie flatter on the treatment table.

RELEASE OF RESTRICTIONS IN MUSCLE AND CONNECTIVE TISSUE

Certain types of massage manually stretch soft and connective tissue, such as skin, muscle, fascia, and scar tissue. After a massage session, the therapist can confirm this by palpation: Shortened muscle fibers or shortened connective tissue fibers will feel longer and more mobile after massage.

INCREASED CIRCULATION OF BLOOD AND LYMPH

Massage stimulates local circulation of blood. Blood vessels in the massaged area dilate and the blood supply to the massaged area increases, as much as tripling after 5 minutes of massage. Cardiovascular surgeon Mehmet Oz verified this effect by massaging the feet of a 16-year-old boy who had acute heart failure and a dangerously enlarged heart. Dr. Oz inserted a mechanical heart pump in the boy's heart as a temporary measure until a heart transplant was available. After the insertion of the mechanical pump, the boy's vital signs began to show that his condition was deteriorating because the pump's blood flow rate was very low (sensors in the pump showed exactly how much blood was being pumped out to his tissues). In desperation, Dr. Oz began to massage the boy's feet; as he rubbed and squeezed the boy's feet, the boy's blood flow rate began to rise. When massage was stopped, the rate would drop; when resumed, the rate would rise. After 45 minutes, the boy's blood flow rate finally stayed at a healthy level, and Dr. Oz was able to stop massage.[12]

The therapist can confirm the increase in blood flow by comparing the temperature of an area before and after massage with the hands—it will feel warmer, reflecting an increased flow of warm blood. The therapist can also confirm increased circulation by observing local color changes. For example, in a bedridden child or a child confined to a wheelchair, legs that are darker or dusky red will quickly become a more normal pink with a few minutes of Swedish massage. Sores, which are also dusky red, will quickly become a more normal pink after a few minutes of Swedish massage is applied to the general area of the sore. In certain areas of the body, such as the tops of the feet, veins refilling with blood can be seen after a compression stroke has momentarily interrupted the blood flow.

In adults, massage also enhances circulation of lymphatic fluid. Although research has not been done on the effects of lymphatic flow in children, firsthand observation confirms that massage moves lymphatic fluid. For example, children with swelling in the legs have decreased edema for 1 hour or more after 15 minutes of Swedish massage. This can be verified by visual inspection or by measuring the limb with a measuring tape.

There is a great deal of anecdotal evidence indicating that hands-on craniosacral therapy can affect the circulation of cerebrospinal fluid; at this time, however, no specific research verifies this change. Craniosacral therapy is believed to affect the flow of cerebrospinal fluid by freeing restrictions in connective tissue of the skull, spine, and sacrum, which then alters the rise and fall of cerebrospinal fluid within the meningeal compartment of the brain.[13] Future research will, hopefully, pinpoint the exact mechanisms.

ENHANCED IMMUNE FUNCTION

It seems likely that touch may influence immune function through alterations in the sympathetic nervous system. The stress of being separated from their mothers causes impaired immune function in a variety of young primates, either immediately or when they become adults. Young mammals that have been handled have better immune functions as adults than mammals that have not been handled.[14] Although numerous studies with premature and full-term infants show that massage enhances growth and development, no long-term studies have determined if immune function is improved as well. Two small-scale studies at the Touch Research Institute showed immune function improvement when children received massage. Children with leukemia (average age, 7 years) improved on all blood count measures, including white blood cell count, after a 20-minute massage every night for 30 nights.[15] Field found that teenagers who were HIV-positive had improved immune function after receiving a 20-minute seated massage twice a week for 12 weeks.[16]

OPTIMAL HORMONE LEVELS

Massage affects hormone levels. Small-scale studies at the Touch Research Institute found that premature babies who are massaged gain weight faster, even when they consume the same amount of formula as those who are not massaged, probably because massage stimulates the production of food absorption hormones, such as gastrin and insulin.[17] Healthy, full-term babies receiving effleurage-based massage at bedtime for 2 weeks had increased melatonin excretion at night, resulting in the adjustment of the infants to sleeping during the night and being active during the day sooner than the control infants not receiving massage.[18]

Effleurage-based massage is associated with decreased levels of **cortisol** in both normal, full-term infants and children with asthma, serious burns, bulimia, juvenile rheumatoid arthritis, posttraumatic stress syndrome, and psychiatric problems. Typically, salivary cortisol levels are decreased immediately after therapy sessions; a general decrease in both cortisol and **norepinephrine** then occurs across the treatment period. Another study showed that the blood glucose levels of children who were diabetic fell to a normal level after 1 month of receiving effleurage-based massage from their mothers at bedtime.[19]

PAIN RELIEF

Massage is an effective treatment for many types of pain. Touch Research Institute studies confirm that effleurage-based massage can relieve pain in children with juvenile rheumatoid arthritis and children with severe burns.[20,21] Kubsch et al. performed an experiment with pediatric and adult patients in a hospital emergency department. A 5-minute fingertip massage on or near the site of the patient's pain significantly reduced the amount of pain they experienced. Their blood pressure and heart rates were also lowered.[22]

In another study, connective tissue massage and mobilization was effective in resolving the diffuse, persistent pain of **reflex sympathetic dystrophy** in 4 of 5 girls. The girls were placed on a program that included self-massage, at least 3 times a day, and weight-bearing and range-of-motion exercises. Immobilization, the most common treatment for this condition, is of little benefit in resolving pain.[23]

The author has observed that Swedish massage relieves musculoskeletal pain in children with cerebral palsy, muscular dystrophy, polio, and spinal cord injuries. Massage therapists Dianne and Richard Keene have used a combination of techniques, including Swedish, acupressure, reflexology, craniosacral, and myofascial release, to help relieve the severe headaches experienced by their son Tim, who has hydrocephalus.[24]

IMPROVED RESPIRATION

Massage encourages full and effortless respiration. Twenty minutes of effleurage-based massage given by mothers to their children with asthma every night at bedtime for a 1-month period resulted in fewer asthma attacks and increased peak air flow and forced expiratory flow rates.[25] A pilot study by the Office of Education in Santa Cruz, California, found significant improvement in asthma symptoms in disabled children who received 8 weekly sessions of Jin Shin Do.[26] Children with cystic fibrosis had improved air flow readings after 1 month of effleurage-based massage.[27] After a massage session, the therapist can both feel and see an improvement in respiration: the amount of ribcage expansion can be felt with the hands before and after massage and the amount of expansion can be seen before and after massage.

RELAXATION

Gentle touch is the foundation of every massage and bodywork technique. If it is perceived as safe and nurturing, it encourages a relaxation response through its effect on the autonomic nervous system. In a classic study in a hospital shock-trauma unit, Lynch et al. found that simple touch had dramatic effects on the heart rate and rhythm of both adults and children. This touch was simply the taking of a patient's pulse for 3 minutes without conversation. Certain patients for whom these effects were seen were in comas or near death.[28] Another study found that preschoolers fell asleep faster and slept longer at naptime after receiving effleurage-based massage, presumably because they were more relaxed.[29]

Field found significant decreases in anxiety in studies with children with asthma, bulimia, severe burns, diabetes, juvenile rheumatoid arthritis, posttraumatic stress disorder, and psychiatric problems. These studies showed that effleurage-like stroking—as briefly as 15 minutes daily for 1 month—improved sleep patterns in sexually and physically abused children and in children and teens with psychiatric problems.[17]

The Santa Cruz Office of Education study found significant new signs of relaxation in 25 disabled children who received sessions of Jin Shin Do, including decreased insomnia, fewer temper tantrums, reduced body tension in gross motor activities, less frantic verbalizing, and more relaxed facial expressions.[26] In Eugene, Oregon, similar results were found in an acupressure project modeled after the Santa Cruz Jin Shin Do pilot study. Profoundly retarded and emotionally disturbed children were treated with a 30- to 45-minute acupressure session, twice a week for 6 weeks. Students showed improved relaxation during sessions and improvements in tension levels, body awareness, and class responsiveness.[30]

SENSORY STIMULATION

Massage can stimulate the nervous system; it is particularly important for children who are immobilized or otherwise lack normal tactile experiences. Massage strokes and passive movements help inform the child's brain about the many different qualities of her skin, such as its temperature, flexibility, and thickness. During massage, she also receives information about her body's position in space, its muscle tension, its movements, and its relationship to other people and objects in the environment. Point of Interest Box 1–2 illustrates that tactile stimulation can be crucial for normal development.[31]

Early sensory experience can have a profound impact on how the brain develops; there are probably measurable increases in brain growth for children who receive sufficient sensory stimulation over those who do not. Experiments with animals reared as pets, compared with animals reared in isolation, show that the pet's brains are heavier, thicker, and contain as many as 25% more **synapses** per neuron.[32] Tactile experiences must occur to normally develop those neurons, which are sensitive to tactile stimulation. Tactile stimulation in adulthood does not cause changes in brain growth because the most critical periods of brain growth are complete by age 7 (Land P, PhD, University of Pittsburgh, personal communication, January 2003).[33]

EMOTIONAL EFFECTS OF MASSAGE

RELIEF FROM PSYCHOLOGICAL DISTRESS

Caring human touch has an extraordinary power to soothe, reassure, and relieve anxiety. Triplett and Arneson studied nurses attempting to comfort hospitalized children (newborn to age 4). When the chil-

POINT OF INTEREST BOX 1–2
Effects of Extra Touch and Stimulation for Deprived Children

In 1990, massage therapist Faustine Settle spent 1 month as a volunteer in an orphanage in Nicoresti, Romania, where 115 multihandicapped orphans, ages 9 months to 16 years, lived. Conditions were extremely deprived, with a ratio of orphans to caregivers of 30:1. Economic conditions were so bad that no diapers were available and the orphanage was insufficiently heated. Prior to the winter of 1990, about 20 children died each year. During that winter, volunteer health professionals from abroad began arriving to take care of the children's needs. Their diagnosis of the cause of the high death rate in the orphanage was that the children were experiencing a failure to thrive due to touch deprivation and malnutrition.

Volunteers provided nurturing touch, including rocking, holding, and stroking. The room where Settle gave massages had to be locked while she worked with specific children because children were so drawn to the human contact that massage offered; she and other volunteers found that children screamed only when their work was finished and they put them down. Volunteers also treated infections, rashes, and fractures. Malnutrition was not addressed; children were not given more or better food. Only one child died that year. Because blood samples were not taken from the children, it is not possible to ascertain exactly what changed. However, because the children's nutrition was not improved, other profound physiologic changes evidently accounted for the decrease in the death rate.[31]

In 2000, pediatric nurse and massage therapist Diane Charmley volunteered in an orphanage in Romania. Her team of volunteers did daily massage with the children there. The volunteers also increased the amount of stimulation the children received in other ways, such as putting mirrors in the cribs to give the children something to look at, and moving them around instead of keeping the children in one place all day. Ms. Charmley did developmental testing with the children before and after massage and stimulation was offered; within 2 weeks, she found a marked improvement in their social behavior—they were much less apathetic and much more interactive (Charmley D, RN, personal communication, October 2002).

dren were distressed and crying, they were usually quieted with a combination of verbal comfort (talking or singing) and tactile comfort (patting and rocking). Children who received talking or singing but were not touched, rarely quieted quickly. Of those who received verbal and tactile comfort, 88% stopped crying after 5 minutes, compared with only 12% of the children who received verbal comfort alone.[34]

The need for tactile comfort is so strong in states of distress that children may instinctively try to comfort themselves with touch if there is no one else to give it to them. Family therapist Helen Colton treated an adult client whose mother had abandoned her at an orphanage when she was a small child. To comfort herself as a child, and later as an adult, she would hug herself and rock back and forth, repeating "I'm all I've got, I'm all I've got."[35] Field et al. found that after a 30-minute effleurage-based backrub for 5 days, teenagers in a hospital psychiatric ward were less anxious, slept better, and had lower cortisol and norepinephrine levels.[36] Another small Touch Research Institute study found that effleurage-based massage decreased anxiety and situational depression in children with posttraumatic stress disorder following Hurricane Andrew.[37]

THE IMPORTANCE OF CARING TOUCH

Robert Coles describes the power of touch to provide comfort and stability. He witnessed the courage of black children and their parents during the struggle for school integration in New Orleans in 1961. He was profoundly moved by the strength the young students showed as they faced white mobs. A mother of one child described her daughter's response to the school day: "My child comes home from school, and she's heard those white people shouting. She's not going to show them she's scared, not for a second, but she is scared, I know she is. And the first thing she does is come to me, and I hold her. Then she goes to get her snack, the Oreos and juice, and she's back, touching me. I'll be upset myself, so, thank God, *my* mother is still with us because I go to her, and she'll put her hand on my arm, and I'm all settled down again, and then I can put my hand on my daughter's arm! Like our minister says, the Lord touches us all the time, if we'll just let Him, and He works through each of us; so when my mother puts her hands on me and I put my hands on my child—it's God giving us strength."[38]

Touch between parents and children communicates caring, builds trust, and affirms their biologic connection. When touch is withheld during infancy or childhood, the effect on the emotional life of the individual may be profound and long lasting. Pediatrician Maurice Rosenthal interviewed 25 mothers of babies with eczema, as well as a control group of 18 mothers of babies without eczema. A significantly higher proportion of the babies with eczema had not received adequate physical contact, such as cuddling, and were often left to "cry it out" when there was nothing obviously wrong with them. Rosenthal felt that in certain predisposed infants, eczema was an indication that their needs for touch had not been met. A sudden decrease in physical contact—caused by abrupt cessation of breast-feeding, a maternal health problem, or the loss of someone to help with the baby—was followed rapidly by eczema in many cases.[39]

A 2½-year-old girl was referred to psychiatrist Philpe Seitz because she had been pulling her hair out for a year and was completely bald on one side of her head. The girl had been breast-fed for her first 2 weeks of life, then her mother abruptly stopped. She was then fed with a bottle and, later, solid foods. At 18 months, a punitive toilet training program was begun, including spankings and scolding. At this point, the girl began to refuse all solid foods, insisting on milk from a baby bottle. When feeding, she pulled hairs out of her scalp and rolled them against her upper lip and nose while the bottle was in her mouth. She stopped rolling the hairs the moment the bottle was removed from her mouth. On examination, the mother's nipples were found to have a ring of long, coarse hairs around them. When the girl was given a rubber nipple for her baby bottle that had a ring of coarse human hairs attached, she completely stopped pulling out her hair when feeding. Under stress, this small child had attempted to comfort herself by reproducing, as best she could, the exact type of tactile comfort she had received in only her first 2 weeks of life. The breast-feeding had clearly had a profound influence on her.[40] Biggar, after detailed observations of 94 3-month-old infants with their mothers, found that, when mothers consistently disliked having physical contact with their infants, those children were found to be unusually angry and aggressive at age 1 year.[41]

In a classic paper published in 1960, pediatric psychiatrists Kulka et al. observed that acute early tactile deprivation caused increased muscle tension in infants and might lead them to rock, bang their heads, or make other types of repetitive movements in an attempt to satisfy their own tactile and kinesthetic needs. Severe tactile deprivation as an infant may lead to hyperactivity or depression in childhood. Kulka treated a 7-year-old girl who was brought for psychiatric treatment because she was "bizarrely jumpy" and disturbing to the rest of her class in school. She was born premature; bottle fed; and, when her mother went back to work when the child was 5-weeks old, she was placed in a variety of homes. Her mother admitted she was not ready for the child and could not bear physical contact. Kulka treated children with similar histories by "babying" them—the child was allowed to sit on the therapist's lap, nurse from a baby bottle, ask to be rocked, and given soft toys to cuddle.[42] A similar approach was used by Zerbe when treating a 17-year-old female college student for bulimia. The student had not had a calm, soothing, or involved mother who cared for her, and, consequently, she lacked the capacity to soothe herself or provide nurturance. She was given a small, furry bunny to hold during times of stress and was instructed to remember her therapist's concern for her.[43]

Pediatric psychiatrists Shevrin and Toussieng, who worked with severely emotionally disturbed children who were deprived of tactile stimulation during infancy, concluded that when there is a disturbance in tactile stimulation during infancy, children may deny their need for touch and begin to avoid physical contact altogether, keeping a physical distance from others or creating an elaborate fantasy life. When touched by a person they had affection for, they had tremendous emotional conflict over the touch, both craving it and fearing it. One patient was a 15-year-old girl who was hospitalized when she threatened to kill her mother and herself. She had been raised on a rigid timetable and, if she was not scheduled to be picked up and fed, left to cry for long periods. At age 1, she began rocking in her crib (a common way to compensate for the lack of tactile stimulation). On the recommendation of her pediatrician, her legs were then splinted to her crib for 1 week. During psychotherapy, she expressed conflict over touch and recoiled from the mere memory of having accidentally touched her therapist. At one moment when she felt warm feelings for her therapist, she reached out and touched him but then backed away in fright, saying she would kill him. Then she tried to choke him. She also told him, "You should stay away from me because I am glass and would break if you touched me."

A fearful, suicidal, severely asthmatic 9-year-old boy would remain close to his therapist, yearning for contact but ready to flee if touched. His mother had never received much attention from her parents and remembered being repulsed by sitting in her mother's lap. The boy's surroundings had been made as sterile as possible, and he was touched only when unavoidable. His mother was afraid of touching her son and avoided kissing him. He was 7-months-old before being touched by his father. After working with such severely disturbed children, Shevrin and Toussieng concluded that severe conflict over lack of tactile stimulation could be resolved only through a long and arduous therapeutic process.[44]

STRESSORS IN THE LIFE OF THE MODERN CHILD

Contemporary American children should be experiencing lower levels of stress than in the past. Consider the many improvements in pediatric health. Until about 200 years ago, three-fourths of all children died before age 5, mostly of infectious diseases. Vaccines, antibiotics, and public health measures, such as pu-rification of drinking water and pasteurization of milk, have greatly reduced common pediatric illnesses and mortality rates.

The decreased amount of hard physical labor is another major improvement. Previously, children as young as age 6 or 7 were believed capable of working like adults and traditionally shared the burdens of unremitting domestic and agricultural labor. Child abuse and exploitation were common, and children were exposed to adult realities, such as sexuality and death. Around the end of the eighteenth century, Western society saw the rise of a new attitude toward children. Childhood was now considered a special stage in life, with attributes such as innocence, imagination, and closeness to nature. Conscientious parents struggled to preserve their children's innocence, shelter them from life's ups and downs, and keep childhood a carefree "golden age." Child labor laws were passed in the 1920s that prevented children from having to do so much physical labor. Modern conveniences made day-to-day life easier for all ages.

Childhood should now be much less stressful. Technology, however, has proved to have both benefits and drawbacks in modern society. The stressors discussed above have been replaced by psychological stressors. Social changes have caused parents to change their view of childhood and how children should be raised. Increasing numbers of parents now believe that children need an adult understanding of reality to prepare them to survive in an increasingly complex and uncontrollable world. Many parents no longer try to shield their children from adult realities such as violence, cruelty, sexuality, war, and natural disasters. Even those who would like to shield their children from these realities find it difficult to do so when both parents must work full-time and the extended family is no longer available to help care for children. Exposing children to adult realities before they are developmentally mature enough to handle them, however, can be highly stressful.[45]

Children are also treated more like adults; they are given far more choices that formerly would have been the prerogative of adults, such as choosing their own food, mealtimes, clothing, and entertainment. Having so many choices is a different type of stressor because, although children may seem mature enough to make decisions that once were made for them, too often this is not the case. Psychologist David Elkind, author of *The Hurried Child*, believes the new realities that send both parents into the workplace should not blind us to children's built-in limitations of responsibility, achievement, and loyalty. He feels it is important to recognize that children have special intellectual, emotional, and social needs that are not met when they are "turned loose" to care for themselves.[45] According to psychiatrist and eating disorder specialist

Katherine Zerbe, the end of family mealtimes and group dining experiences in college can contribute to the development of eating disorders. When children are left to fend for themselves, the responsibility of eating properly proves too great for most of them.[43]

Pediatrician Benjamin Spock stated that, although human beings do make some adjustment to stress, he felt children being brought up with these new stresses would become harsher, more intensely competitive, and more greedy.[46] Specific new stresses affecting children today are listed below.

Greater Exposure to the Adult World's Problems at Earlier Ages

The average American child watches 5 hours of television a day.[47] Violence, adult sexuality, crime, natural disasters, and other adult realities are readily accessible to children watching television. On September 11, 2001, and many times in the succeeding days, children watching television were repeatedly exposed to scenes of the World Trade Center collapse, with graphic images of destruction and death. Preschoolers have particularly highly active imaginations and may be more prone to worry after such exposure, but all children are susceptible to free-floating anxiety after being exposed to films or television programs they are not emotionally prepared to handle.[45,47]

As a representative of UNICEF, James Garbarino interviewed Kuwaiti children at the conclusion of the Gulf War in 1991. These children had been traumatized by firsthand exposure to Iraqi atrocities. Surprisingly, a follow-up study conducted 1 year later by psychologists Kathi Nader and Robert Pynoos revealed that more children were traumatized after the war was over by secondhand exposure to Iraqi atrocities on videotape as part of a Kuwaiti government political education campaign.[48]

According to psychologist Elkind, exposure to television represents a unique type of stress for children. "Television forces children to accommodate a great deal and inhibits the assimilation of material. Consequently, the television child knows much more than he or she can ever understand. This discrepancy between what children know and what they can process is the major stress of television."[45] Watching television also precludes free active play, one of the best ways for children to relax.

Television, however, is only one element of our media-saturated culture. Much of the music children listen to undermines impulse control through the glamorization of sex and drugs. These are messages to which children are particularly susceptible at an age when loss of impulse control can have disastrous consequences. The entertainment industry deliberately markets violent music, movies, and video games to underage children.[49]

Intense Media Pressure for Children to Be Thin

Media pressure to be thin is stronger now than at any time in the last two decades.[50] The ideal body type is now at the thinnest 5% of a normal weight distribution.[51] Typical beauty contestants and models weigh 13–19% below normal healthy weight.[52,53] Children's books have progressively portrayed girls as thinner over the last 80 years; no such trend has been seen for boys.[54]

Deterioration of Family Support

Children in America have been deeply affected by changes in the structure and living arrangements of the nuclear and extended family. Separation and divorce now affect 1 of 3 marriages.[45] In 1970, 85% of all children lived in a household with married parents; however, by 1993, this number dropped to 71%.[55] The amount of time parents spend with their children dropped 40% between 1965 and 1989.[56] Parents are working more and have less time for child rearing than in the 1970s and 1980s.[45] Because of the highly mobile American society, extended family members are often not geographically close enough to help single and working parents by spending time with their children. Many children spend more and more time alone or with their peers than ever before.

James Alan Fox, dean of Northeastern University's College of Criminal Justice, believes that the unraveling of the American family is responsible for much of the increase in juvenile violence (see page 15). According to Fox, "Too many parents are going off to work or otherwise ignoring their children before they've bonded. Without some substitute to become a child's emotional anchor, such as a grandparent, child-care provider, or family friend, the child is not going to be getting strong antiviolent messages and television may become the child's primary socializer." He stresses the need for both a national system of day care and for more and better schoolteachers to essentially fill the place of absent parents.[57]

High Incidence of Child Maltreatment (Physical and Sexual Abuse)

Each year, child welfare agencies in the United States receive more than three million allegations of childhood abuse and neglect, and collect enough evidence to confirm more than one million cases. In 2,000 to 3,000 of those cases, the child dies as a result of the abuse. Long-term effects of mistreatment include physical, emotional, and psychological problems.[58]

Loss of Religious Beliefs and the Support of Religious Communities

The impact of religious life, which has been a positive socializing source in the lives of American children for generations, has been declining since the 1960s. After a review of more than 50 national polls, time diaries, and surveys, sociologist Robert Putnam concluded that church participation (including not only attending church services but also participating in church-related activities, such as youth groups) has fallen by about 30% in the last generation. The number of children ages 3 to 12 and those in high school involved in church activities has declined significantly, and the number of incoming college freshman with no religious affiliation has increased.[59]

Increased Competition and Decreased Playtime

Parents are under more social pressure to enroll children in organized sports and other activities that may not be age-appropriate. Psychologist Davis Elkind believes there is little value and considerable risk in engaging young children in organized team or individual sports until, at least, age 6 or 7. Children may be forced into activity that is simply too much for their stage of body development. According to child psychiatrist Elizabeth Guthrie, "The entire specialty of pediatric sports medicine owes its existence to our allowing our children to 'overdo' it with sports."[60] Many parents feel pressured to enroll their children in an increasing number of activities, so that even an activity that the child enjoys may lose its appeal as it becomes part of a tightly packed schedule. Rather than letting children play, these types of activities transform play, nature's way of dealing with stress, into work.[45]

There is also increased pressure on many children to perform academically at an early age. For example, more children are taking college entrance exams at earlier ages. More than 172,000 students in eighth grade or lower took SAT or ACT college entrance exams in 2001, up 19% since 1996.[61] These tests are designed for high school students and, although occasionally appropriate for the younger child, they are great sources of stress for most children.

Educator and therapist Maureen Murdock, who teaches guided relaxation to her students, tells how children really feel when coping with a high-pressure lifestyle. "In an exercise that I once did with my third-grade class about what they didn't like in their lives, the symbol that appeared in all of their drawings was a ticking alarm clock. When I asked them to elaborate about the clock, typical responses were: 'I hate rushing from school to soccer practice' 'I never have any time to just sit'; 'I don't get enough time to play with

my friends because my mom has to pick me up early so she can go someplace else.' In a similar exercise with older students, one commented: 'I thought teachers would let up on the work during senior year, but we have more than ever. I have no time for my friends.'"[62]

Inadequate Child Care

Today, more than 60% of mothers with a child younger than 2 years of age are employed. More than 3 million children have mothers who returned to work before their child was 1 year old.[63] Entering high-quality day care is associated with greater cognitive, emotional, and social competence in middle childhood and adolescence; however, many studies have found that the majority of American day care services are either mediocre or poor.[64]

The economic environment also contributes to the plight of America's children. In many of today's families, both parents must work full-time, and so children are often far less supervised than only a few generations ago.

Poverty

One of five children in America today lives in poverty. A child growing up in poverty is more likely to experience abuse, neglect, malnutrition, homelessness, and substandard day care. Factors such as poor diet, poor health care, and higher stress levels lead to worsened health in poor children.[65] Childhood poverty also places young people at risk for a range of long-term psychosocial problems, including failure in school, teenage pregnancy, crime, and drug abuse.

THE BEHAVIORAL EFFECTS OF STRESS ON THE MODERN CHILD

What evidence is available that indicates these new forms of stress are taking a toll on American children? A review of statistical data on the social and psychological problems involving children shows that many of them are becoming more common. In the past, most children did not encounter many of these problems before adulthood; as the problems become more common, they are altering the nature of childhood itself (Table 1–1).

High School Dropout Rates

In 1999, one of five teenagers aged 15 to 18 dropped out of school before graduation. Those with the lowest family incomes were five times as likely to drop out of school as those with the highest family incomes.[66]

TABLE 1–1   CHILD STRESS SCALE: LIFE EVENT SCORES (IN LIFE CHANGE) BY AGE GROUP

Life Events	Preschool	Elementary	Junior High	Senior High
Beginning nursery school, first grade, seventh grade, or high school	42	46	45	42
Change to a different school	33	46	52	56
Birth or adoption of a sibling	50	50	50	50
Sibling leaving home	39	36	33	37
Hospitalization of sibling	37	41	44	41
Death of sibling	59	68	71	68
Change of father's occupation, requiring increased absence from home	36	45	42	38
Loss of job by a parent	23	38	48	46
Marital separation of parents	74	78	77	69
Divorce of parents	78	84	84	77
Hospitalization of parent (serious illness)	51	55	54	55
Death of a parent	89	91	94	87
Death of a grandparent	30	38	35	36
Marriage of parent to stepparent	62	65	63	63
Jail sentence of parent for 30 days or less	34	44	50	53
Jail sentence of parent for 1 year or more	67	67	76	75
Addition of third adult to family (e.g., grandparent)	39	41	34	34
Change in parents' financial status	21	29	40	45
Mother beginning to work	47	44	36	26
Decrease in number of arguments between parents	21	25	29	27
Increase in number of arguments between parents	44	51	48	46
Decrease in number of arguments with parents	22	27	29	26
Increase in number of arguments with parents	39	47	46	47
Discovery of being an adopted child	33	52	70	64
Acquiring a visible deformity	52	69	83	81
Having a visible congenital deformity	39	60	70	62
Hospitalization of yourself (child)	59	62	59	58
Change in acceptance by peers	38	51	68	67
Outstanding personal achievement	23	39	45	46
Death of a close friend (child's)	38	53	65	63
Failure of a year in school		57	62	56
Suspension from school		46	54	50
Pregnancy in unwed teenage sister		36	60	64
Becoming involved with drugs or alcohol		61	70	76
Becoming a full-fledged member of a church/synagogue		25	28	31
Not making an extracurricular activity you wanted to be involved in (e.g., athletic activity or band)			49	55
Breaking up with a boyfriend or girlfriend			47	53
Beginning to date			55	51
Fathering an unwed pregnancy			76	77
Unwed pregnancy			95	92
Being accepted to a college of your choice				43
Getting married				101

This scale measures the amount of life change experienced by a child. Each type of life change requires a certain amount of social and psychological adaptation, which is stressful to the child. This scale is not an exact predictor of illness, because different children react differently when confronted with life change. It also does not measure subtle, but real, sources of stress in a child's life, such as poverty, dysfunctional family dynamics, loss of a pet, or school failure. In general, the more significant life change a child has experienced, the greater the child's susceptibility to illness. When children with acute or chronic physical or mental illness are studied, they are consistently shown to have had two to three times the amount of stressful events experienced by control groups of healthy children.

Between the ages of 4 and 6, the average child's total life stress score is approximately 75; between the ages of 9 and 12, the average score is approximately 100; and between the ages of 14 and 16, the average score may approach 200. If a child scores higher than these averages, she may be at risk of physical or emotional health problems.

Adapted from Heisel J, et al: The significance of life events as contributing factors in the diseases of children. *Behavioral Pediatrics*, 83:119-123, 1973

Increased Rates of Juvenile Crime

There has been a sevenfold increase in serious assaults committed by juveniles in the United States since World War II. Juvenile arrests for possession of weapons, aggravated assault, robbery, and murder rose more than 50% from 1987 to 1996. The rate of violence increased most in inner cities and among black males.[48] Experts believe many factors are involved, including widespread availability of guns, increased exposure to violence in the media, and less family support for children.[45] Television violence is responsible for up to 15% of all aggressive behavior in children.[48]

High Rates of Substance Abuse

The average age American children begin drug use is 12 years. The popularity of certain illegal drugs changes; for example, in 2002, use of marijuana declined and illicit use of prescription drugs OxyContin and Vicodin increased—but illicit drug use remains high. In 2002, 24% of eighth graders, 44% of tenth graders, and 53% of twelfth graders reported past use of some illicit drug. Also in 2002, 47% of eighth graders, 66% of tenth graders, and 78% of twelfth graders reported use of alcohol.[67] One national survey reported 39% of surveyed high school seniors had been drunk in the last 2 weeks. Alcohol-related accidents are the leading cause of death in teenagers.[68]

Increased Rates of Severe Depression

Signs of severe depression are more common in teenagers than in adults, and an estimated 8% of teenagers suffer from severe depression. The onset of depression is occurring earlier in life today.[69] Approximately one-half to one million prescriptions for antidepressants are written for American children and teenagers every year, and the number is growing. Even those psychiatrists prescribing antidepressants are undecided about their use.[60]

Increased Suicide Rates

The suicide rate among children ages 10 to 14 is 1.2 per 100,000. The teenage suicide rates were stable from 1900 to 1955 when they began to rise dramatically, from 4.5 per 100,000 in 1900 to 13 per 100,000 in 1992. Suicide is the third leading cause of death in teenagers. The strongest risk factors for attempted suicide in youth are depression, heavy use of alcohol or other drugs, and aggressive and disruptive behavior.[70]

Increased Sexual Activity

Sexual activity is beginning at younger ages, increasing risks of pregnancy and sexually transmitted diseases, including AIDS. About 50% of teenagers have sexual intercourse before graduating from high school. The United States has the highest teen pregnancy rate of any developed country, with more than 800,000 teenage girls becoming pregnant each year.[71]

High Rates of Eating Disorders, Including Anorexia Nervosa and Bulimia

One of 10 teens struggles with an eating disorder; 90% of teens with eating disorders are girls.[51] Many girls in primary grades are already trying to diet and, by fourth grade, 40% or more girls say they diet at least occasionally. Many of these young females may not have full-blown eating disorders, but are at risk of having poor nutrition at a time when their bodies are growing and they need optimum nutrition. Surveys taken in Ohio, Iowa, South Carolina, and Arizona show that 25–40% of primary grade girls and boys are worried about being "too fat." Researchers at University of South Carolina identified children as young as age 9 with severe eating disorders.[72-75] Many parents are deeply concerned about the long-term effects these fears may have on their daughters' health and happiness. The book *One Hundred and One Ways to Help Your Daughter Love Her Body* addresses these concern with ideas about how to teach young girls to "have an internalized image of their bodies as whole and wholesome, rather than a package of distorted parts that must be dressed up and displayed to their best advantage."[76] The first suggestion is for parents to massage their daughters, beginning when they are infants.

High Rates of Type A Behavior

Although no statistics are available on the incidence of type A behavior in children, many child specialists, including pediatricians, child psychologists, and educators, are alarmed by what they perceive as significant increases over the last two decades (see Point of Interest Box 1-3).[45] Pediatrician Steven Shelov believes that recent changes in the American value system foster negative type A behavior, including how the American culture defines success by the amount of material possessions and money one has, new pressure to enroll children in early educational and extracurricular activities, and the tendency to hurry children out of childhood too early. Children who by temperament are susceptible to this type of message may become driven and competitive at an early age. In contrast, type A behavior is lower in cultures that emphasize harmony, loyalty, and cooperation as part of their definition of success.[77] Exploiting values that lead to type A behavior, Bonne Bell Cosmetics Company markets a shower gel to teens called *Hyper*, with the motto, "I feel...like going sixty miles an hour."[78]

POINT OF INTEREST BOX 1–3
Type A Behavior in Children

Type A behavior is a cluster of certain behavioral traits, including impatience, restlessness, repressed hostility, and an excessive competitive drive. Persons with type A personalities walk fast, talk fast, and tend to do more than one thing at a time (such as simultaneously reading, eating, and watching TV). Their high tension level is revealed by rapid eye blinking, knee jiggling, and finger tapping. They have rapid and forceful speech patterns, and interrupt others frequently in conversation. These behaviors may cause them to become isolated from others. Type B personalities, by contrast, are easygoing, work without agitation, and relax without guilt. Often, they are actually more efficient than type A personalities.

The development of heart disease has been directly linked to type A behavior.[79] Type A patterns are usually established in childhood and persist into adulthood.[80] Cardiologist Meyer Friedman, who first coined the term *type A behavior,* has concluded that deep-seated insecurity is the root cause of the behaviors. He believes that this insecurity is most commonly caused by a failure to do well in school and that this insecurity causes the person to constantly compete against others.[81]

For children, the major drawbacks of type A behavior are social isolation and a greater probability of having heart disease when they are adults. As high cholesterol is a significant risk factor in the development of heart disease, the elevation in blood cholesterol levels found in both children and adults with this behavior pattern is worrisome. One study found that children, ages 10 to 17, who are type A personalities had higher blood cholesterol readings than type B children.[82]

A Duke University Neurobehavioral Diabetes Program study investigated whether diabetic children with type A personalities have a different physiologic response during times of stress than those with type B personalities. Type A and type B children played Super Breakout, a demanding video game, and then researchers tested their blood glucose levels. In general, the type A children showed an increase in blood glucose, while the type B children did not.[45]

Increased Attention Deficit and Hyperactive Behaviors

Prescription of Ritalin to treat hyperactivity increased six-fold between 1971 and 1989 and several hundred-fold from 1995 to 2000. Many child psychologists and medical professionals believe Ritalin is increasingly prescribed for children with attentional and hyperactive behavior caused by stress rather than by a true neurologic dysfunction.[45,83] Ritalin is also being prescribed for younger and younger children.[84] For more information, see Chapter 6, page 165.

High Incidence of Psychosomatic Illness

Many American children suffer stress-related health problems at some point during their childhood. Pediatricians report an increase in stress symptoms in children, including headaches and stomachaches.[45]

CHILDREN'S BODILY RESPONSE TO STRESS

Although children encounter different types of stress than those affecting adults, their physiologic response to stress is the same. In the fight-or-flight response, the body's different systems react in various ways.[85] Even exposure to maternal stress hormones in utero can cause the child's body systems to react both physiologically and behaviorally (see Point of Interest Box 1–4).

- Adrenal glands release cortisol, an anti-inflammatory hormone. Continued high levels of cortisol hamper the immune system's ability to fight both minor and major illnesses, probably by destroying immune cells. It can also corrode connective tissue, leading to weakness in muscles, tendons, fascia, and ligaments, with an increased risk of injury. High levels may lead to damage in the brain, causing memory lapses, anxiety, a decreased attention span, and an inability to control emotional outbursts. The adrenal glands also release adrenalin hormone. Elwood et al. examined urine samples taken from children under both stressful and nonstressful circumstances. The samples revealed that under the stress of waiting to give a presentation in front of a class, 83% of girls and 89% of boys had a significant hormonal response, such as increases in adrenalin and noradrenalin.[90]
- The thyroid gland secretes the hormone thyroxin, which speeds up the body's metabolism. Excess thyroxin can lead to shaky nerves, insomnia, and exhaustion.
- Endorphin, a painkilling hormone, is released in greater than normal amounts by the brain. Eventually endorphin supplies are depleted and pain tolerance decreases.
- The entire digestive tract shuts down: the stomach and the large intestine virtually stop their secretions and movements, diverting blood to the skeletal muscles. Continued shutdown can lead to digestive discomfort such as cramps, nausea, bloating, and diarrhea.

- As described in Case Study 1–1, the secretion of hydrochloric acid in the stomach is affected by stress.
- The blood sugar level rises and, to metabolize it, the pancreas produces more insulin. Chronic elevation can cause one to crave sugar. Diabetes can be initiated or aggravated by excessive demands on the pancreas to produce insulin.
- Cholesterol flows from the liver into the bloodstream. Sustained high levels can cause deposits of cholesterol to accumulate in the blood vessels, leading to arteriosclerosis and heart disease.
- The heart beats harder and faster. On a long-term basis, this can lead to high blood pressure, increasing the risk of stroke and heart attack. Male newborns who are circumcised without anesthetic have measurable increases in heart rate and blood pressure for hours following the circumcision.[92] Preschoolers who have been assigned stressful tasks show measurable increases in both heart rate and blood pressure.[93] Even an isolated stressful event may cause marked increases in heart rate and blood pressure for an extended time. For example, three small girls suffered an extremely frightening event. One night, tied up and threatened with a gun by two gunmen who had broken

POINT OF INTEREST BOX 1–4
Exposure to Stress Hormones May Begin Before Birth

Babies born of mothers who have experienced severe psychological stress during pregnancy show delays in early motor development and such behavioral disorders as excessive anxiety and crying, hyperactivity, and a lower tolerance for frustration. By comparing the behavior of infants whose mothers had high stress during pregnancy with mothers who had high stress during the first year of the baby's life, Weinstock demonstrated that these behaviors are linked to prenatal life and are probably are caused by the maternal stress hormones released during stress at critical periods of fetal development. These findings have been confirmed in experiments with monkeys and rodents.[86]

Zuckerman found a significant association between maternal depression and low birthweight, poor growth, and behavior problems and speculates that maternal depression may make the child more likely to suffer from depression.[87,88] Intense anxiety during pregnancy is also associated with a wide range of difficulties, including low birthweight, newborn respiratory illness, and certain physical defects such as cleft palate and **pyloric stenosis**.[89]

CASE STUDY 1–1

STUDY OF HYDROCHLORIC ACID IN A HOSPITALIZED CHILD

Monica was born with her esophagus completely closed as a result of a birth defect. At 4 days of age, she had corrective surgery to make a temporary passage from her stomach to the surface of her abdomen. An opening was made on her abdomen that allowed her to be fed through a tube that went into her stomach. (At 20 months of age, she would have a permanent passage constructed under her sternum, between her esophagus and her stomach.) Because of family, personal, and financial stresses, Monica's mother was unable to adequately care for her, and the infant was twice hospitalized for a failure to gain weight. When she was admitted to the hospital for the second time, Monica was 15 months old; however, as a result of neglect and malnourishment, she was 8 to 12 months less developmentally mature compared with the average child her age. At 15 months for example, most children can crawl, walk, and kick a ball, and they are also learning how to do new actions such as how to go up and down a steep hill. By contrast, Monica was unable to sit up or even turn over in bed. She remained in the pediatric ward for 11 months until she gained sufficient weight to be ready for and recuperate from surgery and was physically fit enough to return home. While she remained in the hospital, she was studied by having gastric juice withdrawn from her stomach and her emotional states noted at the same time.

Researchers found that the rate at which her stomach secreted hydrochloric acid was intimately related to her behavioral and emotional states. Higher levels of physiologic activity (more active interactions with the environment) were paralleled by higher amounts of hydrochloric acid being secreted. For example, acid secretion was:

- at its very lowest level while she was sleeping
- slightly higher when she was awake but depressed
- still higher during states of irritation, displeasure, contentment, and joy
- at its highest level when she was in a state of rage, which was accompanied by loud crying, high-pitched wailing, screaming, and sobbing

Similar differences were found in Monica's heart and respiratory rates; during a period of depression, they became lower and, when she was angry and irritated, both markedly increased. After her surgery. Monica learned to stand, walk, and feed herself. She was then discharged home to her family, but remained significantly less mature in development compared with the average child her age.[91]

into their apartment, they witnessed the shooting of an older sister. When the girls were seen at a hospital psychiatric clinic the next day, they sat quietly and showed no outward signs of stress. However, their heart rates were still more than 100 beats per minute and their blood pressure rates were high.[94] For some children, the rise in blood pressure may be permanent. Cardiologist Samuel Mann has treated adults whose hypertension is not lowered by medication and lifestyle changes and found that it can be caused by unresolved emotional pain or trauma during childhood. Addressing these emotions has permanently lowered their hypertension.[95]

- All five senses become temporarily more acute, but repeated stress will eventually cause the senses to "burn out" and become less efficient. With chronic stress, the ability to concentrate is greatly diminished.
- Muscle tension increases, resulting in feelings of tension and stiffness, decreased freedom of movement, and, at times, muscular pain, such as muscle contraction headaches or stomachaches. The child finds it increasingly difficult to relax when not under stress.

THE EFFECT OF LIFE STRESS ON CHILDREN'S HEALTH

Each child has an Achilles heel, an organ which responds to stress and creates symptoms which become the outlet for any unusual or excessive pressures in the child's life. It is important for adults to realize that children rarely 'fake' symptoms when they are overwhelmed by stress. Many symptoms arise as a way of coping with tension and are based on the normal stresses of growing up.[96]

—*T. Berry Brazelton, MD*

Brazelton believes that when a child's stress load overwhelms his or her capacity to cope, the child may develop physical, emotional, or mental illness. The response to overwhelming stress is highly variable and may not only cause current symptoms, but also exacerbate illnesses that were already present (for example, a child with epilepsy might have increased seizures at a time of stress). Stomachaches, headaches, allergic reactions, and increased susceptibility to colds and flu are minor and extremely common signs of stress.[45,96] The wide range of major health problems associated with stress are as individual as the child herself. These problems may occur in any body system; the most common ones are identified in Checklist Box 1–1. As explained in Point of Interest Box 1–5, children may make improvements in many of their health problems by tapping the interconnection between their minds and their bodies.

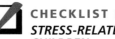

CHECKLIST BOX 1–1
STRESS-RELATED HEALTH PROBLEMS IN CHILDREN

- ☐ cardiovascular system: migraine headaches and hypertension
- ☐ gastrointestinal system: ulcerative colitis, diarrhea, persistent vomiting, **encopresis**, recurrent abdominal pain, obesity, and anorexia nervosa
- ☐ respiratory system: asthma and chronic coughing
- ☐ urinary system: bedwetting and urinary frequency
- ☐ neuromuscular system: muscle contraction headaches and tics
- ☐ central nervous system: epileptic seizures
- ☐ skin problems: warts, habitual scratching, and anxiety-produced hives
- ☐ **conversion reactions**: hysterical disorders of motor function, including paralysis, blindness, back pain, dizziness, and hallucinations

Schaeffer C, Hillman H, Levine G: *Therapies for Psychosomatic Disorders in Children.* San Francisco: Jossey-Bass, 1979, p xiii-xx

Roghman examined the relationship between stress and illness in families with children younger than the age of 18. Mothers recorded both upsetting events and illnesses occurring in their families during 1 month. These records indicated that the likelihood of children developing fevers, colds, or other minor illnesses increased by 50% after a stressful event.[100]

For 4 decades, stress research has consistently shown a link between childhood stress and childhood illness. Heisel et al. studied children with major physical illnesses and found that their illnesses began after they had experienced twice the stress of control populations of healthy children.[101] Mutter and Schleifer studied children who were admitted to the hospital for acute illnesses, such as meningitis and asthma, and found that they had been exposed to more life stress in the previous 6 months than a control group of well children. In addition, the families of the sick children were less able to function well, so that there were less resources to enable the children to cope with stress when it did arise.[102] Greene et al. found that teenagers with recurrent somatic complaints with no organic cause reported higher amounts of life stress than those who had pain with an organic cause or those who had an acute minor illness.[103] The effects of stress may be cumulative. Major traumas in the first 4 years of life predispose a child to psychological problems when stressful situations occur in the teen years; having lived through two or more major family problems, such as divorce, loss, death, or separation, as a younger child increases the likelihood that a teenager

POINT OF INTEREST BOX 1–5
Mind-Body Approaches to Children's Stress-Related Health Problems Can Help Children Influence Their Physiology

In recent years, mind-body approaches have successfully helped children cope with organically caused diseases, stress-related health problems, and chronic conditions. When sensitively adapted to their needs, massage and bodywork techniques can be one of these mind-body techniques that are effective for children. By teaching children greater awareness of their bodies and how to consciously relax during massage sessions, children learn how to feel and control some internal body processes.[97]

Many problems have shown improvement with mind-body techniques, including learning disabilities; hyperactivity; emotional problems, such as phobias and test anxiety; and physical problems, such as tension headaches, asthma, and burn pain. Medical hypnosis has helped children to control many types of pain; make dental work more tolerable; recover from stress-related health problems; and improve chronic health conditions, such as cystic fibrosis, Tourette's syndrome, and head injury; and relieve pain and discomfort during a terminal illness.[98]

Children have also demonstrated that they can learn to increase their body awareness and control their muscle tension through biofeedback,[98] visual imagery,[62] hatha yoga,[99] and relaxation of different muscle groups.[98] Use of these mind-body techniques clearly shows that children are capable of influencing their own physiologic processes, if given the tools to do so. For example, psychologist Robert Hill has trained 11-year-old boys, using biofeedback, to consistently raise the temperature of a single finger to 103° to 104° F.[83]

When sensitively adapted to their needs, massage and bodywork techniques can be one mind-body technique that is effective for children. By teaching children not only greater awareness of their bodies, but also how to consciously relax during massage sessions, they learn how to feel and control some of their internal body processes.

even within the same family, children may suffer different types of stress-related health problems. For example, Powell et al. treated 13 children, ages 3 to 11, whose growth was severely delayed: all were 30–66% of the expected height for their ages (see Figure 1–4). All had bizarre eating and drinking behaviors, and 11 of 13 had delayed speech. There was evidence of extreme neglect in all families, and malnourishment and physical abuse in many. Immediately or soon after being admitted to a convalescent hospital, all the children grew rapidly, at a much greater than normal growth rate for children their age. They received no medication or psychiatric treatment; tender loving care in the hospital was sufficient to start their growth again. The growth retardation observed in these children was caused by decreased growth hormone secretion, which was directly linked to their emotional deprivation.[106] However, not all of the children in

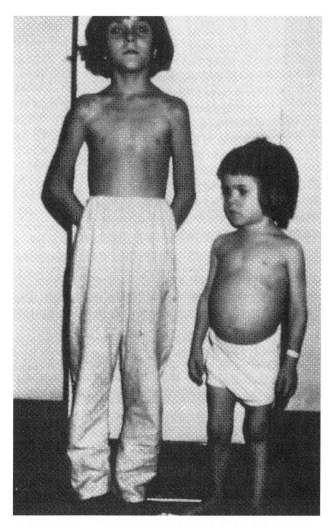

FIGURE 1–4 ■ Two 7-year-old girls. The girl on the left is of normal size for her age; the one on the right has growth retardation caused by extreme emotional neglect. Reprinted with permission from: Proffit W, Fields H: *Contemporary Orthodontics*. St. Louis: Mosby, 2001, p 54.

will have psychological problems.[104] A high level of stress in childhood, particularly child abuse, also increases the likelihood of suffering from chronic pain as an adult.[105]

A child's response to stress depends on a number of different factors, including his or her individual temperament and particular Achilles heel, how emotionally healthy their families are, and what kind of coping skills and support they have. Interestingly, each family experienced growth retardation: in some families, it occurred in only one of the siblings. Even with two children with the same parents and the same home environment, it is not possible to predict which body system will be their Achilles heel.[93] If treatment for children with this type of growth retardation is delayed, or if children are returned to their homes without any improvement in the home environment, the long-term effects also include poorer language development, poorer verbal abilities, less social maturity, and a greater incidence of behavior problems.[107]

A more common symptom of stress overload is psychosomatic musculoskeletal pain. Sherry et al. reported on 100 children with musculoskeletal pain who were evaluated at a major pediatric rheumatology referral center and were found to have no organic disease. The typical child was a 13-year-old girl who had had severe pain for at least 1 year and who had been under a great deal of stress from school, family, or her own expectations. Only 8% of the children's families were emotionally healthy, and the children had been in psychologically stressful environments long before the onset of their pain. Most were in stressful family roles or had recently experienced major life events, such as a death in the family, frequent moves, or a parent with a major illness; 41% had experienced some type of trauma. After intensive physical therapy and psychotherapy, almost all the children became symptom-free and fully functional, which verified that their symptoms were not organic.[108]

LONG-TERM EFFECTS ON CHILDREN OF LOCALIZED TRAUMA OR PAIN

Massage therapists commonly find muscular tension in specific areas that have been contracted for many years; this is one of the major challenges of doing massage with adults. It often originates in the body's emergency response to injury. For example, if the jagged ends of a fractured femur are moved, they could lacerate the femoral artery and cause a child to bleed to death in a short time.[96] Movement of the fractured bone could also cause further damage to already injured soft tissue; therefore, when muscles around the fracture site spasm, they are preventing harmful movement. This reaction is dysfunctional, however, when muscles remain contracted after the bone is set and heals. A defensive reaction—fear of having the area retraumatized—can cause surrounding muscles to contract even when the fracture has healed. Deep tension and restriction remain and become the norm. The child (or adult) may have no idea of the connection between the original trauma and the present discomfort and pain. A memory of the original pain or trauma in the area may occur when the muscles in the area are deeply relaxed during a massage session; this indicates that there is still significant guarding even though the injury happened long ago.

Many patterns of chronic muscle tension in specific areas originate when there is localized trauma or pain in infancy or childhood. An example from before birth is the baby who was pricked in the neck by a needle while his mother was undergoing amniocentesis during the eighth month of pregnancy. At 16 months, spastic neck muscles around the area that was pricked pinned his head to one side and he could barely crawl.[109] It has been observed that babies in the neonatal intensive care unit come to know who takes blood samples and can be seen tensing their legs and feet when that person arrives. If blood samples are taken from a baby's feet over a long period, the baby's feet may become tense and hypersensitive (Fronzuto J, RN, neonatal intensive care, personal communication, December 1992). Children who have been intubated repeatedly often carry such deep tension in their throats that they resist swallowing and require special therapy. For example, the author treated a premature infant who was intubated immediately after birth. At home with her family and with no other physical problems, she still had to be fed through a stomach tube at age 3 because she refused to swallow solid food. Medical examinations could find no physical reason for her inability to swallow with ease.

Craniosacral practitioner and teacher Hugh Milne described a 40-year-old woman attending a craniosacral therapy class, who had experienced headaches from unknown causes for many years. When her sphenoid bone was touched gently by another student during class, the woman began to scream repeatedly, "She's pressing too hard," as she remembered her mother repeatedly squeezing her head with a great deal of pressure before age 5. As the craniosacral therapy released both her cranial restriction and the emotions associated with her pain, the woman reported that the feeling of head pressure she had experienced since the original trauma was permanently gone and that she felt an enormous weight was lifted from her psyche.[111] The author treated a 30-year-old woman who had been born with an incompletely developed hip socket. At age 10, she had radical, experimental surgery on the hip joint. During the 2 weeks she was hospitalized, her parents were not allowed to visit her, and she felt terribly abandoned. After four sessions of Swedish massage and myofascial release on her hips and legs, including the surgical scar itself, she began to have nightmares about her stay in the hospital and not being able to see her parents.[110]

Sustained contraction of a muscle, as might happen when a child is in pain, can cause the development of a myofascial trigger point, which could lead to chronic discomfort or pain. Aftimos treated a 7-year-old girl with two trigger points in the sternal division of one sternocleidomastoid muscle. The girl was experiencing pain and limitation of motion in her neck and ipsilateral cheek and eye from the trigger points. They had developed secondary to pain and irritation from an enlarged and painful tonsillar lymph node when she had an upper respiratory infection. He also treated a 10-year-old boy with severe flank pain caused by a trigger point in the ipsilateral external oblique muscle, which developed from splinting the chest wall when he had pneumonia. Dr. Aftimos treated both children when they were sick—before they developed the trigger points and pains. He later treated the trigger points with vapocoolant spray and stretching, which completely resolved their pain.[7]

Exposure to significant pain in infancy or early childhood may have another effect as well—it can alter the child's (and later, the adult's) perceptions and reactions to pain. Porter et al. reviewed the research on the long-term effects of pain in infancy and concluded that children who experienced the chronic stress and repeated physical pain of a neonatal intensive care unit will react with more anxiety and stress and will feel more pain when given vaccinations than children who were not in a neonatal unit. They are likely to have this reaction of increased anxiety and stress in any situation in which they will have to experience pain. Many nurses and doctors who work in prenatal intensive care units are deeply concerned about the long-term effects of the pain and invasive procedures the infants must undergo. The majority of the tactile interactions for infants in intensive care are clinical in nature, such as endotracheal suctioning, insertion of intravenous lines, heel pricks, and arranging respirator tubes, and many of these interactions are painful. Porter concluded that anesthetic should be given before painful procedures to prevent these long-term effects.[111]

Similar conclusions have been drawn from animal studies. Newborn rat pups stimulated with painful stimuli four times a day have significantly lower pain thresholds compared with rats that received repetitive nonpainful stimuli during the same period. During adulthood, pain-stimulated rats had an increased preference for alcohol, increased anxiety, and defensive withdrawal behavior. It seems that, once activated during sensitive periods of development, the adrenocortical system may behave differently in reaction to subsequent stress. The nervous system may be structurally and functionally changed as a result of early pain and stress, so that specific populations of synapses may be stimulated and others destroyed. Gray et al. reported on a study that compared the response of two groups of infants to a standard heel lance procedure. One group of infants wore only a diaper and laid on their mother's bare chests, and the infants in the other group were swaddled and lying in a crib. After the painful heel stick, the infants in skin-to-skin contact with their mothers cried 82% less, grimaced 65% less than the swaddled infants, and did not have the extreme increase in heart rate of the swaddled infants.[112] Based on these results, it appears that a combination of careful use of anesthesia and skin contact (including massage) in the neonatal intensive care unit could be the ideal intervention to alleviate stress and to prevent future anxiety regarding pain.[112,113]

MASSAGE THERAPY AS AN APPROACH TO CHILDREN'S STRESS-RELATED HEALTH PROBLEMS

Although stress may be at the root of many childhood health problems, it can also worsen those problems with an organic cause. Almost any condition which a child suffers can be worsened if he or she is under a lot of stress. For example, stress may truly be the basis of a child's struggles with muscle contraction headaches or stomachaches; in this case, regular massage can help release tension and reverse this problem. Asthma and epilepsy, however, are not caused by stress, but may be significantly worsened by it; children with asthma and epilepsy may have fewer attacks or seizures when their tension levels are lower. Massage does not deal with the cause of the stress; however, it can be tremendously supportive by enhancing the child's fundamental internal physiologic processes, helping her release tension, and helping her feel nurtured and supported. Feelings of isolation and loneliness, which are often part of the child's stress, are combatted by sensitive and caring touch. More than receiving simply a clinical regimen of proscribed massage strokes, that touch has the capability to affect a child on an emotional and psychological level. By teaching the child to relax through the basic and advanced relaxation sequences, children will not only feel less tense, but learn that they have a measure of control over their physiology. Many specific massage treatments for stress-related health problems are found in Chapters 5 and 6. In Chapters 4 and 5, the reader will learn specific techniques that can ease pain, treat soft-tissue dysfunction, and stimulate normal physiologic processes. In Chapter 6, the reader will learn how relatively simple massage techniques can be specifically used to treat a variety of childhood disabilities, increasing their comfort, improving their mobility, and stimulating their normal physiologic processes.

INCREASED PERCEPTUAL FEEDBACK AS A BENEFIT OF MASSAGE

In addition to its physiologic and emotional benefits, massage therapy also provides children with perceptual feedback, which is essential to the development of a healthy body image.

THE IMPORTANCE OF A HEALTHY BODY IMAGE

Body image is a person's "mental picture" of his or her body (see Figure 1–5). This mental representation of the physical self is made up of the perceptions of the body's individual parts and planes, and also its size, weight, shape, boundaries, and relationship to the rest of the world.[114,115] Each person's body image develops from her unique physical, emotional, and cultural experiences.

Body image is central to the sense of self and self-organization. Children need a distinct and relatively stable body image to perceive themselves and others accurately and to interact well with their environment. A distinct body image is necessary for good balance, good spatial orientation, and precision of move-

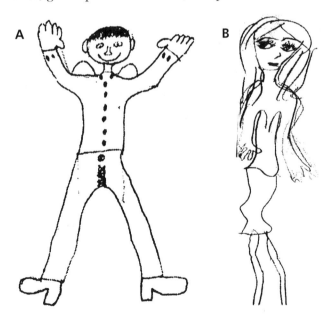

FIGURE 1–5 ■ Self-portraits by two children. Having a child draw a self-portrait is one way to assess her body image; the drawing can indicate how well the parts, planes, and boundaries of her body are perceived. Drawing A is by a healthy 9-year-old boy. Drawing B is by a 12-year-old girl with schizophrenia. Blaesing S, Brockhause J: The development of body image in the child. *Nursing Clinics of North America*, 7:603-604, 1972.

ment. A child with a vague body image may be clumsy because she is unable to orient herself in space or in relationship to other objects.

The definiteness of children's body boundaries, or how well defined and structured they perceive their bodies to be, is basic to their identity. Children with vague, indefinite, or distorted body images may not actually know where their bodies start and where they stop and exactly where the rest of the world begins. Their body images are like a distorted reflection in a fun house mirror, with some of their body parts blackened out, which may lead to high anxiety and low self-esteem. According to psychiatry professor David Krueger, "Individuals who have an inauthentic image of their bodies typically describe the sense of never having lived in their own bodies, of never having inhabited them. Their bodies never seem to be their own; their bodies do not become integrated as a seamless aspect of the self. In some instances eating, exercise, or other self-stimulating physical activities are attempts to create a sensory bridge to feeling and inhabiting one's body."[116] Because the definiteness of the child's body boundaries is basic to her identity, if she has an indefinite or weak sense of her boundaries—that is, she lacks a clearly defined line between herself and the rest of the world—she will feel incapable of protecting herself. Intimacy, which involves some boundary loss, may seem frightening. A child with a weak body image may be threatened by normal attempts to interact with her physically or socially. Or she may have a tendency to slap, punch, push, or otherwise intrude upon others to show affection. If, however, she has a sense of her body boundaries being too strong, she will feel safe letting her feelings out but she may also feel lonely and numb.[117] Weak or distorted body images can be caused by a number of different factors, including:

- Negative touch experiences, such as physical abuse (see Chapter 6, page 157).
- Touch deprivation. Healthy touch experiences during childhood are perhaps the single most important contributor to a healthy body image.
- Problems with neurologic development. These may result in weak or poorly developed neurologic functions, such as the ability to distinguish the various nuances of touch or the ability to develop proprioception from the information coming into the brain.[118]
- Stress and strife. Chronic conflicts may lead people to develop rigid personality styles, which can manifest as rigid body posture and armor-hard body boundaries. Psychologist Wilhelm Reich believed that parents who emphasize inhibition

and self-control raise children with this type of boundary.[43] Such people may be attracted to thrill-seeking behavior, alcohol abuse, or drug abuse to increase the intensity of their sensations.

Many aspects of a child's body image can become distorted, including her size, weight, shape, body parts, the distinctness of her body boundaries, and her distance from other people and objects. For example, we have all experienced a change in our perceived size when we stand beside a particularly large or small person. Lack of body awareness or misperceptions of the body may be noted during massage therapy. For example, many people have little or no awareness of muscular tension, even in tight areas. Others appear to conceive of their bodies as almost two-dimensional—they are aware of the front and back aspects of their bodies, but they have little awareness of the sides of their bodies. Or, some people may be aware of the upper part of their bodies, but have little true awareness of their lower bodies; some are aware of the right side but not the left side.

Anorexia nervosa is an extreme example of severe body image distortion; in fact, it is defined as *a disturbance in the way in which one's body weight, size, or shape is experienced.*[43] An anorexic girl may refer to herself as plump or fat when others see her as skeletal. A study of 214 anorexic and/or bulimic young women found that 75% of them were not able to correctly estimate the size of their body parts. When asked to estimate the size of their biceps, calves, thighs, waist, abdomen, hips, and bust, 75% perceived the parts as one-tenth to one-third larger than the actual size. By contrast, a control group of women without eating disorders rarely estimated the size of their body parts incorrectly by more than one-twentieth of the actual size.[119] Anorexia most often develops from an overwhelming importance being given to one's physical appearance, profound body dissatisfaction, and a deep conviction of physical defect.[120] The emaciated teenage girl who looks in the mirror and sees a fat person lacks a healthy body image to help ground her in reality.

Can touch therapy play an essential role in building that healthy body image? Studies of adult women with anorexia nervosa have found that they have a strong desire for nurturing touch and that they feel that they were deprived of touch as children.[121] A small study of young women with anorexia found that the women had less dissatisfaction with their bodies after effleurage-based massage performed twice a week for 5 weeks.[122] Hopefully, this research will be conducted with children as well as adults and that it will show that massage can have a more powerful effect if administered earlier in life.

HOW A HEALTHY BODY IMAGE DEVELOPS

The foundation for a healthy body image is developed during infancy. Childhood and teenage experiences then continue to shape its development.

Infancy

At birth, infants possess a fairly well-developed capacity for registering and associating sensory impressions received through contact with other human beings. Touch is the most mature of the senses at birth; babies can feel much better than they can see, hear, or even taste.[123] The construction of body image begins in the first few days of life, as infants interact with people and objects in their environment. They begin to have a variety of new tactile experiences not experienced in the womb, including different temperatures, new movements, the handling by different people, and the textures of fabric and skin. They also process the input of sound, taste, movement, and vision. Their body image gradually builds from these different sensations. During this period, adequate somatosensory stimulation and tactile stimulation, in particular, are critical for developing a healthy body image. Rocking, holding, and massaging are excellent ways to meet this need. Bathing or swimming are also excellent because water exerts pressure in all directions to provide one type of tactile stimulation to the skin and the temperature of the water adds another type.[117] Each touch stimulates a mental image of the area touched and, eventually, the cumulative effect of these mental images is the ability to localize the body parts and their functions.[124] When infants lack adequate sensory stimulation, especially that of touch and movement, their body image as children will be weak and possibly distorted. As noted earlier, they will be anxious and have difficulty forming normal emotional attachments to significant others and their ego development will be impaired.[125]

A variety of circumstances increase the likelihood that an infant will be touch-deprived. One is a tendency for the infant to be hypersensitive to all stimulation. Brazelton studied a group of infants who had no identified physical problems who were, however, difficult to nurture because of their hypersensitivity. As one attempted to rock them gently, they stiffened, arched away, and sometimes had a series of bodily startles that resulted in inconsolable crying. If one looked in their faces or talked to them, they looked frightened and turned away. Such infants are difficult for even the most well-intentioned parents to care for. The parents may begin to pull away from the infants, interacting with them less and less as their attempts to nurture and comfort repeatedly fail. The infants do not receive the one thing that might normally coax them out of their hypersensitivity—loving touch—and their hypersensitivity may never be overcome. Through no fault of the parents, this hypersensitivity may lead to a type of touch deprivation. Brazelton found that these babies could be reached if parents learned to change their approach by slowing down, cutting down on stimuli during interactions, and dealing with their baby in a low-keyed manner. For example, feeding time needed to be in a dim, quiet room with other stimulation avoided during the feeding process, including singing to or playing with the baby.[96]

Other circumstances might cause an infant to be touch-deprived: a mother with too many small children to care for; a mother who becomes seriously depressed or ill; a mother who has to return to work without having high-quality day care; an anxious and self-involved mother who cannot adequately respond to her infant's specific needs for comforting and feeding; and major stress or upheaval in a family.

Psychiatrist Katherine Zerbe, who specializes in the treatment of eating disorders, believes that failure to care adequately for the infant not only causes a false or distorted body image but that, in a peculiar way, eating disorders may be an attempt to self-cure such early touch deprivation.[43] Baby monkeys used in classic touch deprivation experiments by Harlow could see, hear, and smell their mothers but not touch them. As a result of this bizarre experience, when the baby monkeys became adults they had such distorted body images that they sometimes mutilated themselves or stared at body parts as if they were foreign objects.[126]

At the other extreme from deprivation, excessive intrusion into the infant's boundaries can cause problems as well. Physical or sexual abuse can weaken the sense of the body being whole (see Abuse section, Chapter 6, page 157). The invasiveness and use of physical restraint in some medical procedures can also affect body image. The result may be that the child has a weak sense of her body as a private domain.[127]

Early Childhood

During the toddler stage, the body image continues to develop and parental attitudes continue to make an indelible impression on the child's concept of himself, his body, and its functions. How children are touched when sick, what kinds of games parents play with them, how they are dressed, toilet trained, and so on, all contribute to the formation of body image.

As children develop in size, shape, and motor skills, their body image is continuously reshaped. During the preschool years, a child's body image becomes clearer and more conscious. Because preschoolers are gaining an awareness of a separate self inside a body that belongs to them, they may feel more anxious about getting hurt or being in a situation in which they might experience pain.[128] At this stage, however, they are not as worried about how their bodies appear to others as might be older children. Nonetheless, if there is conflict with adults about any specific body area, a body image distortion may develop; for example, if there is parental conflict about touching the genitals, a body image distortion can develop in the genital area.[117]

Middle Childhood

During middle childhood (ages 6 to 12), children begin to compare their bodies with those around them as they learn how to interact with others. Cultural attitudes begin to influence the child's body image (see Point of Interest Box 1-6). For example, in a culture in which plumpness is taken as a sign of health or prosperity, a naturally chubby girl will be treated differently than in a culture in which thinness equals beauty. If they have been teased because they look different, children who are disabled may see their bodies as ugly or deformed. A large study of body image attitudes found that childhood teasing about appearance led to a negative body image and a tendency to develop an eating disorder.[129]

Adolescence

The onset of adolescence confronts all children with the task of revising their body image. The personal frame of reference that they have developed has to be reconstructed to accommodate the many normal changes in body structure and function that occur at a dramatically rapid rate.[127] These rapid physical changes lead the teenager to be more self-conscious and increasingly preoccupied with their body image and the question, "Am I normal?" The young teenager's concern with body image is characterized by a preoccupation with self, uncertainty about appearance and attractiveness, frequent comparison of his or her own body with those of other teenagers, and increased interest in sexual anatomy and physiology.[127] Dieting, exercise, and cosmetic surgery, such as liposuction and breast enhancement surgery, are becoming increasingly common in teenage girls[130] and may be used to help make the body fit the cultural ideals.

By the end of adolescence, the major concern with body image has largely abated—growth is no longer proceeding at such a rapid rate and teenagers have integrated their physical changes into their body image.[128] Cultural and parental attitudes toward the body continue to influence the older teenager's body image. A poll of 33,000 women found that women with mothers who were more critical of their appearance were more likely to have a negative body image.[131]

POINT OF INTEREST BOX 1–6
Cultural and Parental Attitudes about a Child's Body Influence Her Body Image

Fortunately, Natasha N., age 6, has a mother who is not preoccupied with how her daughter fits the cultural standard. One evening when taking a bath, Natasha looked down and complained to her mother that her thighs were too fat. This striking statement by a 6-year-old occurred after Natasha had been teased by a friend at school about her weight. Slightly plump, Natasha worried that she had disappointed her parents and had not lived up to their expectations of what she should be. She asked solemnly why her mother's legs were more slender than hers.

One could infer that Natasha was trying to identify with her mother and, perhaps, compete with her a bit, too. Natasha's mother was attuned to these and other issues at hand: she recognized the growing preoccupation of young children, like her daughter, with the cultural stereotype and with the shape of their own bodies. She reassured Natasha that, as she grew to womanhood, her figure would change: the "fat" that she was seeing would be redistributed on her body and used to feed her children. This sensitive mother then empathetically explained, "Someday you will need some fat to feed your little ones just as I fed you. It's not bad for little girls or women to have fat on their bodies. They need this fat because it will later be put to good use and keep them healthy."

Natasha was unconvinced. For quite some time, she continued to complain to her mother about her "fat legs." Because of what Natasha had seen in the media and heard discussed by her friends, her mother had to spend a great deal of time educating and reassuring her daughter about what was normal. Peer attitudes, originating and reinforced by cultural views, were not easily overcome, even by this sympathetic and involved parent.[43]

THE ROLE OF MASSAGE IN THE DEVELOPMENT OF A HEALTHY BODY IMAGE

Massage Provides Perceptual Feedback

There are at least four different kinds of nerves of the skin in all mammals. Just under the epidermis, nerves that end in Meissner corpuscles are responsible for sensations of itching and light touch. Deeper within the dermis are insulated fibers that innervate the pacinian corpuscles; these onion-layered miniorgans allow perception of pressure. Ruffini corpuscles, deeper in the dermis, respond to heat in one temperature range, while Krause end bulbs pick up temperature changes at another range.

Uninsulated nerves that terminate at the dermal-epidermal junction are the nerves predominantly responsible for detecting subtle pressure changes at the skin surface. The deeper nerves, well-insulated with myelin, have more weighty functions, including the perception of pressure, deep pain, and temperature changes. In aggregate, it is these nerves that give us our outer sense of self and provide sensations of impending forces that may injure us severely.[132]

—*Mark Lappe, MD*

All humans need a certain amount of tactile stimulation to maintain a healthy body image. Without any perceptual feedback, we soon experience serious distortions of our body image, such as changes in the perceived size or weight of different parts of our body. Massage is a rich source of perceptual feedback that can stimulate the various nerves in the skin and construct a realistic, well-defined body image. Massage techniques can give children a tremendous amount of information about their bodies. For example, a long effleurage stroke from the hand to the shoulder and back can tell a child exactly how long and how wide the arm is, in effect creating an outline of the area for the brain. Varying amounts of pressure provide gradations of feedback to pressure receptors in the skin and muscles. Direct pressure techniques, such as ischemic compression and acupressure, give feedback on density and tension of muscle tissue. Tapotement can give the child a sense of the solidity of different areas of the body. Range of motion techniques can give the child information about how the bones relate to each other and how heavy the parts of the body are. Stretches can give a sense of the length and plasticity of muscle tissue. Positional changes during massage, such as lying on the side, can give an awareness of more than just the front or the back of the body. The temperature of the therapist's hands and the massage oil or cream provides thermal feedback as well.

The Touch Research Institute found that Swedish massage given twice weekly to teenage girls who were hospitalized for bulimia led to a less-distorted body image after 5 weeks.[17] Infant massage instructor Helen Rowe tells of a similar success with a 7-year-old girl with a thyroid disorder. The child was the size of a 3-year-old, and, when someone drew around her body on butcher paper, she was upset to see just how small she was. After receiving infant massage techniques, however, she remarked that she felt much taller.[133] Massage is physically pleasurable and leaves a strong impression in the child's mind because pleasurable touch enhances the perception of the touched part.[127]

The Santa Cruz California Office of Education pilot study found significant improvement in body image in many of the 25 children who were disabled who received 8 weekly sessions of Jin Shin Do (see Figure 1–6). One boy became more aware of the difference between his right side and his left side. Another had increased internal awareness of his body, with improvements in his ability to control his movements.[26]

Massage Reinforces Body Boundaries

Self-touching is one common way that people reinforce their body boundaries; it tells the self "the edge of me is there and intact." The patient cited earlier is an example of how a child used self-touching to comfort herself and reinforce her boundaries.[35] Nursing professor Irene Riddle suggests that when restraining children in the hospital, positioning them so that they can self-touch can be an important way of validating

TT's Drawing of himself February 9, 1981

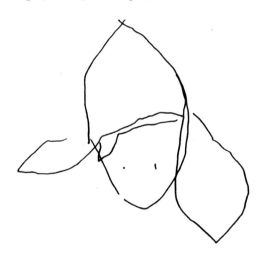

TT's Drawing of himself May 8, 1981

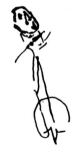

FIGURE 1–6 ■ Body image before and after eight sessions of acupressure. Self-portraits provide many indicators of self-esteem, as well as motor control. This 6-year-old boy was in a special education program; he had aphasia and gross and fine motor coordination problems. His second self-portrait indicates that his body awareness has noticeably increased. Reprinted with permission from: St. John J: *High Tech Touch: Accupressure in the Schools.* Novato, CA: Academic Therapy Publications, 1987, p 66.

their boundaries.[127] Massage can reinforce the child's boundaries in much the same way, as the repeated laying on and taking off of the hands increases awareness of their edge—where the body stops and the world begins.

Massage Enhances a Sense of Body Intactness

Riddle recognized the need for touch to enhance the child's sense of body wholeness. She felt that confinements, restraints, extensive bandages, traction, and casts all limit the child's mobility and may seriously decrease the tactile, kinesthetic, and visual perceptions he needs to define his body boundary and his location in space. Riddle called for nursing intervention to be specifically designed to provide the child with adequate perceptual feedback. She felt that this principle could be incorporated into the caring process through the use of touch, through encouragement of the full range of passive movements, and by whatever active movements the child was capable of. Simple games such as "Where's your leg? Here's your leg!" "Where's your foot? Here's your foot!" when carried out with the daily bath could also help a child maintain a sense of intactness even when immobilized.[127] Those who work with children who are blind or visually impaired recommend lots of tactile stimulation to help the children develop a healthy body image.[134]

Massage Shows Respect for the Child's Body

Riddle points out that, in many health care settings, children are not afforded the same respect as adults, and she believes that children can never learn to respect their bodies unless they are first shown that respect.[127] Susan Thompson, a massage therapist who was born with a cleft palate, illustrates the impact on her body image from the medical care she received. "My earliest memories of touch are unpleasant ones. I have effectively blocked out many details of my 17 operations, but can clearly remember the nauseating smell of ether, the painful removal of stitches from my lip and nose, and the anger and humiliation I felt at being physically restrained with wooden arm splints tied down to my bed. Touch became associated with a sense of bodily invasion." Many years later, Hakomi bodywork helped her to restore respect for her body.[135]

During massage, show respect for the child's body by obtaining her permission to be massaged, giving her privacy, and protecting her from being inappropriately exposed. By listening carefully to what she prefers in terms of strokes and pressure and avoiding the areas where she clearly does not want to be touched, the therapist teaches the child that she has the right to have her bodily needs met, that she can have control over her body, and that she can set appropriate boundaries.

REVIEW QUESTIONS

1. Identify five scientifically validated physiologic effects of massage with children that can also be confirmed by firsthand observation.

2. Explain how massage and nurturing touch can benefit a child emotionally.

3. Discuss the major stressors affecting American children today and the evidence that a high stress level is affecting them in various ways.

4. Discuss the physiologic effects of the fight-or-flight response to stress.

5. Explain how massage therapy can help treat high levels of stress and stress-related health problems in children.

6. Give five examples of pain or trauma to a specific area of the body that can cause muscular shielding in a child.

7. Give five examples of mind-body approaches to addressing a child's physical and emotional problems.

8. Discuss the importance of the body image to a child's personality.

9. Discuss the normal development of a healthy body image. What can disrupt this normal development?

10. Explain how massage can enhance the development of a healthy body image.

REFERENCES

1. Fritz S: *Mosby's Fundamentals of Therapeutic Massage*. St. Louis: Mosby-Year Book, 1995, p 79-88

2. Prentice W: *Therapeutic Modalities for Allied Health Professionals*. New York: McGraw Hill, 1998, p 412-415

3. Tappan F: *Tappan's Handbook of Healing Massage Techniques: Classic, Holistic, and Emerging Methods*. New York: Prentice Hall, 1998, p 21-33, 43-47

4. Travell J, Simons D, Travell J: *Travell and Simon's Myofascial Pain and Dysfunction: The Triggerpoint Manual*, vol. 1, Upper Body. Baltimore: Lippincott Williams & Wilkins, 1999

5. Temerlin MK, et al: Increased mothering and skin contact on retarded boys. *American Journal of Mental Deficiency*, 71:890-894, 1967

6. Schulz RL, Feitis R: *The Endless Web: Fascial Anatomy and Physical Reality*. Berkeley, CA: North Atlantic Books, 1996, p 14-15

7. Aftimos S: Myofascial pain in children. *New Zealand Medical Journal*, 9:440-441, 1989

8. Fine P: Myofascial trigger point pain in children. *Journal of Pediatrics*, 111:547-548, 1987

9. Bates T, Grunwaldt E: Myofascial pain in childhood. *Journal of Pediatrics*, 22:4, 1952

10. Prudden B: *Pain Erasure the Bonnie Prudden Way*. New York: Ballantine, 2002

11. Hernandez-Reif M, et al: Cerebral palsy symptoms in children decreased following massage therapy. *Journal of Early Intervention* (in press)

12. Oz M: *Healing from the Heart: A Leading Heart Surgeon Explores the Power of Complimentary Medicine*. New York: Dutton, 1998, p 106-109

13. Upledger J: *Research and Observations Support the Existence of a Craniosacral System*. Palm Beach Gardens, FL: Upledger Institute, 1995

14. Reite M: Effects of touch on the immune system. In Gunzehauser N: *Advances in Touch: New Implications in Human Development*. Johnson and Johnson Consumer Products, 1990, p 22-29

15. Field T: *Touch Therapy*. Edinburgh: Churchill Livingstone, 2000, p 214

16. Field T: HIV teenagers show improved immune function following massage therapy. *International Journal of Neuroscience*, 106:35-45, 2001

17. Field T: Massage therapy for children. *Journal of Developmental and Behavioral Pediatrics*, 16:105-110, 1995

18. Ferber S, et al: Massage therapy by mothers enhances the adjustment of circadian rhythms to the nocturnal period in full-term infants. *Journal of Developmental and Behavioral Pediatrics*, 23:410-415, 2002

19. Field T, et al: Massage therapy lowers blood glucose levels in children with diabetes mellitus. *Diabetes Spectrum*, 10:237-239, 1997

20. Field T, et al: Juvenile rheumatoid arthritis benefits from massage therapy. *Journal of Pediatric Psychology*, 22:607-617, 1997

21. Hernandez-Reif M, et al: Children's distress during burn treatment is reduced by massage therapy. *Journal of Burn Care and Rehabilitation*, 22:191-195, 2001

22. Kubsch S, et al: Effect of cutaneous stimulation on pain reduction in emergency department patients. *Complementary Therapies in Nursing and Midwifery*, 4:25-32, 2000

23. Dietz F, Mathews K, Montgomery W: Reflex sympathetic dystrophy in children. *Clinical Orthopedics and Related Research*, 258:225-231, 1990

24. George T: With his parents' touch. *Massage Magazine*, January/February:44-48, 2000

25. Field T: Children with asthma have improved pulmonary functions after massage therapy. *Journal of Pediatrics*, 132:854-858, 1998

26. St. John J: *High Tech Touch: Acupressure in the Schools*. Novato, CA: Academic Therapy Publications, 1987, p 52-58

27. Hernandez-Reif M, et al: Cystic fibrosis symptoms are reduced by massage therapy intervention. *Journal of Pediatric Psychology*, 24:183-189, 1999

28. Lynch J, et al: Effects of human contact on the heart activity of curarized patients in a shock-trauma unit. *American Heart Journal*, 88:160-169, 1974

29. Field T, et al: Preschool children's sleep and wake behavior: Effects of massage therapy. *Early Child Development and Care*, 120:39-44, 1996

30. Newsletter of the Northwest Acupressure Institute, Eugene, OR, Spring 1987

31. Settle F: Muzica, da? My experience in a Romanian orphanage. *Massage Therapy Journal*, 30:64-72, 1991

32. Greenough B, Black JE: Induction of brain structure by experience: Substrates for cognitive development. In Gunnar MR, Nelson CA: *Minnesota Symposia on Child Psychology*, vol. 25. Hillsdale, NJ: Earlbaum, 1992, p 155-200

33. Land P, et al: Early experience of tactile stimulation influences organization of somatic sensory cortex. *Nature*, 326:694-696, 1987

34. Triplett J, Arneson S: The use of verbal and tactile comfort to alleviate distress in young hospitalized children. *Research in Nursing and Health*, 2:17-23, 1979

35. Colton H: *The Gift of Touch*. New York: Seaview/Putnam, 1983

36. Field T, et al: Massage therapy reduces anxiety in child teenager psychiatric patients. *Journal of the American Academy of Adolescent Psychiatry*, 131:125-131, 1992

37. Field T, et al: Alleviating posttraumatic stress in children following Hurricane Andrew. *Journal of Applied Developmental Psychology*, 16:37-50, 1996

38. Coles R: Touching and being touched. *The Dial*, Public Broadcasting Publication, December, 1980, p 29

39. Rosenthal M: Psychosomatic study of infantile eczema. *Pediatrics*, 10:581-592, 1952

40. Seitz P: Psychocutaneous conditioning in the first two weeks of life. *Psychosomatic Medicine*, 12:187-188, 1950

41. Biggar M: Maternal aversion to mother-infant contact. In Brown C, ed: *The Many Facets of Touch—The Foundation of Experience: Its Importance Through Life, With Initial Emphasis for Infants and Young Children*. Skillman, NJ: Johnson and Johnson Baby Products Company Pediatric Round Table Series, 1984, p 15

42. Kulka A, Fry C, Goldstein F: Kinesthetic needs in infancy. *American Journal of Orthopsychiatry*, 39:562-571, 1960

43. Zerbe K: *The Body Betrayed—A Deeper Understanding of Women, Eating Disorders, and Treatment*. Carlsbad, CA: Gurze Books, 1995

44. Shevrin H, Toussieng P: Conflict over tactile experiences in emotionally disturbed children. *Journal of the American Academy of Child Psychology*, 1:564-569, 1972

45. Elkind D: *The Hurried Child: Growing Up Too Fast Too Soon*, ed. 3. New York: Perseus Publishing, 2001

46. Spock B, quoted in Zill N: Children under stress. *U.S. News & World Report*, October 27, 1986, p 64

47. Pruitt D: *Your Child: What Every Parent Needs to Know about Childhood Development from Birth to Preadolescence*. New York: Harper Collins, 1998, p 110-111

48. Garbarino J: *Lost Boys: How Our Sons Turn Violent and How We Can Save Them*. New York: The Free Press, 1999, p 107

49. Grossman D: *On Killing: The Psychological Cost of Learning to Kill in War and Society*. Boston: Little, Brown, 1999, p 314

50. Berg F: Television ads promote dieting. *Healthy Weight Journal/Obesity and Health*, 7:106, 1993

51. Berg F: *Children and Teens Afraid to Eat: Helping Youth in Today's Weight-Obsessed World*. Hettinger, ND: Healthy Weight Network, 2001, p 21, 43

52. Rubinstein S: Is Miss America an undernourished role model? *JAMA*, 283:1569, 2000

53. Berg F: Thin mania turns up pressure. *Healthy Weight Journal/Obesity and Health*, 6:l83, 1992

54. Oswalt R, Davis J: Societal influences on thinner body size in children. *Proceedings of the Eastern Psychological Association*, Philadelphia, PA, April 1990

55. Statistical Abstract of the United States, 114th ed., Washington, DC: Department of Commerce, 1994

56. Louv R: *Childhood's Future: New Hope for the American Family*. Boston: Houghton Mifflin, 1990, p 15

57. Carton B: Young Guns. *Boston Globe*, June 7, 1999, p B2

58. Burg F, Wald E, Ingelfinger J, Polin R: *Gellis and Kagan's Current Pediatric Therapy*. Philadelphia, PA: W.B. Saunders, 1999, p 406

59. Putnam R: *Bowling Alone: The Collapse and Revival of American Community*. New York: Touchstone, 2000, p 70-73

60. Guthrie E: *The Trouble With Perfect: How Parents Can Avoid the Overachievement Trap and Still Raise Successful Children*. New York: Broadway Books, 2002, p 80, 93

61. Zaslow J: When little kids take big tests. *Time Magazine*, March 11, 2001, p 71

62. Murdock M: *Spinning Inward: Using Guided Relaxation with Children for Learning, Creativity and Relaxation*. Boston, MA: Shambahla, 1987, p 22

63. U.S. Bureau of the Census, 1997

64. Berk L: *Infants and Children, Prenatal through Middle Childhood*. Needham Heights, MA: Allyn and Bacon, 1999, p 235

65. Behrman R, Kliegman R, Jenson H, eds: *Nelson Textbook of Pediatrics*. Philadelphia, PA: W.B. Saunders, 2000, p 134

66. High School Dropout and Completion Rates 1972-1999, National Center for Education Statistics. Available at: http://nces.ed.gov/pubs2001/dropout. Accessed January 2003

67. National Institute on Drug Abuse: High School and Youth Trends in Drug Use. Available at: http://www.nida.nih.gov/Infofax/HSYouthtrends.html. Accessed January 2003

68. Oster G: *Helping Your Depressed Teenager: A Guide for Parents and Caregivers*. New York: John Wiley and Sons, 1991, p 14-15

69. National Institute of Mental Health: Depression in Children and Teenagers. Available at: http://www.nimh.nih.gov/publicat/depchildresfact.cfm. Accessed January 2003

70. National Institute of Mental Health: Suicide Facts. Available at: http://www.nimh.nih.gov.reaearch/suifact.htmath. Accessed January 2003

71. Centers for Disease Control and Prevention: Nation and State-Specific Pregnancy Rates Among Teenagers 1995-1997. Available at: http://www.cdc.gov.mmwr/preview/mmwrhtml/mm4927a7.htm. Accessed January 2003

72. Smolak L, Levine M: Toward an empirical basis for primary prevention of eating problems with elementary school children. *Eating Disorders*, 2:293-307, 1994

73. Gustafson-Larson AM, Terry RD: Weight-related behaviors and concerns of fourth-grade children. *Journal of the American Dietetic Association*, 8:818-822, 1992

74. *Food Nutrition News*, 65:4, 1993

75. Nichter M, Park S: Body image and weight concerns among African American and white adolescent females. Anthropology Department, Tuscon, AZ: University of Arizona, 1994

76. Richardson B, Rehr E: *One Hundred and One Ways to Help Your Daughter Love Her Body.* New York: Harper Collins, 2001, p xvi

77. Shelov S, Kelly J: *Raising Your Type A Child: How to Help Your Child Make the Most of an Achievement-Oriented Personality.* New York: Simon and Schuster, 1991, p 76

78. Bonne Bell Company, Lakewood, OH, http://www.bottledemotion.com

79. Friedman M: *Type A Behavior: Its Diagnosis and Treatment.* New York: Plenum Publishing, 1996

80. Hunter S, et al: Tracking of type A behavior in children and young adults: The Bogalusa Heart Study. *Journal of Social Behavior and Personality*, 6:71-84, 1991

81. Friedman M, quoted in Rosch P: Social support: the supreme stress stopper. *Newsletter of the American Institute of Stress*, 1997, p 7

82. Hunter S, et al: Type A coronary-prone behavior pattern and cardiovascular risk factors in children and teenagers: The Bogalusa Heart Study. *Journal of Chronic Diseases*, 35:613-621, 1982

83. Hill R, Castro E: *Getting Rid of Ritalin: How Neurofeedback Can Successfully Treat Attention Deficit Disorder Without Drugs.* Charlottesville, VA: Hampton Roads Publishing, 2002, p xii, 16

84. Stolberg S: Preschool meds. *New York Times Magazine Supplement*, November 17, 2002, p 58-61

85. Sapolsky RM: *Why Zebras Don't Get Ulcers: An Updated Guide to Stress, Stress-Related Disease, and Coping.* New York: W.H. Freeman, 1998

86. Weinstock M, et al: Does prenatal stress impair coping and regulation of the hypothalamic-pituitary-adrenal axis? *NeurolScience Biobehavioral Review*, 21:1-10, 1997

87. Zuckerman B: Maternal depression: a concern for pediatricians. *Pediatrics*, 79:111-115, 1987

88. Zuckerman B, et al: Maternal depressive symptoms during pregnancy and newborn irritability. *Journal of Developmental and Behavioral Pediatrics*, 11:418, 1990

89. Hoffman S, Hatch M: Stress, social support, and pregnancy outcome: a reassessment based on research. *Pediatric and Perinatal Epidemiology*, 10:380-405, 1996

90. Elwood S, et al: Catecholamine response of children to a naturally occurring stressor situation. *Journal of Human Stress*, Winter:154-161, 1986

91. Engel GL, et al: A study of an infant with a gastric fistula. I. Behavior and the rate of total hydrochloric acid secretion. *Psychosomatic Medicine*, 18:374-398, 1956

92. Anand K: The biology of pain perception in newborn infants. In Tyler D, Krane E, eds: *Advances in Pain Research Therapy.* New York: Raven Press, 1990, p 113-155

93. Boyce, et al, cited in Olness K, Kohen D: *Hypnosis and Hypnotherapy with Children.* New York: Guilford Press, 1996, p 326

94. Brownlee S: The biology of soul murder. *U.S. News & World Report*, November 11, 1996, p 71

95. Mann S: *Healing Hypertension—Uncovering the Secret Power of Your Hidden Emotions.* New York: John Wiley and Sons, 1999

96. Brazelton TB: *To Listen to a Child: Understanding the Normal Process of Growing Up.* Reading, MA: Addison-Wesley, 1984, p 9, 10, 29, 125

97. Ireland M, Olson M: Massage therapy and therapeutic touch in children: state of the science. *Alternative Therapies*, 6:54-63, 2000

98. Olness K, Cohen D: *Hypnosis and Hypnotherapy with Children.* New York: Guilford Press, 1996, p 178-79

99. Sumar S: *Yoga for the Special Child.* Chicago, IL: Special Child Publications, 1998

100. Roghman KJ: Daily stress, illness, and use of health services in young families. *Pediatric Research*, 7:520-526, 1973

101. Heisel J, et al: Significance of life events as contributing factors in the diseases of children. *Journal of Pediatrics*, 83:119-123, 1973

102. Mutter A, Schleifer M: The role of psychological and social factors in the onset of somatic illness in children. *Psychosomatic Medicine*, 28:333-343, 1966

103. Greene J, et al: Stressful life events and somatic complaints in teenagers. *Pediatrics*, 75:19-22, 1985

104. Dumont L: *Surviving Adolescence: Helping Your Child Through the Struggle to Adulthood.* New York: Villard Books, 1991

105. Goldberg R, et al: Relationship between traumatic events in childhood and chronic pain. *Disability and Rehabilitation*, 21:23-30, 1999

106. Powell GF, et al: Emotional deprivation and growth retardation simulating idiopathic hypopituitarism. *New England Journal of Medicine*, 276:1271-1278, 1967

107. Oates RK, et al: Long-term effects of non-organic failure to thrive. *Pediatrics*, 75:36-40, 1985

108. Sherry D, et al: Psychosomatic musculoskeletal pain in childhood: Clinical and psychological analyses of 100 children. *Pediatrics*, 88:1093-1099, 1991

109. Verny T: *The Secret Life of the Unborn Child.* New York: Delta Books, 1981, p 210

110. Milne H: *The Heart of Listening.* Berkeley, CA: North Atlantic Books, 1995, p 393

111. Porter F, et al: Long-term effects of pain in infants. *Journal of Developmental and Behavioral Pediatrics*, 20:253-261, 1999

112. Gray L, et al: Skin-to skin contact is analgesic in healthy newborns. *Pediatrics*, 105:14-20, 2000

113. Sparshott M: Psychological function of the skin. *Paediatric Nursing*, April:22-23, 1991

114. Grogan S: *Body Image: Understanding Body Dissatisfaction in Men, Women, and Children.* London and New York: Routledge, 1999

115. Cash T, Pruzinsky T: *Body Image: A Handbook of Theory, Research, and Clinical Practice.* New York: Guilford Press, 2002

116. Krueger D: Psychodynamic approaches to changing body image. In Cash T, Pruzinsky T: *Body Image: A Handbook of Theory, Research, and Clinical Practice.* New York: Guilford Press, 2002, p 463

117. Blaesing S, Brockhause J: The development of body image in the child. *Nursing Clinics of North America*, 7:597-607, 1972

118. Bluestone J: Course syllabus 2001. Get a HANDLE on

Neurodevelopmental Disorders: Observational Assessment and Drug-Free Treatment. HANDLE Institute, Seattle, WA

119. Horne R, Van Vactor J, Emerson S: Disturbed body image in patients with eating disorders. *American Journal of Psychiatry*, 148:211-215, 1991

120. Garner D: Body image and anorexia nervosa. In Cash T, Pruzinsky T: *Body Image: A Handbook of Theory, Research, and Clinical Practice*. New York: Guilford Press, 2002, p 463

121. Gupta M, Gupta A, Schork N, Watteel G: Perceived touch deprivation and body image: some observations among eating disordered and non-clinical subjects. *Journal of Psychosomatic Research*, 39:459-464, 1995

122. Hart S, et al: Anorexia nervosa symptoms are reduced by massage therapy. *Eating Disorders*, 9:289-299, 2001

123. Weiss S: Parental touch and the child's body image. In: *The Many Facets of Touch—the Foundation of Experience: Its Importance through Life, With Initial Emphasis for Infants and Young Children*. Skillman, NJ: Johnson and Johnson Baby Products Company Pediatric Round Table Series, 1984, p 2

124. Krueger D: Psychodynamic perspectives on body image. In Cash T, Pruzinsky T: *Body Image: A Handbook of Theory, Research, and Clinical Practice*. New York: Guilford Press, 2000, p 32

125. Blaesing S, Brockhause J: The development of body image in the child. *Nursing Clinics of North America*, 7:597-607, 1972

126. Harlow H: The nature of love. *American Psychologist*, 12:573-685, 1958

127. Riddle I: Nursing intervention to promote body image integrity in children. *Nursing Clinics of North America*, 7:651-661, 1972

128. Neinstein L: *Teenager Health Care: A Practical Guide*. Baltimore: Lippincott Williams & Wilkins, 1996, p 42-43

129. Fabian R, Thompson JK: Body image and eating disturbance in young females. *International Journal of Eating Disorders*, 8:63-74, 1999

130. Gerhart A: More young women choose surgical perfection. *Washington Post*, June 23, 1999

131. Wooley SC, Kearney-Cooke A: Intensive treatment of bulimia and body-image disturbance. In Brownell KD, Foreyt JP, eds: *Handbook of Eating Disorders: Physiology, Psychology, and Treatment of Obesity*. New York: Basic Books, 1986, p 476-502

132. Lappe M: *The Body's Edge: Our Cultural Obsession with Skin*. New York: Henry Holt, 2001, p 61

133. Massaging the handicapped child. *Tender Loving Care*, 4:2, 1988

134. Scott E, Jan J, Freeman R: *Can't the Child See? A Guide for Parents and Professionals About Young Children Who Are Visually Impaired*, ed. 3. Austin, TX: Pro-Ed, 1995, p 36

135. Thompson S: AboutFace, facial sculpting, and healing touch. *Touchstone, the Journal of the Oregon Massage Therapists' Association*, p 7, Summer, 1992

NOT A MINIATURE ADULT: THE UNIQUE DYNAMICS OF PEDIATRIC MASSAGE

2

The transformation of a human being from a tiny infant to a full-grown adult is a complex, sophisticated process. At each stage of transformation, however, obstacles may arise that can interfere with children becoming adults who are at home in their bodies, free of musculoskeletal pain and with a healthy attitude toward touch. These obstacles include emotional trauma, injuries, and physical or emotional abuse. Sensitive caring massage can go a long way towards helping children heal their negative effects and develop in a healthy way. In this chapter, we look at normal child development to give you an understanding of how children can be helped by massage during different developmental stages. We begin by describing the major musculoskeletal differences between a child's body and an adult's body and continue by discussing each unique stage of pediatric growth and development. We conclude the discussion with ideas on how to customize massage therapy to individual children and how to prepare to work with children, including taking a pediatric medical history.

POINT OF INTEREST BOX 2–1
Typical Vital Signs for Various Stages of Childhood[1,2]

Pulse or Heart Rate

1. Infant: 160
2. Preschool child: 120
3. School-age child: 100
4. Teenager: 80

Systolic Blood Pressure

1. Infant: 80
2. Preschool child: 90
3. School-age child: 92
4. Teenager: 100

Respiratory Rate

1. Infant: 40
2. Preschool child: 30
3. School-age child: 18
4. Teenager: 12

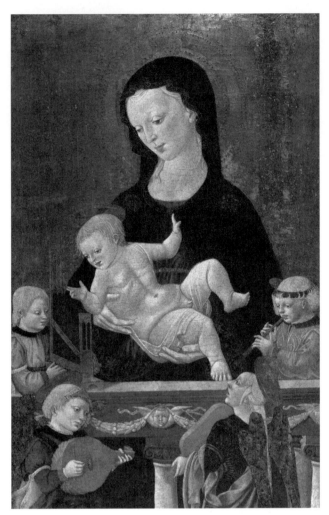

FIGURE 2–1 ■ An Infant Depicted as a Miniature Adult. This medieval depiction of Jesus as an infant looks incongruous to the modern eye because the artist really portrayed a miniature adult. The features that we recognize as characteristic of an infant, such as a disproportionately large head and soft facial features, are not depicted here. Until he reaches adulthood, the muscles of the chest, abdomen, legs, and feet will not really be this well defined, nor will the bones of his lower extremities be so stout and well developed. "The Virgin and Child with Angels," c. 1450, by Apollonio de Giovanni. Courtesy of the Fogg Art Museum, Harvard University Art Museums, The William M. Prichard Fund. Photo by Rick Stafford.

THE GROWTH AND DEVELOPMENT OF CHILDREN

During the childhood years, body tissue grows far more rapidly than that of an adult. Together with physical growth, major advances occur in such areas as coordination, strength, self-control, reasoning, and the ability to relate to others. Maturation happens in a fairly predictable sequence of developmental leaps, as children's bodies, minds, and abilities develop and expand (see Figure 2–3). New abilities develop in each stage of childhood, based on those skills that have already developed. For example, children must learn to crawl before they can walk, and to walk before they can run. Although children are natural candidates for sensitive, caring massage, they may present the therapist with different needs at different ages. Also, child development does not always fit into neat categories; at any given time, a child may be ahead of the average development in some areas and behind in other areas. However, thinking this way about childhood is useful to begin to make sense of the many different things that happen as a child grows.

THE FIRST 3 YEARS OF LIFE— A BRIEF REVIEW

Although this book does not discuss infant massage, a review of the first 3 years of life is necessary to understand the foundation of childhood growth and development. Development is defined as *the acquisition and refinement of different skills.*

Physical Development

During the first 3 years of life, children's bodies grow and develop rapidly in many amazing ways. By the end of the first year, a child weighs three times as much as at birth; the head has grown as much as it will for the remainder of childhood.[3,17] By the end of the second year, a child's brain has tripled in weight, as the nerve cells, which formed before birth, are sculpted by experience and interconnections continue to multiply.[18] This rapid growth and maturation of the brain is reflected by major leaps in all areas of development.

Much of the newborn skeleton is immature at birth; the pelvis and legs are still primarily cartilage, the baby's vertebrae are all the same shape, and the skeleton is made up of 330 separate bones.[19,20] However, by the end of the third year, the spine, femurs, tibiae, and the arm and hand bones are nearly twice as long as at birth.[20] Due to this rapid bone growth, a child's height increases an average of 10 inches a year. By contrast, even at the peak of height growth during puberty, children grow only about 4 inches a year.[17] This growth process continues until the child reaches full height— in the middle or late teens (Figure 2–3).* In the first 3 years, not only has bone growth continued at a rapid pace, the extreme flexion typical of full-term babies

---

*Ossification of the skeleton takes place gradually. The baby's vertebrae begin to shape individually, and the 330 bones of the infant skeleton eventually fuse, becoming the 206 bones of the adult skeleton.[5]

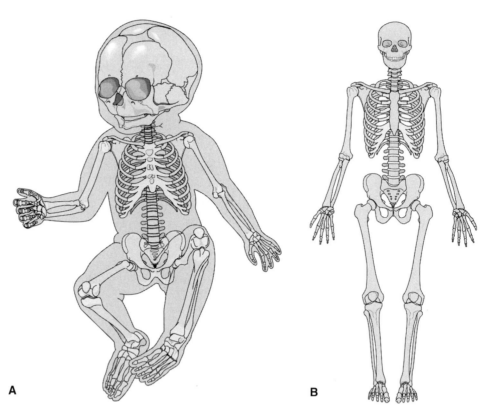

FIGURE 2–2 ■ Newborn Skeleton Versus Adult Skeleton. Note the dramatic differences in the shape, number, and degree of ossification of bones between the newborn skeleton **(A)** and the adult skeleton **(B)**. LifeART images, ©2004, Lippincott Williams & Wilkins. All rights reserved.   **A**   **B**

has also decreased because they are no longer folded up in utero and they begin to creep, crawl, and walk.[21] By age 3, children may have already acquired significant musculoskeletal issues as a result of their position in utero, the birth process, infections, and injuries. These issues may be the precursors of postural problems and soft-tissue pain (see Point of Interest Box 2–2, page 39).

Motor Development

During the first 3 years, acquisition of motor skills also proceeds with great speed. Children have progressed from being virtually helpless—unable to raise their heads or roll over—to small people who can walk, run, throw overhand, dress themselves, pedal a tricycle, and control their bowels and bladder. They are capable of many activities requiring eye-hand coordination, such as stacking cubes and drawing circles. Visual motor skills have progressed from the infant's initial ability to barely fix on and follow a bold bright object, to now being able to use both eyes together, locate objects in space, follow moving objects (and move the eyes without moving the head), and perceive depth. Visual acuity (sharpness) at birth was 20/600; some children may reach 20/20 by age 3, but many will not see that well until age 5.

Cognitive Development

During the first 3 years, children make major advances in cognitive development. As newborns, their activities were mostly reflexive; as their brains developed, they progressed to simple repetitive behaviors, imitative behavior, and questioning. By age 3, children are curious and enjoy novelty; they begin to develop a sense of self as they are increasingly able to differentiate themselves from their environment. They begin to use language and symbols to represent their environment, and can "pretend" play. During these years, they come to perceive the outer boundaries of the body more specifically and their internal states as separate from their external body boundaries.

Emotional and Social Development

With consistent loving care from a mother or mother substitute, children form deep emotional attachments, which are the basis of healthy emotional relationships in adulthood. During the first 3 years, they also form an awareness of themselves as separate from others. They begin to have stranger anxiety (the fear of unknown adults) and also fear separation

A

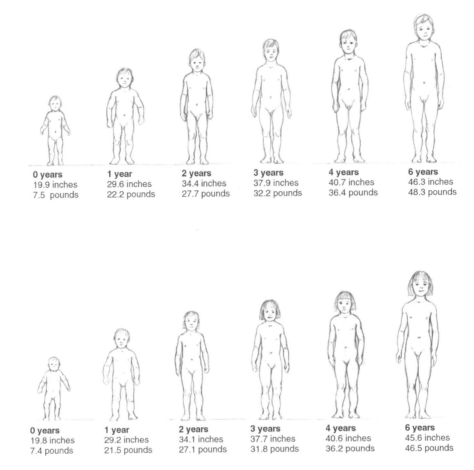

0 years	1 year	2 years	3 years	4 years	6 years
19.9 inches	29.6 inches	34.4 inches	37.9 inches	40.7 inches	46.3 inches
7.5 pounds	22.2 pounds	27.7 pounds	32.2 pounds	36.4 pounds	48.3 pounds

0 years	1 year	2 years	3 years	4 years	6 years
19.8 inches	29.2 inches	34.1 inches	37.7 inches	40.6 inches	45.6 inches
7.4 pounds	21.5 pounds	27.1 pounds	31.8 pounds	36.2 pounds	46.5 pounds

FIGURE 2–3 ■ Stages of Physical Growth During Childhood, From Birth to Age 18. These numbers are averages for American children. A boy's development is shown in the top row; a girl's development in the bottom row.

from their parents. Their language development proceeds at a great pace as well. By age 3, most children have all of their basic language skills. They progress from having no speech and communicating only by crying to speaking their full name, using three-word sentences, and even using the future tense.

Behavior regression is one indicator that children younger than age 3 are under high levels of stress; they regress to behaviors that belong to an earlier, outgrown stage of development. Under high levels of stress, toddlers may regress to infantile behaviors. They may begin sucking their thumbs, after having stopped for months, or begin crying uncontrollably; become hypersensitive to noise; or have nightmares or other sleep problems.

THE PRESCHOOLER—AGES 3 TO 6

Physical Development

Children become taller and heavier during the preschool years, but not as rapidly as before. Between the ages of 3 and 6, the average child grows 3 inches and gains 3 to 5 pounds per year.[18] During these years, children's trunks and legs grow longer, their shoulders grow lower and broader, their necks lengthen, and their chests gradually broaden and flatten. Bowlegs and knock-knees are common until age 5. Joint hypermobility, which is normal at birth, begins to decrease and continues to do so throughout childhood.[22] As infants and toddlers, children breathed mostly with their diaphragm and only minimally

B

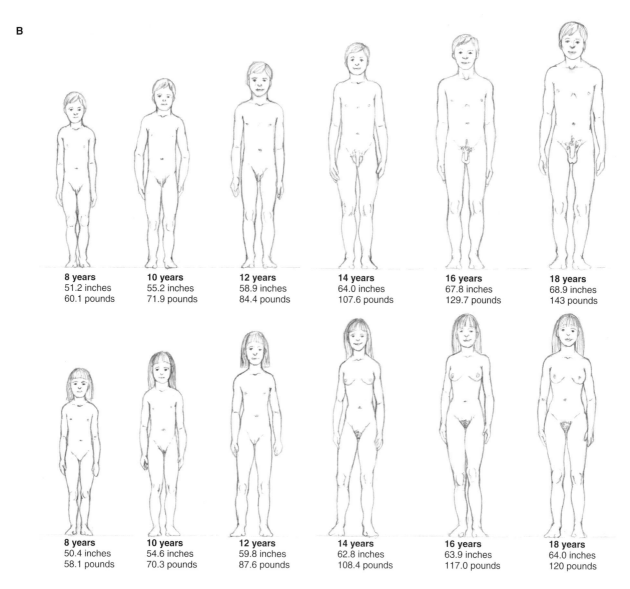

8 years	10 years	12 years	14 years	16 years	18 years
51.2 inches	55.2 inches	58.9 inches	64.0 inches	67.8 inches	68.9 inches
60.1 pounds	71.9 pounds	84.4 pounds	107.6 pounds	129.7 pounds	143 pounds

8 years	10 years	12 years	14 years	16 years	18 years
50.4 inches	54.6 inches	59.8 inches	62.8 inches	63.9 inches	64.0 inches
58.1 pounds	70.3 pounds	87.6 pounds	108.4 pounds	117.0 pounds	120 pounds

FIGURE 2–3 ■ (Continued)

with their chest wall muscles; now they begin to breathe with both.

- The average 3-year-old child weighs 31 pounds and stands 37″ tall.
- The average 4-year-old child weighs 36 pounds and stands 41″ tall.
- The average 5-year-old child weighs 38 pounds and stands 44″ tall.
- The average 6-year-old child weighs 41 pounds and stands 46″ tall.

Motor Development

From ages 3 to 6, most children are able to move around with increasing confidence and competence; they continue to make advances and refinements in gross motor skills, such as running, climbing, and walking. When running, a 3-year-old may have difficulty turning corners and stopping quickly and may often fall down; by age 6, the same child can run in a faster and more controlled way and seldom falls down. Three-year-olds can sit on a riding toy and push it with their feet; by age 6, they can ride a small bicycle.[18] They continue to improve at fine-motor skills such as drawing and dressing themselves. Visual skills requiring the coordination of the two eye muscles continue to develop, but the average child's visual system is not yet mature enough for sustained close tasks such as reading.[23]

Cognitive Development

During the preschool years, children are increasingly able to acquire knowledge and beliefs about their environment, interpret sensory events, and register and receive information from memory. They also begin to reason and understand symbols and images. They have an increased ability to process and express information, to problem-solve, to remember, to concentrate, and to understand. They have no sense of time and do not yet have a complete understanding of the concepts of left and right. Children love imaginative play, such as playing "dress-up" in which they take different roles, and may play happily for long periods. This type of play helps develop both cognitive and motor skills.

Emotional and Social Development

Preschoolers continue to move toward a less egocentric view of the world and begin to have a sense of limits and consideration for others. They begin to learn to repress and control their aggression, but still act impulsively much of the time and are in the early stages of learning self-discipline.

The preschooler is not particularly worried about his appearance; however, children of this age often feel anxious about getting hurt. Fear of injury may start with images of being broken, damaged, or having lost a part of themselves. Adhesive bandages are beloved by this age group because they provide a tactile and visual reinforcement of body boundaries, which preschoolers feel are threatened after injuries. Preschoolers may also focus intensely on potential pain, such as going to the doctor for immunizations.[24] Children who experienced an unusual amount of pain during infancy may exhibit greater anxiety about potential pain.[25] Preschool children may still have stranger anxiety but, in general, they are now less worried about being separated from their parents.

The use of language continues to become more complex and sophisticated; preschool children are able to make longer and more complete sentences and use many more words. (The average 6-year-old has a vocabulary of more than 2,000 words.) However, they are still not fully capable of articulating their feelings.

Under stress, preschoolers may become irritable, anxious, or overly fearful. Common behaviors include uncontrollable crying, an exaggerated fear of being alone, anger, and eating or sleeping problems.

THE SCHOOL-AGE CHILD—AGES 6 TO 12

Physical Development

During middle childhood, children continue to grow in a variety of ways. Slowly but steadily, they grow taller and heavier. The skull and brain grow slowly because they are already at virtually their full size. During these years, the bones continue to lengthen, broaden, and become ossified; however, they are still weaker than mature adult bones. Muscles continue to grow larger and stronger as well. Growth is not steady and there may be growth spurts followed by plateaus.[17] As the bones grow, a child's height increases about 2 inches a year.

The "growth spurt" of puberty, a period of fast growth that continues for 2 to 3 years, begins at the end of this stage of childhood; at about age 10 for girls and age 11 for boys. It accounts for about 25% of the final adult height and 50% of the adult's ideal body weight.[17] During a growth spurt, a child may grow as much as 4 inches a year.

- The average 8-year-old child weighs 59 pounds and stands 51" tall.
- The average 10-year-old child weighs 71 pounds and stands 55" tall.
- The average 12-year-old child weighs 86 pounds and stands 59" tall.

Motor Development

Because children's muscle strength doubles during their school-age years, they can handle greater physical demands in athletic activities; however, they can be easily injured because their bones are not yet fully ossified and their immature muscles can be strained or torn. With brain development and plenty of practice, they continue to gain more control over their movements. Their greater precision of movement and coordination leads to gains in balance, agility, and reaction time. Posture improves and children are steadier on their feet. Fine motor skills, such as model building, drawing, and writing, also continue to improve.

Cognitive Development

During middle childhood, the brain continues to mature. Although its size increases only slightly, myelinization and lateralization of the cerebral hemispheres continues. Children begin to develop a better understanding of cause and effect, and their language abilities and communication abilities also continue to develop.[18] Their ability to localize and communicate physical symptoms is not yet well developed; however, the therapist who hopes to get a complete verbal description of symptoms will probably be frustrated.

Emotional and Social Development

As they mature, school-age children become increasingly independent from their parents, but they still need and want parental authority to help them cope with their expanding environment. Peers become more important to them, and children begin to try out their skills in comparison with their peer groups. They play primarily with same-sex friends, and best friends are important. During these years, children begin to develop a greater understanding of right and wrong and their ability to control their impulses continues. They are also increasingly able to relate to new adults without fear.

Signs that school-age children are under high levels of stress include behavioral problems, such as excessive worrying, irritability, not attending to school or friends, and withdrawal from others. Physical manifestations can include headaches, stomachaches, insomnia, and loss of appetite.

BOX 2–1

MUSCULOSKELETAL DIFFERENCES BETWEEN CHILDREN AND ADULTS

Children are truly not just miniature adults; the human body is not fully mature until about age 20. Here are some of the differences the hands-on therapist will encounter between the bones and soft tissue of children and those of adults:

- When infants are born, their cranial bones are not fused; instead, the bones are separated by gaps, or soft spots, called fontanels. This allows for significant molding to take place during the birth process. During the first 2 years of life, the fontanels gradually close and sutures are formed that permit the skull to expand easily as the brain grows. The cranial sutures do not firmly unite until about puberty. Sutures are not completely calcified, even in the adult, but contain collagen, elastic fiber, blood vessels, and nerve fibers.[3,4] Unlike the adult skull, the shape of the skull in childhood is so changeable that it may be permanently altered by the application of force.*
- Compared with the prominence in the adult face, a child's face and jaw are relatively underdeveloped at birth. This makes it easier for the head to pass through the birth canal. As a result, there is a greater growth of facial structures than of cranial structures during childhood—the face increases in size to a greater extent than does the rest of the skull.[9]
- The child's periosteum is thicker, stronger, and more biologically active than the adult's.[10]
- Until **ossification** is complete, a child's bones are not as hard or dense as an adult's bones (see Figure 2–4). For example, the cranial bones at birth are the consistency of a paper milk carton.[11] Because children's bones are not as strong as adult bones, they are more prone to fractures; adults are more likely to have soft tissue injuries, such as ligament sprains or dislocations.[10] However, a child's fractures heal more rapidly as a result of a more active periosteum and a more abundant blood supply to the bone. The younger the child, the more rapid the healing.[10]

- Children are more flexible than adults and have joints that are hypermobile compared with adult joints. Because the child's spine is more mobile than an adult's, a force that could cause a spinal cord injury in an adult may not injure a child. Instead, the force can be more easily dissipated over a greater number of segments, and the spine will "give" rather than break.[12] Children's tendons, muscles, and ligaments gradually become more rigid as they grow, and the greater range of motion of most joints will gradually disappear. An infant's backs and hips bend so much, for example, that they can bend over from a sitting position and lie across their straightened legs. During early childhood, young children can still touch their toes with their legs straight but they are not able to bend as far forward. By adulthood, many will find it difficult to touch their toes at all. True **hypermobility**, however, is present in only a small percentage of children.[13]
- From birth, a child's skeletal muscles become progressively stronger until about age 20; they gain weight at about the same pace. Their strength remains at that level for 5 to 10 years and gradually decreases throughout the rest of life.[14]
- Children begin to develop measurable muscle tightness as they grow. Increasing height and weight are correlated with an increasing incidence of muscle tightness in the triceps, rectus femoris, tensor fascia latae, thigh adductors, hamstrings, quadratus lumborum, trunk erectors, levator scapulae, upper trapezius, hand flexors, and finger flexors. This muscle tightness increases from ages 8 to 16 and then usually remains constant. It does not decrease unless it is treated with stretching exercises or other therapy. Children who are not physically fit have more muscle tightness.[15]
- Children's muscle tissue is not as dense as that of adult's and, therefore, requires less pressure. However, their muscles are not fragile; children can tolerate and enjoy firm pressure.

(continued)

---

*The skull during infancy and young childhood is mobile and will change shape in response to pressure, both external and internal. In many places around the world including Europe, Africa, and North and South America, people have taken advantage of the mobility of an infant's skull to intentionally alter its shape for aesthetic reasons. (The skull has been purposely deformed.) Tying hard, flat objects to the front and/or the back of the skull flattens the frontal and occipital bones; wrapping the head with tight cloth bands produces a circular depression around the entire circumference of the skull. Inadvertent deformities occur as well; for example, wrapping an infant in a hard cradle board puts pressure

on the lower occiput, causing it to flatten.[5,6] The success of the "Back-to-Sleep" SIDS prevention program, which warns parents to always place newborns on their backs when putting them to sleep, has increased the number of flat spots occurring on the occiput.[7] Deformities also occur when torticollis causes an infant or child to sleep with the head turned in one direction, which places the face and skull under constant pressure.[8] The cranial bones grow in response to internal pressure, as well; the entire top of the skulls of children with **hydrocephalus** is enlarged as the bones grow to accommodate the increased intracranial pressure.[9]

MUSCULOSKELETAL DIFFERENCES BETWEEN CHILDREN AND ADULTS (*Continued*)

- Normal body posture is different for children than for adults. The typical child ages 2 to 3 years has a protruding abdomen and a mild lumbar lordosis (swayback). By age 6, with increased strength of the abdominal and other muscles, there is less lordosis. Newborns are top-heavy because of their proportionately larger head and because their center of gravity is at the xyphoid process. By late childhood, with increased growth of the extremities, their center of gravity shifts to the upper, anterior edge of the first sacral vertebrae.

- A child's body is smaller than an adult's. An effleurage stroke, performed with the whole palm on an adult, may need to be done with only the fingertips in a small area on a child.
- A child's skin is softer and more mobile and sensitive than an adult's skin. However, it is extremely strong. The skin of a child can withstand over 25 pounds of force applied laterally before tearing.[16]

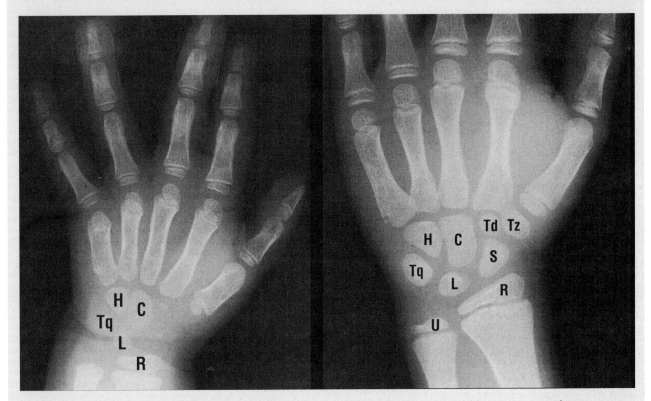

FIGURE 2–4 ■ Ossification of the Hand and Wrist Bones in a 2-Year-Old Child and an 11-Year-Old Child. Image courtesy of Dr. D. Armstrong, University of Toronto, Toronto, Ontario, Canada.

THE TEENAGER—AGES 12 TO 18

Physical Development

During the years from 12 to 18, a teenager grows rapidly and is forced to adjust to many physical changes in a short time; body proportions become more and more like those of an adult, and body image undergoes major changes.

As they grow, girls add proportionately more fat; boys, more muscle. Both of their muscles become larger and more developed in response to bone growth. As more and more cartilage becomes bone, the bones also become larger, as well as heavier. The great increases in a teenager's height are a result of

this bone growth, first in the legs and then in the trunk. Teenagers are generally 80% of their adult height when they are 12 years old; by age 17, they have reached 95% of their adult height.[26] The head does not grow much because the brain is already at its adult weight by age 6. At the end of the growth spurt, males will be, on the average, 6 inches taller than females. At the end of puberty, the teenager's original cartilage has been almost completely replaced by bone, and the cartilage cells and the growth plates stop multiplying and disappear.

As their bodies grow, teenagers' proportions become more like an adult. Different parts of the body

(text continues on page 41)

POINT OF INTEREST BOX 2–2
Early Causes of Myofascial Restriction and Myofascial Trigger Points

1. Fascial restriction caused by the position of the fetus in utero.

   In a now-classic study of myofascial restriction, the dissection of the bodies of two infants who had died at birth revealed many of the same restrictions that are common in an adult. Fascial shortness was found along the outside of the legs, as well as a buildup of gnarled fascia along the bottom of the pelvis. Fascial wrappings of individual muscles, such as the pectoralis major and the upper trapezius, had already adhered to the muscles themselves. Tight muscles were found in the lower back as well. R. Louis Schulz, the Rolfer and anatomist who directed the dissection, believes that these restrictions were primarily caused by the infants' position in utero (Schulz RL, personal communication, May 2001).

   "Around the sixth month of pregnancy, size limitations in the uterus become a factor in the development of fascial patterns. For example, when the legs are folded within the uterus, tension may be created between the kneecap and the hip. Where there is this kind of pressure, the stimulation causes a heavier concentration of fibers, forming a thickened sheet of fascia . . . The child's position in the uterus is, thus, important in its structural development and alignment. Whether the head is to the right or to the left of the knees, where the arms are in relationship to the spine—these factors establish the individual pattern of the vertebral column . . . Such primary rotations are augmented and compensated for by intrauterine limitations during late pregnancy."[1] Based on his expertise as a scientist, as well as a bodyworker, Schulz believes that these rotations in the fetus continue in the structure of the adult. However, this has not been scientifically proven.

   The position in utero may also influence the fascia of the lumbar area. According to Schulz, "The knee-up position in the fetus makes an almost direct line of restriction across the pelvis between the

   (continued)

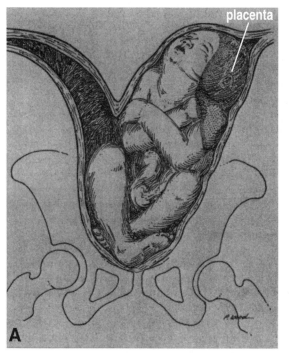

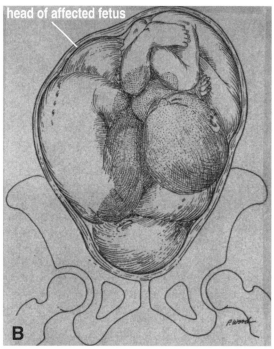

FIGURE 2–5 ■ Uterine malpositioning, leading to premature fusion of the metopic suture, which is between the two halves of the frontal bone at the forehead and normally closes by age 8. In both cases, the sutures closed before birth because the fetal head was positioned so that there was no room for the frontal bones to grow and expand laterally. Both children were born with a triangular configuration of the head, narrow foreheads, ridging where the metopic suture would have been, and close-set, slanting eyes. **A,** The fetal head is tightly impacted together with the placenta in the limited space of the left horn of the mother's uterus. Note the anterior position of the placenta and the constricted position of the fetus' neck. This bicornate (two-horned) uterus is a rare malformation (Drawing based on ultrasound). **B,** The fetal head of the triplet who is head-up is tightly wedged between the hips of the two triplets who are head-down. The mother is a small woman whose uterus is not large enough to accommodate all three triplets without extreme crowding (Drawing based on radiograph). Reprinted with permission from Graham L, et al: Metopic craniostenosis as a consequence of fetal head constraint: Two interesting experiments of nature. *Pediatrics*, 65:1000-1002, 1980.

POINT OF INTEREST BOX 2–2
Early Causes of Myofascial Restriction and Myofascial Trigger Points (Continued)

lower back and the inside of the thigh. This stress line is continuous with the fascial thickening on the small of the back. The combination is a compressed, leaning S-curve between the lower back and the leg. This structure is functional in the womb and as the child crawls. But as the body begins to stand, the shortness is felt as a restriction that inhibits secure upright balance. Gradually, as demand for stable movement increases, this tissue must lengthen or, as is more usual, the growing child finds compensations around the shortness to serve its needs. The lumbar spine may come too far forward or the legs may be pulled up and into the body. There are numerous examples of such restrictions and connections as the child develops in the womb."[1]

2. Myofascial trigger points caused by the fetus's position in utero.

   Long-time myotherapist Bonnie Prudden has found that every newborn has myofascial trigger points, which she believes are largely a result of the effects on the body of the position in utero. She likens this position to "sitting in a chair for 4 straight months with your head tucked between your knees" (Prudden B, personal communication, February 2003).

3. Deformities caused by intrauterine crowding.

   When there is insufficient space for the fetus, a variety of deformities may result, including clubfoot, bowing of the long bones, hip dislocation, and fibrous shortening of the sternocleidomastoid, leading to **torticollis.** An arm that is pressed against the face can prevent the maxilla or mandible from growing normally.[2,3] The legs are usually more tightly constrained than the arms because of their greater size. If the fetus is lying in a transverse or oblique position and there is no room for the fetal head to expand as it grows, some of the sutures may fuse together before birth. In the same way, the crowding of two or more fetuses in the uterus can prevent the head from growing and lead to premature fusing of sutures.[4-6] Crowding can also cause other deformities. For example, the author observed two boys from different sets of twins in infant massage classes. One boy lay under his larger sister in utero; at birth, his second and third cervical vertebrae were fused together and one side of his skull was flattened. The second boy had been side-by-side with his twin sister. A number of ultrasounds in the last months of pregnancy showed that the twins were head down. The boy's head was turned sharply to the left, and he had no room to move his head in any other position. At 3 months, his head was still turned sharply to the left, just as it had been in utero. He never looked

even slightly to the right and resisted any attempt to turn his head in that direction. Physical therapist and Feldenkrais instructor Deborah Bowes treated a baby whose mother was a tiny woman from the Philippines and whose father was a tall, Caucasian man. The baby was too large for her mother's uterus and, for some time before birth, her mouth was compressed against the inside of the mother's pubic bone with sufficient force to leave a dent above her upper lip. After birth, the baby refused to open her mouth and had to be fed through a stomach tube (Bowes D, personal communication, September 1992). Deformities may also be caused by a breech position in utero: an infant may be born with muscular torticollis, scoliosis, hip dislocation, clubfoot, and other musculoskeletal defects.[2,7]

4. Effects of birth trauma.

   Birth trauma may cause trigger points on the head as a result of pressure on the head, particularly during a difficult labor and/or forceps or a vacuum delivery (see Birth Trauma, page 100). Once activated, trigger points may be latent or active, but they never disappear. They may remain as a cause of myofascial tightness and pain throughout life. For example, trigger points in the temporalis, occipitalis, and posterior cervicals, all of which may be caused by birth trauma, are known to induce migraines.[8]

   Traction on the head during delivery may cause strain to the suboccipital muscles, leading to torticollis, scoliosis, asymmetrical muscle development, and head tilting. Breech delivery may also cause damage to the upper trunk of the brachial plexus, as the head is tractioned and tilted laterally to deliver the head (see page 101). Fracture of the humerus or clavicle may occur simultaneously.[7] Due to neck stiffness and pain, infants with suboccipital strain may also be unusually restless or unhappy.[9]

5. Infections and injuries.

   Trigger points in small children may be initiated by upper respiratory and other infections.[10] Injuries, such as falls, may also cause soft tissue problems. For example, the author's son jumped out of a child's backpack at age 7 months and severely sprained his wrist. Toddlers are at risk of injury because they are not aware of potential dangers, such as hot objects, dangerous heights, and other hazards. Among children age 3 and younger, 25% have had more than one injury since birth that required medical treatment.[11] Fractures of the phalanges and metacarapals are common in the first 2 years when the children are learning to walk. Fractures of the tibia are common in the toddler years.[12]

   (Continued)

POINT OF INTEREST BOX 2-2
Early Causes of Myofascial Restriction and Myofascial Trigger Points (Continued)

References

1. Schulz RL, Feitis R, Salles D: *The Endless Web: Fascial Anatomy and Physical Reality.* Berkeley, CA: North Atlantic Books, 1996, p 14–15, 17
2. Saven L: *Textbook of Orthopedic Medicine.* Baltimore, MD: Lippincott Williams & Wilkins, 1998, p 22
3. Long T, Toscano K: *Handbook of Pediatric Physical Therapy.* Philadelphia, PA: Lippincott Williams & Wilkins, 2001, p 8–10
4. Graham, et al: Sagittal craniostenosis: Fetal head constraint as one possible cause. *Journal of Pediatrics,* 95:747, 1979
5. Graham, et al: Coronal craniostenosis: Fetal head constraint as one possible cause. *Pediatrics,* 65:995, 1980
6. Graham, et al: Metopic craniostenosis as a consequence of fetal head constraint: Two interesting experiments of nature. *Pediatrics,* 65:1000, 1980
7. Morrissy R: *Lovell and Winter's Pediatric Orthopaedics.* Baltimore, MD: Lippincott Williams & Wilkins, 2001, p 102, 109
8. Travell J, Simons D: *Myofascial Pain and Dysfunction: The Triggerpoint Manual,* vol. 1, ed. 2. Baltimore, MD: Lippincott Williams & Wilkins, 2001, p 117
9. Rockwell J, DC, quoted in Starlanyl D: *Fibromyalgia and Chronic Myofascial Pain: A Survival Manual.* Oakland, CA: New Harbinger, 1996, p 151
10. Aftimos S: Myofascial pain in children. *New Zealand Journal of Medicine,* August:440–441, 1998
11. Childhood Injury Fact Sheet. National SafeKids. Available at: www.SafeKids.org. Accessed July 2002
12. Ogden J: *Skeletal Injury in the Child.* Philadelphia, PA: Lea and Febiger, 1982, p 4

grow at different rates, which make some children look or feel awkward or gawky. For example, the hands and feet often grow before the hips and shoulders. Some teenagers may go through a period of tripping over their feet or banging into things. Gradually, however, the growth of different parts of the body stabilizes, teenagers become more accustomed to their new form, and their gawkiness disappears.

The growth of reproductive tissue (testes and ovaries) is minimal during childhood; at puberty, there is a huge growth spurt that continues throughout adolescence. Girls begin to menstruate and must cope with breast development and other changes in body shape; boys begin to experience erections, nocturnal emissions, and cracking voices. These developments can cause them to feel anxious or embarrassed.

- The average 12-year-old weighs 86 pounds and stands 59″ tall.
- The average 14-year-old weighs 108 pounds and stands 63″ tall.
- The average 16-year-old weighs 123 pounds and stands 66″ tall.
- The average 18-year-old weighs 132 pounds and stands 67″ tall.

Motor Development

Strength, coordination, and stamina continue to develop as teenage bones and muscles mature. Many athletic abilities peak at age 17 or 18. As a result of this physical vigor, teenagers often have feelings of strength and confidence that are new to them. Unfortunately, these feelings, combined with high energy levels and feelings of invulnerability, make teenagers especially prone to risk-taking. Sadly, injuries are the leading cause of death in this age group.

Although visual motor skills should also be at their peak, one national health survey of 7,000 American youths, ages 12 to 17, found that 12% had moderate to severe eye muscle imbalance in the lateral plane; 1 of 12 had significant eye abnormalities, with the most prevalent problem being **strabismus**.[17] A period of high stress, caused by such events as a death or divorce in the family, a move to a new home, or a negative learning situation in school may precipitate vision problems.[27]

Cognitive Development

Many mental abilities continue to develop during the years from 12 to 18, so that teenagers are increasingly capable of mature memory and attention. Their abilities grow in abstract thinking and problem-solving, and greater sophistication in reading and writing becomes possible. Teenagers become capable of thinking in hypothetical terms and imagining all the possibilities inherent in a situation; however, they continue to have a feeling of invulnerability—bad things happen to others, not to me—which may cause them to be repeatedly at risk.

Emotional and Social Development

The major challenges of the teenage years are:

- To become independent, with one's own identity and sense of self, while still staying related to others. Searching for their own unique identity is part of normal teenage development but, as they move away from what has been their major source of self-esteem—their parents—teens may feel a sense of emptiness.
- To make sense of relationships and the need to feel a sense of belonging and companionship. A

teenager's happiness and psychological well-being is strongly tied to feeling that he has social support and is being included in peer groups. Teenagers also begin to define themselves as sexual beings and begin to explore romantic love.

- To learn how to make appropriate decisions, through trial and error, input from others, and natural consequences.
- To learn how to assume personal responsibility for their actions.
- To adjust to a rapidly changing body.

These are major developmental tasks for any individual and can cause major stress. Most teenagers weather this process well, but approximately 20% of teenagers suffer deeply and experience extreme inner turmoil.[28] Signs of stress may include depression or behavior problems, such as excessive anger, low self-esteem, rebellion, and breaking rules. Bru et al. found that a high level of life stress was significantly associated with increased teenage misbehavior in school, such as bullying, fighting, and disrupting the classroom.[29] Physical manifestations include headaches, stomachaches, insomnia, and loss of appetite. Wide mood swings and ready expressions of anger, coupled with feelings of inadequacy and difficulty asking for help, make parenting the teenager more challenging than with any other age-group.

Teenagers may test authority as a way to better define themselves. Lack of impulse control is still common, but this tends to diminish as they mature.

ADAPTING MASSAGE THERAPY TO CHILDREN OF DIFFERENT AGES

WORKING WITH PRESCHOOLERS

Preschoolers present a real challenge for the hands-on therapist. Because of their stage of intellectual development, it is not always possible to elicit their cooperation with rational explanations of the importance of massage. You will need to use extra patience, playfulness, and understanding to coax them to be still for any time. Any coercion or restraint will not only violate their boundaries, it will prejudice them against you. An example of the worst-case scenario is a preschooler who, accompanied by his mother, visited a well-known Rolfer and ended up crouched under a tabletop, screaming loudly. The Rolfer later admitted that he had no experience with children and, consequently, no idea how to prepare the child for bodywork. The classic advice of Margaret Palmer[30] (see Point of Interest Box 2–3) is still appropriate when working with preschoolers today.

Dr. T. Berry Brazelton[31] tells of receiving a phone call from the mother of 4-year-old Laura, who had a severe

POINT OF INTEREST BOX 2–3
Advice on Massage for Children From 1918

Babies do not always like their toes interfered with, but recourse may be had to the oft-told tale of 'How this little pig went to market, and this little pig stayed home.' It is difficult to get a child of one or two years to lie on its face, so the back has to be done in a sitting position; astride on the lap of the mother or nurse and facing her is a good plan. Young children are happier on the mother's or nurse's lap during a séance . . . The ages of the little patients range from a few weeks to 10 or 12 years. Ten minutes at a time is sufficient for quite a baby; with older children 10 minutes to begin with, then 20, then 30. Thirty minutes is the maximum, 5 minutes of which should be given to the spine, which it is always well to add to the local treatment. . . Delicacy of touch, cheerfulness of manner, and unbounded sympathy are essential qualifications in the masseuse who undertakes the treatment of the little ones.

—*Margaret Palmer (from* Lessons on Massage, *which was published in its fifth edition in 1918. Palmer used Swedish massage to treat children with polio, cerebral palsy, spinal curvature, chorea, rickets, clubfoot, and other orthopedic problems.)*[30]

stomachache. Laura had experienced several severe stomachaches in the last few months, which were cared for by following the advice he gave over the telephone. With this particular stomachache, however, Dr. Brazelton felt he needed to examine Laura personally or she would need to be seen in the hospital emergency department.

"I felt her belly in order to find out where her pain was located. Laura looked at me knowingly as I attempted to distract her from the pain in her belly. On my examining table, she seemed very worried about herself. She whimpered so convincingly that I felt an urgency to help her. Her mother stood watching us, with anxiety in her face. 'She certainly can't be faking. She'd never leave her own birthday party to get you to examine her. She's been looking forward to her birthday for weeks! And she never got to blow out her candles or eat her cake!' At this reminder, Laura's groaning increased in intensity. Even as I came near her, she began to wince and guarded her abdomen. So worried was she, that the muscle wall of her abdomen was too tense for me to palpate it successfully. I could not tell whether it was from pain.

I lifted Laura onto her mother's lap, holding her teddy bear. I told her I wanted to feel his belly too. I asked her to flex her legs up on her abdomen. I put my hand firmly on her belly, but without pressure. Meanwhile, I assured her that I wasn't going to hurt her and that I would see that her bellyache got 'fixed.' She looked at me with anxiety about what I might find. When I listened with my stethoscope, I was reassured. There were bowel sounds all through her abdomen. The gurgles and growls that are a normal accompaniment to bowel activity become decreased or absent in an inflamed or obstructed area. When there is an acute appendix cooking, the bowel sounds will be absent in that area.

I asked her to hold her beloved teddy bear so I could see where his pain was. She assured me he had no stomachache. As she held him, I pressed on his sawdust-filled belly and he let out a squeak. We both laughed, and I pressed him in another spot. No squeak! We both laughed harder. Meanwhile, with the other hand, I had been kneading her belly. As she watched me play with her teddy, couched in the safety of her mother's arms, she had relaxed. As she became distracted, I was able to palpate her abdomen, to reassure myself and her concerned mother that she was all right."[31]

Dr. Brazelton used four principles that are essential when working with preschoolers:

1. Reassurance. Laura was told she was not going to be hurt and that her stomachache would be "fixed." She was able to sit on her mother's lap, a place of great safety.
2. Distraction. Dr. Brazelton was able to distract Laura from his examination of her stomach by playing with her teddy bear. Other ways to distract a child are singing, telling stories, and using toys or other interesting objects to hold the child's attention (see Figure 2–6).
3. Warmth and playfulness. Preschoolers naturally appreciate an adult who is willing to joke and be silly with them. They are reassured and often charmed by an adult who is able to "think like a kid." For example, during the ball rolling portion of massage (Chapter 3), you might be giving a massage and playing a game at the same time, by using a ball that squeaks or has a bell inside it or by using the ball to play a variation of "the eensie-weensie spider."

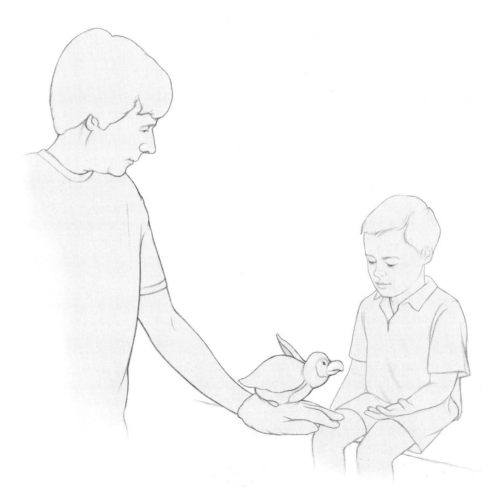

FIGURE 2–6 ■ Toys and other interesting objects can help the therapist win the cooperation of a reluctant child.

4. Sensitivity to the child's feelings. Notice that Dr. Brazelton made no attempt to restrain Laura when she was examined; instead, he found a way to examine her that she could accept without resistance.

Some additional guidelines to make massage therapy more effective with preschoolers include the following:

- Ask parents to bring their children when they are rested. Morning is probably the best time of day. Many children are still taking naps at this age, so be sure to ask parents when the child would normally take a nap.
- Preschoolers will need more familiarity with you and your environment than an adult. Ordinarily, most preschoolers won't be comfortable arriving at a completely unfamiliar place (your office) and having a stranger massage them. Unless you go to their house or they are unusually comfortable with massage and strangers, you may want to have them visit your office for a few minutes before they come in as a patient. Even if they simply come in for 5 minutes, look around, and play briefly, the experience will increase their comfort level immensely; they will not be going to a "strange" place when they return. An ideal situation would be to have them drop in with their mother or father, play with a toy that interests them, and have a snack or pat a live animal, such as a friendly kitten or a nonaggressive dog. (Ask about allergies to cats and dogs before exposing a child to animals.)
- The massage environment should have toys or other objects that are of interest to children, and it should be safe to explore. A variety of massage tools, such as rollers, interesting shaped objects, and tools with different textures, will keep the child interested in what you are doing. Hairbrushes—both soft, baby brushes and the somewhat stiffer adult brushes—are excellent for skin stimulation. All items should be washable and should be washed after each patient.
- A favorite music tape may be brought from home to make children more comfortable. If they have a special comfort object, such as a stuffed animal or blanket, ask the parents to bring it along.
- Modesty is not usually an issue to preschool children; however, you should always ask if undressing is permissible and ask the child's parent to remove the child's clothing. Small-sized drapes may be used, but it is often difficult to keep a drape on wiggly children.
- Because children this age cannot verbalize their feelings as well as older children, you may need to be even more sensitive to nonverbal cues of resistance or pain, including flinching, holding the breath, grimacing, or tensing other parts of the body. If children seem nervous about a stranger touching or examining them, have the parent do as much of the first massage as possible. Begin by teaching the parent some simple massage strokes, avoiding strokes that are painful.
- With rare exceptions, preschool children will not lie still for as long as adults. They have shorter attention spans, and their small bodies do not require as much massage. To encourage them to lay still, take a playful approach as you do the massage; try singing, for example, or playing games or giving them a variety of toys or massage tools to entertain them. Parents are often helpful at knowing what toys their child especially likes or how to keep them amused. Massage therapist and speech/language pathologist Peggy Jones Farlow combines face massage with a game her grandmother played with her as a child. She begins with strokes that go from the child's forehead down to his chin and back up to his forehead several times while saying to the child, "If I lived up here (palms on forehead) and you lived down here (stroke to child's chin), would you come up to see me?" (stroke upward again to child's forehead). I'd come all the way to see you! But first I would go over the mountains (thumbs over eyebrows). I'll slide down this hill (thumbs across the bridge of the nose to the cheeks). Roll down this little hill and up this one (finger rolls downward on upper lip and thumb rolls upward on bottom lip). I'll walk all around the lake (fingertip taps around lips). We can go fishing in the lake (hands make fish-mouth by pulling cheeks together)!" She finishes off the face massage with an ear-rub. "Our ears are used for listening. Sh-sh-sh! Listen. What can you hear?"[32]
- It may not be possible to do specific massage in a small area; children may become bored and suddenly flip over during a massage stroke, so that an effleurage of the back may suddenly become an effleurage of the stomach! To complete a particular number of strokes on a particular area, massage the child for a few minutes, then massage his mother or father for a few minutes, and then massage the child again. Massage therapist Margaret Palmer recommended 10 minutes of massage initially, gradually working up to 30 minutes.[30] The author has found this to be an appropriate guideline for most preschoolers. A full-body Swedish massage for a child may require about 30 minutes, compared with about 60 minutes for a teenager or adult. Extra patience is required for the preschooler. The author did a home visit for a family with a disabled 2-year-old girl

and her three brothers. Because she was only able to be still for 10 minutes, we alternated 10-minute massages: first she was massaged , then one of her brothers was massaged, then she was massaged again, then her mother was massaged and, finally, the little girl received a third 10-minute session.

- Explain what you are doing. Use simple language that children can understand, but do not talk down to them. Studies have shown that children actually have little cognitive knowledge of the body and how it functions until about age 9.[33] Even if children do not fully understand what you are saying, your attempt to communicate shows respect.
- Be sure that any potentially hazardous items, such as Hydrocollator tanks or paraffin baths, are well out of reach. There should be no sharp or breakable objects in the therapy room.
- After receiving a few sessions and becoming familiar with the situation, most preschoolers will be comfortable and happy when they come for their massage session. Make the end of the session more fun for them by giving them a small item, such as stickers, a packet of brightly colored adhesive bandages, bubble wands, or a miniature stuffed animal. Do not give them candy.

WORKING WITH SCHOOL-AGE CHILDREN

Working with school-age children is somewhat different than working with preschoolers; they have a longer attention span and often do not need coaxing to lay still. They are better able to talk about their feelings and can identify areas that are sore or uncomfortable. By this age, children may have more need for massage to help resolve musculoskeletal issues because they are likely to have had more injuries than younger children. Modesty may be more of an issue than for preschoolers.

Guidelines for working with school-age children:

- School-age children are now on a school schedule; the most likely time for their treatments will be after school. After a full day of school and then traveling to your office, however, some children will be overloaded with stimuli. In that case, it will be better for them to arrive a few minutes before their session to allow them to have a few minutes to themselves. This may be accomplished by letting them play quietly in your waiting room with a book or a toy. Or, they may choose to do this in the massage room while the parent receives a short massage.

- Children of this age are more likely than preschoolers to feel comfortable with someone they have never met before; however, it is still ideal for the child and parent to briefly visit the therapist's office before their first appointment. This is especially important if the child is at all apprehensive.
- Toys are not needed to occupy a school-age child as much as a younger child, but objects that are new and interesting, which the child may handle without fear of breaking, will make your office more appealing. The author has a collection of real animal skulls that children may handle; a variety of massage tools; and a collection of balls of different sizes, colors, and textures, including some that make noise.
- It is important to respect a child's modesty. If the child is more comfortable remaining clothed, shorts or bathing suits are good options.
- School-age children often enjoy talking to their therapist, and you may find yourself engaged in interesting conversations. Ask children about family pets, family members, friends, favorite activities, school, what they want to be when they grow up, and other details about their lives. Children have much to offer in their outlook and enthusiasm for the world, and it is great fun to interact with them in this way.
- Children of this age are often intellectually able to understand the benefits of massage, if it is explained to them. They are also old enough to learn relaxation skills.
- Ask the child often about what is the right pressure and type of touch; not only does this make the child more comfortable, it helps him or her have a feeling of control.
- A treatment session may be 30 minutes or more, depending upon the child's attention span and age.
- Joint hypermobility has significantly decreased since the child was a preschooler, but you should exercise caution and not overstretch the school-age child.
- Although their muscle tissue is denser than that of preschoolers, school-age children do not need as much pressure as does an adult.

WORKING WITH TEENAGERS

Although teenagers are more physically and emotionally mature than school-age children, their concerns around their changing body image and sexuality can lead to uncertainty about being touched by a stranger in a personal way. As children grow older, they receive progressively less touch from parents and relatives and, by adolescence, they are receiving

CASE STUDY 2–1

Background

Eleven-year-old Mary has a history of an inherited, nonprogressive muscle disorder (muscular atonia). Similar to muscular dystrophy, this inherited condition causes muscle weakness; however, it is not progressive. Mary's left hip was prone to dislocation from birth. She was in a **spica cast** as an infant and had a femoral **osteotomy** at age 6 to reposition the head of her left femur deeper in the socket. At age 11, she began having problems with left hip pain; a fall appeared to increase her pain and, since that time, Mary had been unable to completely extend her left hip. She could not bear weight on her left foot; when she did, the pain was an "eight" on a scale of one to ten. She was recently seen by an orthopedic surgeon; unaware of just how sensitive her hip was, his examination to determine range of motion was excruciatingly painful. Mary, therefore, tensed her entire leg, and the physician was unable to elicit a full range of motion. Under general anesthesia, when she was not guarding the area, the physician found that her hip did indeed have full range of motion.

Mary had other musculoskeletal problems associated with atonia. Her legs were different lengths as a result of the osteotomy that had never corrected, with secondary scoliosis. She also developed lordosis as a result of compensating for weak pelvic musculature whenever she tried to stand. Although she had no palpable pain around the left femoral head or around the hip socket, she had palpable pain along her hip flexor tendons; specifically, the sartorius and rectus femoris. Her range of motion was: passive flexion of the left hip to about 90 degrees; hip extension was -45 degrees. Mary was referred for massage therapy by her physical therapist to increase her left hip range of motion, stretch a possible hip contracture, and relax the hip joint muscles to decrease pain.

Her mother accompanied Mary for her first visit and all subsequent visits. She entered in a wheeled walker with a seat. She and her mother gave her history. Mary reported pain located in her left groin, near the pelvic insertions of the left adductor muscles. Due to the extreme pain she experienced in the left hip during orthopedic assessments, she was wary of having a stranger manipulate her hip and the surrounding soft tissue.

Treatment

Upon palpation, the therapist found that Mary's left hip adductor tendons were tense and hypersensitive at their medial attachments on the pubic bone, as were her left sartorius and rectus femoris tendons, just distal to the anterior superior iliac spine.

Muscle tone was greater on her noninvolved leg, which she used as a supporting leg when she was not in the wheeled walker. The scoliosis and lordosis were noted as well. Her initial massage treatment consisted of superficial effleurage and petrissage to her legs, hip joints, iliopsoas muscles, and entire back.

The therapist told Mary that she would reduce the pressure at any time Mary felt it was too much, and that Mary should tell the therapist whenever she experienced pain.

No range of motion was attempted during her first visit because of the extreme pain Mary experienced during her orthopedic examination. Her mother was taught how to do superficial effleurage strokes, which she performed at the same time that the therapist was massaging Mary. Mary's mother would do superficial effleurage on one leg, perhaps, as the therapist was doing deeper massage on the other leg. Mary experienced a positive feeling of relaxation after her first session and only mild soreness in the left inner thigh and hip area. Mary had been receiving physical therapy on a regular basis from a female therapist and, because only her mother and a female massage therapist were present during her massage sessions, disrobing was not an issue. Mary was draped for her sessions, with only the treated area exposed.

During the next five sessions, Mary was given a contrast treatment (alternating heat and ice) to the left upper thigh and hip before massage to both relax the muscles of the thigh and hip joint area and to somewhat numb them. In addition, the treatment engaged her interest because it was novel. Her mother assisted in the ice massage portion of the contrast treatment, with considerable joking about the coldness of the ice. Paraffin dips were also used twice on her feet, partly for their therapeutic effect and partly to engage her interest.

After the first two sessions, passive range-of-motion exercises to both hips were added to her treatment. After five sessions, deeper effleurage and petrissage and myofascial release were added to her treatment, always at a depth that Mary could comfortably tolerate. Treatment concentrated on her legs, hip joints, iliopsoas, abdomen, and entire back. Mary was occasionally positioned so that the left hip could be moved in novel ways, stretching tissue that was not being stretched through normal activities such as walking. For example, a small footstool, covered with padding and a sheet, was placed on the massage table, and Mary was positioned across the stool. This position was similar to being on all fours. Her mother supported Mary in this position as she performed active range of motion of her left

(Continued)

CASE STUDY 2–1

(Continued)

hip joint. She received massage of the hip, especially around the hip joint, while her leg was in both internal and external rotation.

After a few sessions, it became obvious to the therapist that Mary's mother was under a continuous high level of stress. She had another child with the same condition and was deeply concerned about her daughter. She often arrived exhausted after a long workday, followed by an hour's drive to the therapist's office. Thereafter, a few minutes were used to give the mother a short massage of the back or neck and shoulders. This massage was done at the beginning of the session and was deeply appreciated by Mary's mother. Mary happily spent that time looking at books or other objects in the therapy room, talking with the therapist and her mother, and playing with a kitten. Then Mary was helped onto the treatment table, and her mother was encouraged to put up her feet and relax while Mary received her massage.

Response

A reduction in the tension of Mary's adductor and hip flexor muscles was observed after two massage sessions; she experienced only slight soreness for a few days postmassage in the area of her left hip. After five treatments, her physical therapist stated that Mary's range of motion in

the left hip had increased by about 30%, and Mary stated that, not only was her pain reduced by about one-third, she could move her left leg more easily and the leg felt "looser." Mary was seen weekly for 10 treatments, then every other week as a maintenance program. Although she had a number of problems that massage therapy was unable to address, such as the scoliosis caused by her leg length discrepancy, her massage treatment not only relieved her pain and increased her range of motion, but taught Mary that she had a right to speak up and tell her doctors and therapists when she was experiencing pain. Her mother learned how to apply simple hydrotherapy and Swedish massage techniques that could be used at home. Mary had also added another caring adult, the therapist, to her support system.

Discussion Questions

1. How was Mary's musculoskeletal system injured or affected by the atonia in her left hip area?
2. What symptoms did Mary have as a result of the atonia in her left hip area?
3. What therapeutic modalities were used, including massage therapy?
4. What personal issues did the therapist need to be sensitive to in addition to the musculoskeletal issues that Mary was being treated for?

---

only a small portion of the touch they received as younger children. (Some touch-starved teens may even become sexually active, when all they really wish for is to be touched or held, rather than to have sex.[34]) For this reason, receiving the amount of touch involved in a massage may be a challenge for them to adjust to. Teenager concern about modesty may be greater than for younger children. Contrary to the understanding of many adults, adolescence can be a very stressful stage of life. Because they are growing and developing at such a rapid rate, teenagers may feel uncomfortable inhabiting their rapidly changing and often unfamiliar bodies. Massage can be an effective tool to help them cope with stress, to become more comfortable in their changing bodies, and to learn to care for their bodies in a healthy way. In addition, teenagers have much to offer the therapist—a unique and fresh slant on life, idealism, and tremendous energy.

Guidelines for working with teenagers include the following:

- Increase the teenager's comfort with the idea of a massage by letting them first watch a session with a parent or friend or by first meeting you and seeing your office. This will not be necessary for all teenagers, but is helpful for those who are tentative. Another option is to first offer the teenager a shorter session in a "safe" body area, such as a massage of the head, neck, and shoulders or the feet and lower legs.
- After taking a medical history, explain to the teen and parent what you plan to do and what you consider appropriate therapy, and ask if all their concerns have been addressed. If the teenager does not want the parent present after the medical history, the parent should remain in the waiting room for the duration of the session. After the first session, it is the prerogative of the family to decide if a parent needs to be there.
- A therapy session may be the same as for an adult; 60 minutes is not too long.
- Holding the teenager's attention to complete

their therapy is not the concern it was with younger children. Offer careful explanations of what you are doing and be available to talk about the stresses in the teenager's life; this is more likely to be brought up in later sessions as the teenager develops trust in you.

- Teenagers may feel uncomfortable with a massage therapist of the opposite sex. When the first contact is made with a parent of a teenager, ask if the teen would prefer a male or a female therapist, and refer to another therapist if appropriate.

- Because concerns about modesty may be greater than with younger children, a special effort should be made to address them. Many teenage clients prefer to remain clothed, especially for the first few massages. Techniques that may be done without disrobing include Swedish massage of the hands, feet, and head; foot reflexology; techniques using rocking, pressure points, compression, or range of motion; and energetic techniques.

- Some teens may be reassured if you are more clinical at first and give a medical explanation of what you are doing. For example, you could use a model of a human skeleton to explain why you are massaging a particular area.

- Stress the relaxation aspect of the massage, and teach a simple relaxation sequence (see Chapter 3). One tremendous postinjury benefit of massage for teens is the opportunity to release tension and guarding caused by pain and discomfort. The author worked with a 14-year-old girl who had dislocated her kneecap doing a kick in karate class. Not only was this injury excruciatingly painful, it also required surgery for knee joint damage. After preparing her knee with an alternating heat-and-ice treatment, effleurage and petrissage strokes were performed around the joint. She was told that the massage would not hurt. She and the author discussed the effect of holding chronic tension in the knee, and she was taught how to visualize healing inside the knee to release tension. The girl was given oil to gently massage into her knee twice a day, partly to stimulate the circulation and partly to help release tension and help her knee feel more like a normal part of her body. This type of treatment can help teach teens to prevent long-term soft-tissue problems by teaching them to recognize and release guarding and tension.

- Painful deep work is not advised unless there is a valid and important reason, which is agreed on by the therapist, teen, and parent. Teens need to know that they do not have to tolerate pain and that they have the right to speak up and tell you how they feel. Tell them that it is fine if they experience a little pain, if they feel that the technique is helping to "work out" tension; however, if the pain causes them to tense other areas of the body (such as gritting their teeth or grimacing), the therapy is not helping them relax.

- Use caution when speaking to a teenager about his or her body. Concern with physical appearance is natural for teens, and tactless or cruel remarks can wound deeply. If, for example, a teenage boy says something derogatory about his "scrawny" appearance, rather than commenting on his external appearance, be supportive of his health and well-being. You might tell him that his internal feelings of comfort and relaxation matter as much as his external appearance and, that after he leaves high school, there will probably be less social pressure about appearance. At the same time, it is a good idea to be positive about the teenager's physical body. Most of them are in glowing health, and it is always possible to find something both honest and positive to say, if only about skin color or texture, muscle tone, or body function. For example, you might comment on the fact that their immune systems are working well or that they are obviously strong and vigorous. Massage therapist Jane Megard teaches teens that those areas of the body that they are not pleased with may hold more tension. She teaches teens to relax those areas, and talks to them about how to love and nurture them.[35]

- Teens who are interested in sports, especially competitive sports, are motivated to heal their injuries and improve their athletic performance and are often excellent candidates for massage.

PREPARING TO WORK WITH CHILDREN

In the previous parts of this chapter, you gained an understanding of the unique stages of pediatric growth and development and how massage therapy can be adapted to each stage. We now turn to specific ways to prepare for giving massages to children. The final section of this chapter covers four topics:

- Establishing ground rules with the parent and child
- Boundary issues
- Taking a confidential pediatric medical history
- What you will need to set up a good massage environment for a child, including necessary supplies

ESTABLISH A SAFE ENVIRONMENT WITH CLEAR GROUND RULES

Many of the principles and ideas in this section are drawn from the experience of Denise Borrelli, PhD

(Borrelli D, Boston, MA, personal communication, February 2003), long-time massage therapist and psychotherapist.

Begin your first meeting with the parent and child by reviewing the parent handout (see Box 2-2). This will help answer any questions and prevent future misunderstandings. For clarity, these issues are expanded here:

1. Age of consent. Patients are not legally considered adults until age 18, unless they have been legally emancipated.

2. Confidentiality is the basis of trust between you and your clients, no matter at what age. However, if a child should divulge any activity that was putting him at risk, from physical danger to drug abuse, it is your responsibility to ensure his safety by informing his parents. If a child has been abused, the same is true. In the extremely unlikely case of a child revealing parental abuse to you, it is your legal responsibility to notify the child authorities or the child's doctor.

3. Preventing the child from experiencing unwanted touch is essential to a healthy therapeutic relationship. To avoid any confusion about those areas where the child does not want to be touched, after the medical history is complete, tell parents where you will be touching the child and what areas are off-limits.

4. You may refuse to treat a child if there are medical contraindications to massage or if you feel you cannot establish a good relationship with the family. Be prepared to refer the child to another massage therapist.

5. Children may or may not want their parent in the treatment room or on the premises when they are being treated. Until at least age 10, a parent should be on the premises. However, many teenagers would be insulted by the idea that they need an adult nearby! After age 10, you, the parent, and the child should make this decision together.

Setting Appropriate Boundaries With Children

When giving massages to children, it is important to realize that the power imbalance between an adult and a child is even greater than the normal power imbalance in a therapeutic relationship between two adults. Professional helping relationships often develop an element of transference, in which the parent-child relationship is unconsciously reestablished. According to physician Eric Cassell, "Tenderness is associated with our parents, and we transfer our permissiveness in this regard to parent surrogates." Healers become parent figures, and we transfer to

---

■ **BOX 2–2**

INFORMATION FOR PARENTS

1. Because your child is younger than 18, you must give your consent for treatment. The only exception is if your child is an emancipated minor.
2. Everything that you and your child tell me is strictly confidential. There are only two possible exceptions to this rule:
   - If your child should tell me something in confidence that I feel is an indication that she is putting herself at physical or emotional risk, I would ask the child to tell you that confidence in front of me; failing that, I would tell you myself.
   - If I need to speak with your child's doctor about medical issues of concern. When you give permission for your child to receive massage therapy, you are also giving me permission to speak with your child's doctor.
3. For their protection, children should already know that no one should touch them in any area that would normally be covered by a bathing suit, with the possible exception of health care providers, and then only with parental permission. After doing your child's medical history, we can discuss where massage strokes are appropriate. Should there be a need to do massage any place that is normally covered by a bathing suit, I will tell you and we can decide together with your child if that is acceptable. To respect your child's modesty, all parts of the body that are not being massaged will be draped with a sheet or towel at all times. (Drapes may not always stay on a wiggly, small child.)
4. As a health care professional, I reserve the right to refuse to treat your child if I feel there are medical contraindications or other problems that rule out my type of therapy. I will be happy to refer you to another therapist or appropriate health care professional, should that be the case.
5. Parents should remain in the treatment room with their child during the taking of the medical history and remain on the premises if the child is younger than age 10. Between the ages of 10 and 18, the parent's presence is optional. If parent, child, and therapist are all comfortable, the parent may leave the premises.

---

them many aspects of the parental role, as well as "the right to lay hands on us, to be tender to us, and to pass through our territorial defenses."[36] Such transference often makes it difficult for adult clients to tell their therapist something they think the therapist may not want to hear, such as "Ouch, I really don't like what you're doing" or "Actually, I hate having my feet touched." When an adult is massaging a child, transference may be even greater, and it may be even more difficult for the child to indicate discomfort or unhappiness. Also, because children are taught to respect adults as authority figures, they may be afraid to speak up when they don't like what the therapist is doing. For this reason, it is vital for the well-being of the child that the parent and therapist respect the child's boundaries and provide an environment where she can safely state her feelings. Part of the value of the massage experience for children lies in teaching them how to interact in a healthy way in a situation where it is possible to have their boundaries invaded. To create a safe, protective environment for both therapist and child, in which there is no danger of the child's boundaries being violated, it is vital for the therapist to be clear about what is appropriate.

If a parent insists that a child receive massage, you may be caught in the middle. Gently, but firmly, let the family know that, if necessary, you will wait to do massage until the parent and child are in agreement. You should never be put in the position of massaging a child against his or her will.

Having the parent present, for at least the first session, helps children feel protected when they are unsure of what to expect from the experience. Basic guidelines for giving children a massage in a way that respects their personal boundaries include the following:

- Explain what you are going to do and why; giving the parent a massage in front of the child is an excellent way to prepare the child for what is going to take place.
- Limit your touch to what has been contracted for by the parent; for example, do not change the diapers of a small child. During the medical history, ask if there is any body area that should be avoided. For their protection, most children should already know that no one should touch them in any area that would normally be covered by a bathing suit, with the possible exception of health care providers, and then only with parental permission.
- It is important to ask verbal or nonverbal permission of the child before touching and whenever resistance is encountered during a massage. Recognize that it may be difficult for the child to say no; ask the parent for feedback occasionally as well.
- Obtain the consent of the child before massaging a new area of the body. For example, ask, "Is it okay if I massage you here?"
- Drape the child carefully, uncovering only the area that is to be massaged, although with wiggly, small children this may not always be possible. Respect the child's modesty and remain alert for nonverbal signs of discomfort when an area is undraped. Ask the child's permission before undraping any area.

Examples of boundary violations with children include the following:

- A young boy is rolling around on the treatment table, and the therapist, who is trying to give him a massage of the back, finds that the child has suddenly rolled onto his back and does not want to turn back over. The therapist insists that the parent turn the child over and hold him still until the back massage strokes are completed. This is a boundary violation. A more positive way to deal with this situation would be to suggest that the parent read to the child and put the book on the table with the pages facing up. If the child wanted to look at the book, he would have to return to a prone position, and the therapist could complete the back massage while the parent kept the child happily distracted. Another positive response would be to massage the child's face or chest until he flipped over again. Alternatively, the parent could offer the child some type of incentive for lying on his belly for 5 more minutes until the therapist completes the massage. Notice that with these better responses, the child has been coaxed, not coerced, and his boundaries have not been violated.
- A 10-year-old boy with cerebral palsy is still in diapers. Before he receives his massage, his father decides that the child should have his diaper changed. He changes the boy's diaper in the therapist's office while chatting with the therapist. The therapist has committed a boundary violation because, although the boy may not realize it, his privacy has been violated. It would clearly be inappropriate for a 10-year-old boy without special needs to have his genitals exposed and this boy should be no different. The therapist should have left the room and allowed the boy to be changed in privacy.

Now for some examples of a successful way to massage a resistant child and not violate his boundaries; one, a short anecdote and, the other, a full case history, which can be found on page 52 (Case Study 2–2).

The author once worked with a 13-year-old boy with severe abdominal pain that had been diagnosed as a stress reaction by his physician (recently, a close family member had died and the boy's parents had divorced). His mother had made his appointment, and he was clearly uncomfortable with the entire idea. He even brought a buddy along for emotional support. He lay down on the massage table fully clothed and was willing to pull up his shirt to expose his abdomen, but no more. He received abdominal massage for 45 minutes, with his mother, his friend, and his little sister present. At the end of the session, he was pleased with how much better his abdomen felt, thanked the author profusely, and left in a positive frame of mind. To insist that his family members and friend wait outside or that he disrobe would have violated his personal boundaries; instead, because his privacy and feelings were respected, his experience was a positive one.

Setting Appropriate Boundaries With Parents

Clear boundaries protect children, parents, and therapists, and will help make the massage experience safe and comfortable. The following guidelines will help you establish and respect personal boundaries:

- Be sure you understand what boundaries the parent feels are appropriate. For example, the author has encountered parents in infant massage classes who felt strongly about not taking off the child's diapers, although the infant massage protocol calls for the diapers to be off. In one class, the mother of an infant flatly refused to remove any of the child's clothes. The therapist can ask about these feelings during the medical history. A tactful way to do this would be to ask the parent what rules the family has about what parts of the body should be covered and what parts of the body need not be covered.
- Remember that you are not a parenting specialist; therefore, giving advice or making value judgments about parenting is not appropriate, even if the parent requests it.
- Refrain from making value judgments about the child's body or personality.

The following are examples of boundary violations with parents:

- A mother of a 4-year-old girl with chronic stomach pain has brought her for a massage. At the conclusion of the massage, she asks the therapist if the child's pain is from emotional stress. The therapist confirms this and gives the mother advice on the family situation that is causing the stress. This is a boundary violation. The therapist should have referred the mother to the child's pediatrician to rule out any organic illness or should have recommended counseling. This does not mean massage is contraindicated; on the contrary, it may be appropriate for relieving the child's pain and releasing emotional stress and tension in the abdominal area. However, the massage therapist does not have the training or the legal authority to diagnose the causes of chronic abdominal pain.
- An anorexic mother brings her young daughter to a massage therapist because she feels that her own anorexia is related to the lack of touch she experienced as a child. She hopes for a better touch experience for her child. The therapist shows her how to massage the child and asks how the mother's anorexia developed and what

her childhood was like. Some of her questions are very personal. This is a boundary violation because the mother was not coming to the therapist for counseling.

TAKING A CONFIDENTIAL PEDIATRIC MEDICAL HISTORY

The client medical history should be filled out by the parents of children younger than age 4; by the parents of children ages 4 to 10, with the help of the children; and by children ages 10 to 18. Inform older children that all information is confidential. Listen carefully to the parents, as well as to their children, and, no matter what their concerns, support them as the expert when it comes to their own child. Credit them with having brought the child to you for massage therapy because of their concern for their child's well-being.

The history-taking process gives the child a chance to observe you from a distance and become more comfortable with you before any hands-on contact. A preschooler will probably be most comfortable on the parent's lap. An older child may be seated comfortably across from you and near the parent. Approach the child from the same height, not from above. For example, if the child is sitting on a chair, kneel on the floor so you are at about the same eye level.

Address as many questions to the child as you can and remember to ask about any concerns or thoughts he might have. However, recognize that children often have difficulty localizing and communicating symptoms. In one study, 25% of children between ages 9 and 16 were not able to provide even one characteristic of their headache, such as whether it was severe, mild, pounding, squeezing, sharp, dull, or throbbing.[37] Therefore, the parent will often need to supply more information, particularly with smaller children. Because children are not skilled at localizing and communicating symptoms, you need to be even more acutely aware of nonverbal communication. The experience of receiving massage therapy may substantially help these children to identify body feelings. A confidential medical history has been provided in Figure 2–7. Readers may photocopy and use this form in their practice without obtaining further permission.

ESTABLISHING A COMFORTABLE MASSAGE ENVIRONMENT

Small children can become more easily chilled than adults because they have a relatively large surface area for their body weight. The treatment room should be kept at a minimum of 70° F. Have chairs for parents or other family members to use and pillows or child-sized chairs for children to sit on. Remove all items that would be dangerous to a small child, such

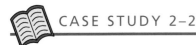

CASE STUDY 2–2

Background
Jane is 11 years old. An American family adopted her at age 5 from an orphanage in Poland. She was brought to a class on massage for children with disabilities because her adoptive mother was concerned about her tactile defensiveness and her inability to form emotional attachments. Her mother hoped that massage would help improve Jane's sleep, help Jane accept touch more readily, and help her be more trusting of others.

Jane and her older sister were left in the care of an aunt when Jane was younger than age 2; both were eventually taken to an orphanage. When she was adopted, Jane had to leave her sister behind; however, 1 year later, the same family adopted her sister, and they were reunited. Jane had endured early separation from her family three times—once from her parents, once from her aunt, and once from her sister. She had not been touched much at the orphanage and, when she arrived in the United States, physical examinations and other touch experiences were extremely difficult for her. Jane is tactile-defensive, has attention deficit disorder, and suffers from severe insomnia (it takes her 2 hours to fall asleep each night). She has a reserved, serious air about her.

Treatment
Jane and her mother came into the classroom the first day and observed the class in session, with children of different ages receiving massage, and Jane was adamant that no one would touch her. Students in the class designed a strategy to coax rather than coerce the girl to participate in any way. One student played with Jane for 2 hours the first day, sharing a variety of puzzles and other toys; they ate snacks together, went outside to watch a mother eagle feed her eaglets, and observed the class. Jane's mother was given a seated massage and did not disrobe, although many of the children were undressed and draped for their massages. Some children were receiving hydrotherapy

treatments as well. Many children and parents came and went that first day, but Jane continued to be adamant that no one was going to touch her.

Response
The next day, Jane arrived in a good mood and ready to play. Again, no one pressured her to receive massage. She played with various toys, ate snacks, and went for a walk outside, accompanied by the student she had made friends with the day before and another child. After walking outdoors, Jane and the other child realized their feet were dirty. The first child had his feet washed and then massaged. Jane decided she should have her feet washed also. As a student was washing Jane's feet off with a washcloth and a towel, Jane asked if the student might "make her feet shiny" too, and the student applied oil and massaged her feet. And that was how she received her first massage.

In a somewhat modified form, the principles of reassurance, distraction, playfulness, and sensitivity that were used successfully with 4-year-old Laura (see page 43) were also successful with Jane. And far more important than receiving any specific massage technique, Jane's boundaries had been respected and she had asked for touch. From that time on, she could begin to receive the benefits of specific massage strokes.

Discussion Questions
1. Why was the simple act of Jane's being able to receive touch more important than any massage technique?
2. What were the simple but appropriate measures taken to win Jane's cooperation in participating in the class? Can you think of any other methods that could have been tried?
3. What would have been some mistakes in trying to approach Jane?
4. What would be a logical next step for performing massage with Jane?

---

as hot water tanks or other heat sources, paraffin baths, sharp objects, and breakable objects.

CHILD-FRIENDLY SUPPLIES

- Toys, stuffed animals, and objects that are interesting and safe for the child to handle. A Raggedy Ann doll is useful to show the child how a leg or arm feels when it is loose and floppy. Preschoolers are often greatly comforted by a favorite object, such as a security blanket or familiar toy, and it may be brought along to make the child feel more secure.

- A variety of massage tools and balls. Let children handle the massage tools and show them how they are used. The balls will also be used for massage. The author has a collection of balls that have different sizes and textures; some have bells inside or squeak when they are pressed, and children enjoy these very much.
- Treatment table or floor pad. Children ages 2 to 4 may prefer to sit on a parent's lap, at least initially. Many small children are better massaged on the floor, as they are more likely than older children to roll off of a massage table. For work-

Confidential medical history for use with a pediatric massage therapy client

Name: _____   Telephone: _____

Address: _____   City: _____ State: _____ Zip: _____

Referred by:_____

Date of birth: _____   Grade in school: _____

Are you currently under a doctor's care? _____   Doctor's name: _____

Birth history:

Premature? _____   Problems? _____

Breech position?_____   Caesarean? _____

Please check if you now have, or ever had, problems with the following:

☐ skin disease   ☐ joint pain or swelling   ☐ other pain

☐ headaches   ☐ contagious illness or disease   ☐ insomnia

☐ epilepsy or seizures ☐ tension or soreness in a specific area   ☐ extra sensitivity to touch or pressure

How is your health in general?

Any chronic health problems?

Any operations in your lifetime?

Injuries:

sprains_____   car accidents _____

broken bones _____   any other major trauma, such as falls or bicycle accidents _____

dislocations _____

concussions or other head injuries _____

Any recent injuries, hospitalizations, or illnesses?

Are you taking any medications?

How much stress have you been under recently?

Where does your body tend to store stress? For example, do you get headaches or stomachaches when you are worried about something?

Is there anything else you would like me to know?

When you receive a massage, you will not be touched in any area that would usually be covered by a bathing suit (shorts for boys, two-piece bathing suits for girls). Is there any other area that you do not want to be touched?

I understand that massage/bodywork is not a substitute for medical examination and treatment. I further understand that massage is for the basic purpose of relaxation, release of muscular tension, and the enhancement of health through increasing circulation and energy flow.

By my signature below, I hereby agree that my child shall receive massage or bodywork from _____, and agree to remain on his/her premises unless that parent, the child, and the therapist are in agreement that the child may remain when the parent leaves.

I hereby give _____ permission to speak with my child's pediatrician if there are any issues of concern.

Signature of Parent or Guardian _____

FIGURE 2–7 ■ Confidential Medical History Form.

ing on the floor, you can use a vinyl or fabric-covered foam pad and cover it with a sheet. These are available in physical therapy catalogs. For older children, use a massage table.

- Have a tape or CD player available. Parents may bring their child's favorite music, which may be played at a low volume during the session.
- Massage lubricants. Use natural oils such as safflower or grape seed oil. Do not use nut-based oils, such as peanut or almond oils. Lotions made from these types of oils are excellent as well. Small children should not be exposed to adult concentrations of essential oils; these should only be used if you have special training on how to use them with children. A small amount of vanilla extract may be added to massage oil for scent; it is not as concentrated as an essential oil. Keep oils and lotions in squeeze bottles because there is a greater likelihood of them being knocked over when working with a small child.
- Linens. It will be helpful to have both adult-sized linens (sheets, blankets, and towels) for teenagers and smaller sheets and blankets for younger children. Use linens, not only for draping, but also for keeping children warm.
- Hydrotherapy supplies. These could include a Thermopore moist heating pad, a hot water bottle, a Hydrocollator steam pack, an ice pack, and small bath towels. If using a Hydrocollator pack, the water tank should be safely out of the way, such as in another room. Use extra caution to ensure that the child is not burned by any heat applications, and inspect the treated area more often than you would with an adult.

The reader has now learned a great deal about the difference between a child's body and an adult's body, and about how children grow and develop physically, emotionally, and cognitively. In addition, the reader has learned how to establish clear boundaries and ground rules to create a safe environment for the child, parent, and therapist and how to take a confidential medical history. Finally, the actual physical items needed to establish an appropriate environment for massaging children have been discussed. In the next chapter, we will turn to the actual techniques of hands-on pediatric massage therapy.

REVIEW QUESTIONS

1. Describe the musculoskeletal differences between a child's and an adult's body. How would you adapt massage strokes to appropriately treat those differences?

2. Compare and contrast the physical and motor development of children during different stages of childhood.

3. Compare and contrast the cognitive development of children during different stages of childhood.

4. Compare and contrast the emotional and social development of children during different stages of childhood.

5. Discuss three different mechanisms by which myofascial restriction and myofascial trigger points may develop in the early years of childhood, and give examples of each.

6. Describe guidelines for winning the trust and cooperation of children during all three stages of childhood.

7. Describe three musculoskeletal differences between children and adults. How would you tailor massage therapy to treat those differences appropriately?

8. Explain the importance of establishing ground rules with the parent and child before treatment. Give three examples of these ground rules from the parent information handout.

9. Describe the process of taking a confidential medical history for a pediatric client.

10. Why is it important to establish and maintain appropriate boundaries with children who are receiving massage and with their parents? Name three ways the therapist can do this.

11. Describe the process of taking a confidential medical history for a child.

12. Describe the ideal massage environment for providing massage therapy to children.

13. Describe the supplies needed for massage with children.

REFERENCES

1. National Center for Emergency Medicine Informatics. Pediatric Vital Signs. Available at: http://www.ncemi.org. Accessed February 2003
2. Pediatric Vital Signs. Available at: http://www.familypracticenotebook.com. Accessed February 2003
3. Nelhaus G: Head circumference from birth to eighteen years: Practical composite international and interracial graphs. *Pediatrics*, 41:106, 1968
4. Upledger J: *Research and Observations Support the Existence of a Craniosacral System*. Palm Beach Gardens, FL: Upledger Institute, 1995, p 5
5. Brothwell D: *Digging Up Bones: The Excavation, Treatment*

and Study of Human Skeletal Remains. Ithaca, NY: Cornell University Press, 1970, p 48

6. Ubelaker D: *Human Skeletal Remains.* Chicago, IL: Aldine Publishing, 1978, p 68

7. Kane AA, et al: Observations on a recent rise in plagiocephaly without syntosis. *Pediatrics,* 19:127-129, 1996

8. Morrissy R: *Lovell and Winter's Pediatric Orthopaedics.* Baltimore, MD: Lippincott Williams & Wilkins, 2001, p 810

9. Proffit W, Fields H: *Contemporary Orthodontics.* St. Louis, MO: Mosby, 2001, p 49

10. Ogden J: *Skeletal Injury in the Child.* Philadelphia, PA: Lea and Febiger, 1982, p 3, 4, 36

11. Gillespie B: *Brain Therapy for Children and Adults: Natural Care for People With Craniosacral, Dental, and Facial Trauma.* King of Prussia, PA: Productions for Children's Healing, 2000, p 101. More information available at: http:// www.healingyourchild.com.

12. Saven L: *Textbook of Orthopedic Medicine.* Baltimore, MD: Lippincott Williams & Willkins, 1998, p 22

13. Gedalia A, et al: Joint hypermobility and fibromyalgia in schoolchildren. *Annals of Rheumatology Diseases,* 52:494-496, 1993

14. Daniels L, Worthingham C: *Muscle Testing: Techniques of Manual Examination.* Philadelphia, PA: W.B. Saunders, 1980, p 3

15. Mackova J: Impaired muscle function in children and teenagers. *Journal of Manual Medicine,* 4:157-160, 1989

16. Lappe M: *The Body's Edge: Our Cultural Obsession With Skin.* New York, NY: Henry Holt, 1996, p 56

17. Neinstein L: *Adolescent Health Care: A Practical Guide,* ed. 3. Baltimore, MD: Lippincott Williams & Wilkins, 1996, p 8, 42, 129

18. Schickendanz J, et al: *Understanding Children and Teenagers.* Boston, MA: Allyn and Bacon, 2001, p 26, 124, 267, 647

19. Schulz R, Feitis R, Salles D: *The Endless Web: Fascial Anatomy and Physical Reality.* Berkeley, CA: North Atlantic Books, 1996, p 25

20. Morrissy R: *Lovell and Winter's Pediatric Orthopaedics,* ed. 5. Philadelphia, PA: Lippincott Williams & Wilkins, 2001, p 50-58

21. Long T, Toscano K: *Handbook of Pediatric Physical Therapy.* Philadelphia, PA: Lippincott Williams & Wilkins, 2001, p 163-164

22. Travell J: *Myofascial Pain and Dysfunction: The Trigger Point Manual.* Vol. 2. Philadelphia, PA: Lippincott Williams & Wilkins, 1983, p 18

23. Grossman M: *Greater Vision.* Los Angeles, CA: Keats Publishing, 2001, p 12

24. Pruitt D: *Your Child: What Every Parent Needs to Know About Childhood Development From Birth to Preadolescence.* New York, NY: Harper Collins, 1998, p 101

25. Porter F, et al: Long-term effects of pain in infants. *Journal of Developmental and Behavioral Pediatrics,* 20:253-261, 1999

26. Wong D, et al: *Wong's Essentials of Pediatric Nursing.* St. Louis, MO: Mosby, 2001, p 530

27. Kavener R: *Your Child's Vision: A Parent's Guide to Seeing, Growing, and Developing.* New York, NY: Simon and Schuster, 1985, p 102

28. Dumont L: *Surviving Adolescence: Helping Your Child Through the Struggle to Adulthood.* New York, NY: Villard Books, 1991, p 40

29. Bru E, et al: Social support, negative life events, and pupil misbehavior among Norwegian teenagers. *Journal of Adolescence,* 24:715-727, 2001

30. Palmer M: *Lessons on Massage.* New York: William Wood, 1918

31. Brazelton TB: *To Listen to a Child: Understanding the Normal Processes of Growing Up.* Reading, MA: Addison-Wesley, 1984, p 128

32. Farlow P: Touch to teach—Massage helps special needs children. *Massage Magazine,* November/December 2000, p 109

33. Blaesing S, Brockhause J: The development of body image in the child. *Nursing Clinics of North America,* 7:597, 1972

34. McNarey E: Touching and teenager sexuality. In: *The Many Facets of Touch.* Skillman, NJ: Johnson & Johnson, 1984, p 86

35. Megard J, quoted in Sinclair M: Teenworks: Easing the transition to adulthood. *Massage Magazine,* July/August:63, 1999

36. Cassel E: *The Healer's Art, A New Approach to the Doctor-Patient Relationship.* Cambridge, MA: MIT Press, 1985, p 15

37. Stafstrom C, et al: The usefulness of children's drawings in the diagnosis of headache. *Pediatrics,* 109:460, 2002

SUGGESTED READINGS

1. Wong D, et al: *Wong's Essentials of Pediatric Nursing.* St. Louis, MO: Mosby, Inc., 2001

2. Berk L: *Infants and Children: Prenatal Through Early Childhood.* Boston, MA: Allyn and Bacon, 1999

3. Schickendanz J, et al: *Understanding Children and Teenagers.* Boston, MA: Allyn and Bacon, 2001

PEDIATRIC MASSAGE AND HYDROTHERAPY TECHNIQUES

KEY POINTS

After completing this chapter, the student will be able to:

1. Understand the rationale for using Swedish massage, relaxation techniques, passive range-of-motion exercises, and skin stimulation with children.

2. Perform basic and advanced relaxation techniques prior to and during massage sessions.

3. Give a child a full-body Swedish massage that incorporates relaxation techniques, passive range-of-motion exercises, and different types of sensory stimulation.

4. Adapt massage techniques to individual children.

5. Explain how hot and cold applications affect the body.

6. Give examples of specific hydrotherapy treatments and understand what each is used for.

This chapter describes a variety of massage techniques that are especially appropriate for children. You will learn how to give a child a full-body Swedish massage, how to teach children to consciously relax, and how to perform a variety of hydrotherapy treatments.

SUITABLE TECHNIQUES FOR CHILDREN

Many of the same techniques that are useful for adults are also appropriate for pediatric massage; however, they may need to be modified for a child's physical, emotional, and cognitive differences. In this section, we discuss this modification of basic Swedish massage strokes, as well as the use of passive range-of-motion exercises and other specific techniques.

WHY USE SWEDISH MASSAGE WITH CHILDREN?

Swedish massage incorporates gentle passive touch, superficial fluid techniques (superficial effleurage), percussion strokes, deep neuromuscular techniques such as petrissage, and passive range-of-motion techniques. It is relaxing, readily accepted by children, easy to learn, and easy to teach to parents. It is also versatile enough to be effective for a wide variety of problems, from touch issues to physical therapy needs. One particular advantage of using Swedish massage strokes, as opposed to many other styles of bodywork, is that they give both you and the child specific feedback about the child's soft tissue. With it, you will both be able to feel the mobility of the skin, the length and tonicity of muscles, adhesions if they are present, the relationship of different muscles and fascial tissue to each other, and the relationship between bones and the soft tissue overlying them.

In this pediatric version of Swedish massage, special techniques for sensory stimulation and relaxation training have also been incorporated. Emphasis has been placed on using great care so that children do not experience pain, and on constantly giving children choices about how they are massaged.

You should practice the whole-body sequence until the sequence and timing of the strokes are second nature to you. At that point, you will have not only the basic pediatric massage skills, but also an understanding of how to vary massage according to an individual child's needs and according to your own intuition and creativity. Simple variables that allow you to individualize Swedish massage to suit different children are: the sequence in which different areas of the body are massaged; which layer of tissue you are working with; the amount of pressure you use; how much time you spend on each area of the body; the speed at which you do the strokes; how many times you do each stroke; and how you make transitions between different strokes. Over time, you will naturally develop your own style and will quite naturally weave techniques from other forms of massage and bodywork into your massage treatment to achieve particular goals with an individual child.

Lyse Lussier, a Canadian therapist from Montreal, has aided children with a wide variety of problems through the use of Swedish massage. During almost two decades of experience, she has worked with many normal healthy children, including her own, and with children facing many serious illnesses and disabilities. She has treated children in all stages of cancer, including immediately after diagnosis; during hospitalization for stressful treatments, such as bone marrow transplants; during recuperation at home from various treatments; during cancer reoccurrences; and during the terminal stages of the illness. She has also treated children undergoing renal dialysis and kidney transplants, children who are totally paralyzed, and children who are comatose and in long-term care. Her massage treatments have eased both physical distress (such as pain, nausea, and discomfort from being immobilized) and psychological distress (such as anxiety, lack of stimulation, insomnia, and feelings of isolation). Although Ms. Lussier occasionally incorporates other bodywork techniques, such as polarity therapy or craniosacral therapy into her practice, the basic modality that she uses is Swedish massage (Lussier L, personal communication, November 2002).

CONTRAINDICATIONS TO PEDIATRIC MASSAGE

Although massage with children is safe, contraindications must always be observed. Specifically, do not massage skin that has sores, cuts, burns, boils, or infectious rashes such as scabies. Do not massage inflamed joints, tumors, or any undiagnosed lumps. In the event of injuries (such as severe bruises, joint sprains, fractures, or dislocations) or medical conditions, consult with the child's doctor before you begin massage. Endangerment sites that should be avoided unless otherwise specified include the back of the knee, the xyphoid process, and the inner elbow. If a child is acutely ill, especially if his or her body temperature is elevated, massage is contraindicated.

BASIC MASSAGE STROKES

Basic massage strokes include passive touch, effleurage, petrissage, friction, and tapotement.

Passive Touch

Softly lay your warm, relaxed hands on the child's body and keep them still for about 30 seconds or more (see Figure 3–1). This meditative beginning is used to initiate touch in a gentle, noninvasive way. The warmth of your hands helps give passive touch a relaxing and nurturing feeling.

Effleurage

Effleurage strokes are done entirely with the palmar surface of your hands (see Figure 3–2). Rather than attempting to move deep muscle masses, your hands flow over the body contours, molding to them. Effleurage movements are smooth and continuous, and their effect is soothing and relaxing. Effleurage also increases lymph flow and aids venous flow. By using variations based on the amount of pressure and the direction and the speed of the stroke, effleurage is well suited for many different purposes. For example, if effleurage strokes are done slowly, they are sedating; rapid effleurage strokes are far more stimulating. Light (or superficial) effleurage has a different effect than deep effleurage. For example, at the beginning of the massage of each part of the body, light effleurage accustoms the child to being touched by you, helps you evaluate both the child's tissue and her response to being touched, and warms and relaxes the area. Deep effleurage, which may be used when the area is thoroughly relaxed and warmed, releases tension in deep muscles.

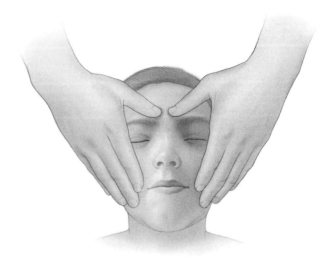

FIGURE 3–1 ■ Passive Touch.

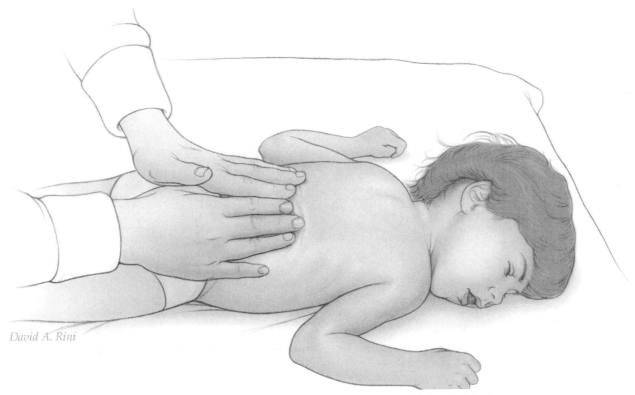

David A. Rini

FIGURE 3–2 ■ Effleurage. Notice that the entire palmar surface of your hands is in contact with the child's body.

Both superficial and deep effleurage can help increase a child's awareness of body boundaries (Chapter 1) by, in effect, outlining different body regions. An effleurage stroke of the arm, which goes from the hand to the top of the arm, sends a different message than an effleurage stroke that continues on to circle around the top of the shoulder. The first effleurage gives the child the sense that the arm stops just below the shoulder joint, whereas the second effleurage, by including the top of the shoulder, gives the child the message that the arm is longer and that the shoulder is an integral part of the arm.

Petrissage

Petrissage, which comes from the French word for kneading, is actually a category consisting of many different strokes that press, roll, squeeze, lift, wring, or knead soft tissue. Unlike effleurage, there is minimal sliding over the skin. Petrissage can release deeper tension than effleurage strokes, increase local circulation, help free adhesions and separate muscle fibers, and increase a child's awareness of the thickness and texture of deeper muscle layers. Because petrissage is a deeper stroke, it should not be attempted until the child is able to tolerate both light and deep effleurage. When doing petrissage, you should observe the child for any nonverbal signs of resistance, as well as ask

the child if the stroke is acceptable. The three variations of petrissage strokes are raking, kneading, and thumbstroking.

Raking

Raking is done on the back, arms, and legs. The fingers are curved and stiffened so that the hand looks like a garden rake (see Figure 3–3). Raking is begun at the top of the back or limb. The fingertips of one hand are dragged, with medium pressure, a short distance downward so that the fingers "rake" the tissue, then one hand is lifted off and the other hand does the same raking motion. Let the rakes overlap and work gradually down to the bottom of the area.

Kneading

Using medium pressure, grasp and lift a handful of flesh between the thumb and fingers of one hand (see Figure 3–4). Do not pinch, just squeeze gently. Slowly release as the other hand grasps the same tissue; lift and release it in turn. Continue with alternating hands.

Thumbstroking

This stroke covers smaller areas in a specific and thorough way, and may help you discover small areas of deep tension that cannot be as readily felt with effleurage. The area is stroked first with the flat of one thumb and then with the flat of the other

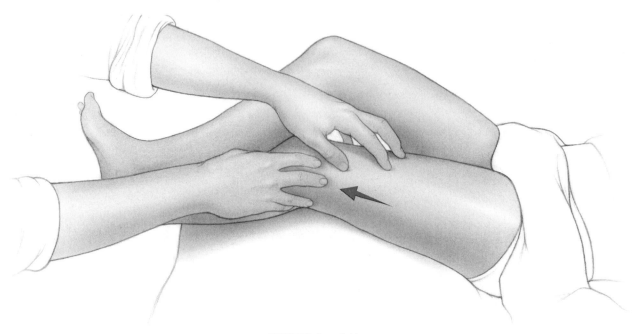

FIGURE 3–3 ■ Raking.

thumb (see Figure 3–5). Let these small pushes or strokes overlap slightly and move in the direction specified for each part of the body. Use medium to firm pressure.

Friction

Friction strokes are performed by placing the palms of your hands against the surface of the skin and rubbing briskly (see Figure 3–6). This gives a sensation of warmth to the area. In classic Swedish massage, both superficial and deep friction may be used; however, pediatric massage typically calls for only superficial friction. In this book, it will only be used on the hands, feet, and chest.

Tapotement

Tapotement (from the French word for tapping) is a series of brisk, rapid blows applied with alternating hands that are parallel to each other. It is primarily used to stimulate nerve endings. It should always be done after the child's tissue is warmed with, at least, effleurage and, perhaps, other strokes as well.

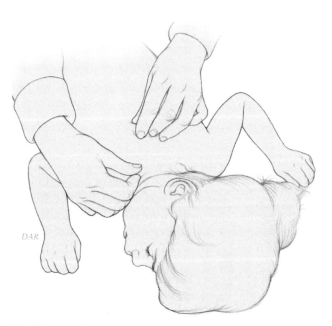

FIGURE 3–4 ■ Kneading.

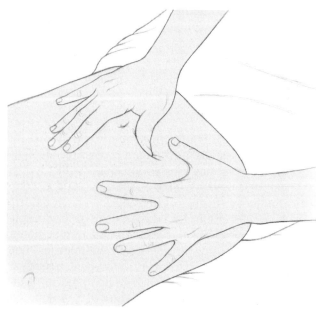

FIGURE 3–5 ■ Thumbstroking.

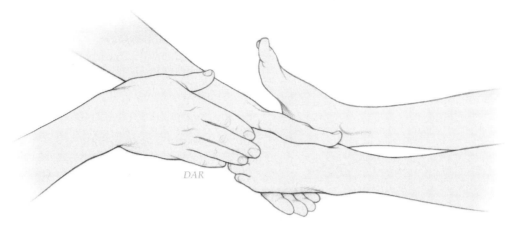

FIGURE 3–6 ■ Friction.

In pediatric massage, tapotement can provide additional sensory stimulation at the end of the massage on any part of the body. Most children enjoy tapotement if it is done in a light, playful way—during cupping of the chest, if the child is asked to exhale and make a loud noise, the resulting sound is often a source of great amusement. Do not use tapotement over kidneys, bony prominences, the popliteal or antecubital areas, throat, breasts, or abdomen. The variations of tapotement include tapping, pincement, and cupping.

Tapping

Tapping consists of quick, light, alternating taps of your fingertips on a small portion of the child's body (see Figure 3–7).

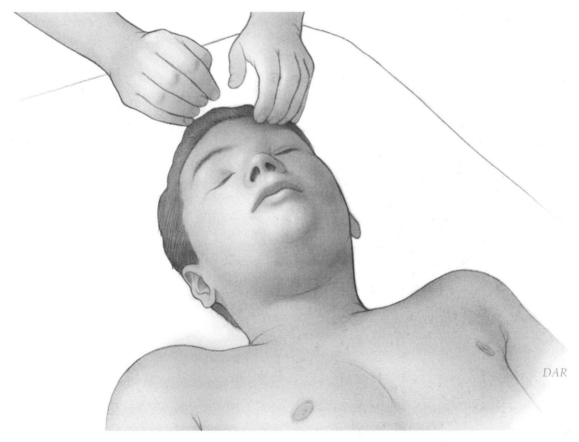

FIGURE 3–7 ■ Tapping.

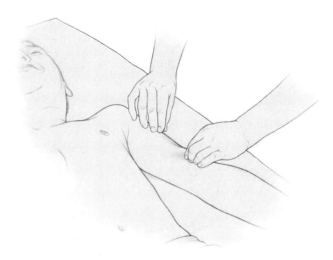

FIGURE 3–8 ■ Pincement.

Pincement

Pincement (from the French word for pinching) is when the skin is picked up or "pinched" lightly and rapidly with alternating hands, using the thumb and first two fingers of each hand (see Figure 3–8). Think of lifting the skin rather than pinching it.

Cupping

To perform cupping, rapidly alternate cupped-hand movements with both hands (see Figure 3–9).

This movement is not only used to stimulate nerve endings, but to break up congestion when a child has a chest cold, pneumonia, or cystic fibrosis. Use caution so that the child does not receive too much pressure or feel that he or she is being beaten.

PASSIVE RANGE OF MOTION

During passive range-of-motion exercises, you move each of the child's joints through its full comfortable range of motion. The child remains totally passive and motion only occurs within the joint as a result of the outside force from the therapist. Range-of-motion exercises are done to maintain or increase joint motion, as well as to stretch other tissue that surrounds the joints. When they are not regularly moved through their full range of motion, by activity or by someone else helping them move, joints can lose their flexibility and even develop contractures. In addition, muscle tension, adhesions, and trigger points may decrease range of motion at a joint.

When to Use Passive Range-of-Motion Exercises

You can use passive range-of-motion exercises initially to evaluate a child's joint flexibility. In addition to being useful for assessment, passive range-of-motion exercises are valuable for treatment. They are an excellent tool to help you pinpoint where children

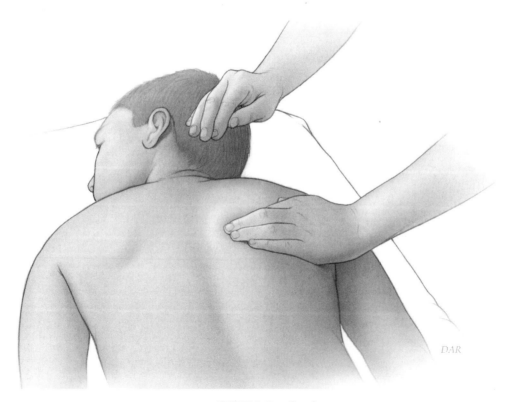

FIGURE 3–9 ■ Cupping.

hold muscular tension. They also help maintain joint flexibility when children are immobilized by injury, illness, surgery, or paralysis. When children are not using all joints freely, they should have regular, passive range-of-motion exercises. For example, when a girl is using crutches to walk, she is not going to be swinging her arms back and forth as a child will normally do when walking, and her shoulder joints are going to be supporting part of her body weight in a way that they would probably never do otherwise. The girl is at risk of accumulating both extreme muscle tension and the loss of some range of motion in her shoulder joints. She would benefit from regular, passive range-of-motion exercises to help her maintain full range of motion in her shoulders and to release tension in the surrounding muscles.

It is important to understand that children have greater movement in most of their joints than adults do. A classic study, which compared the range of motion in an adult's joints and a child's joints, found that many pediatric joints had about 10% more movement than those of adults. The greatest differences between adult and pediatric joint movements were found in backward extension and outward rotation of the shoulder, radial deviation of the wrist, internal and external rotation of the hip, and plantar flexion of the ankle.[1]

The range-of-motion exercises you will be learning in this chapter are not for the purpose of treating tightness or limitation of range caused by dysfunction in the joint itself. Instead, they will be used to:

- Help children learn to relax a specific area of the body by surrendering its weight to you. Many adults have a great deal of difficulty relaxing in this way. An extreme example of this is an adult who is supine on a treatment table with his or her head held stiffly, unaware that his or her muscles are contracted. Because this adult is truly unaware of the muscle tension, it may not be possible for him or her to receive some of the benefits of massage. For example, he or she may never be able to relax, have his or her neck muscles fully stretched, or to fully perform range-of-motion exercises. By teaching a young person to relax an area when it is moved by another person, you teach an important lesson that may prevent the type of chronic contraction described for adults.
- Help you pinpoint where a child holds muscular tension.
- Build the child's trust and acceptance of a different kind of touch, during which the child learns to be totally relaxed and passive.
- Increase the child's body awareness. Sensory nerve endings in the joints that respond to mechanical pressure (mechanoreceptors) are

responsible for much of an individual's balance, **proprioception,** and kinesthetic awareness. Range-of-motion exercises stimulate these receptors and help the child feel these sensations: the weight of the body part as the child lets you lift it; the feeling inside the joint as the bone ends are pushed together and apart; how large the body part is as it moves through space; and the stretching or the resistance to stretching of soft tissues around the joint, such as the muscles, tendons, fascia, and joint capsules. This resistance may be partially caused by muscle tension and/or adhesions.

How to Perform Passive Range-of-Motion Exercises

When integrated with massage strokes during a session, passive range-of-motion exercises are not only relaxing and therapeutic, they make a treatment more varied and interesting. Here is how to do them:

- Do these exercises in a playful fashion, singing as you do them or moving in time to a nursery rhyme. Children may find it uproariously funny to have their hands "accidentally" hit you in the face during a movement of the shoulder joint!
- Each time you finish massaging a part of the body, do the range-of-motion exercises for that part. Do all the joint movements with the child in the supine position, except hip extension and knee flexion and extension, which need to be done in the prone position. Do each movement three times.
- Gently pick up the limb or body part, fully supporting its weight. Use a firm, comfortable grip. Use good body mechanics to prevent excessive reaching. Ask the child to let the body part rest in your hands and be heavy.
- Move the body part smoothly, slowly, and rhythmically. Jerky or fast movements can cause the child to tense the area.
- Avoid moving or forcing a body part beyond its existing range of motion. Muscle strain, pain, or injury could result.
- If the child tenses during the movement, stop temporarily while you ask the child to relax and let the body part rest in your hands. Should there be any pain associated with the movement, try it again but do not move the body part as far. If there is still pain, discontinue the motion.
- If the amount that the joint can move seems less than normal, move it even more slowly through its potential range; have the child relax whenever you find restrictions or if the child is tensing. Do not use force. Point of Interest Box 3-1 describes how to determine when a joint has reached the end of its normal range of motion.

CASE STUDY 3–1

Background

Joe Polk was born with arthrogryposis (definition, *condition of curved joints*) in 1998. A child with this condition has multiple limb contractures that are present at birth, often accompanied by hip dislocation, clubfoot, and muscular atrophy. Arthrogryposis is not inherited and its cause is unknown. One theory holds that arthrogryposis is caused by a virus contracted by the mother during pregnancy; the muscles are affected so that they do not develop properly, and the fetus does not move in utero. A child with this condition typically has severe joint restriction and deformities. Those afflicted with this disability have stiffness, varying degrees of difficulty with motion, and pain. Correction of clubfeet and hip and knee contractures usually begins soon after birth, with casts and/or range-of-motion exercises and, possibly, surgery. Some children with arthrogryposis may be able to walk and, if so, they may have varying musculoskeletal restrictions, including limitations in the various joints. Often they will require a wheelchair. When adults, their condition usually deteriorates as multiple contractures, stiffness, and pain increasingly limit their activity.[2]

When Joe Polk was born, his arms were straight and rigid, his wrists were fixed in full flexion, and his ankles were severely twisted (see Figure 3–10). His mother, a critical care nurse, remembers that his pulses were weak and the circulation in his hands was so poor that, when she would try to do even minor

movements with his wrists, his hands would turn purple. Trying to hold Joe during breast-feeding was like "trying to hold a bowling ball." His feet were so contracted that they were twisted up to his stomach. His family was told that due to his condition, he would never use his hands and would need seven or more operations on his upper and lower extremities. This included surgery to remove his pectoralis major and implant it in place of his biceps, which would have fixed his arm in a flexed position; surgery on his feet to reset the bones in their proper position; and serial casting to correct his foot contractures.

Joe had foot surgery and serial casting on his feet, which involved having a new cast put on every week for 5 months; however, his parents were reluctant to have major surgery on his arms.

Treatment

Joe was fortunate to be born in a family in which his mother, Mary Polk, was a critical care nurse with special training in Swedish massage and reflexology. Joe was an alert and strong baby, but somewhat irritable as he was continually frustrated by not being able to move. Joe's mother began on the day he was born to give him daily massages and range-of-motion exercises. She massaged Joe while he was in her lap, using Swedish massage strokes on his entire body. She used firm pressure, especially around his joints, and also did foot reflexology. She did passive range-of-motion exercises and stretched his contracted tis-

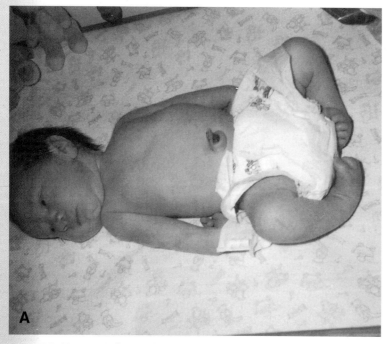

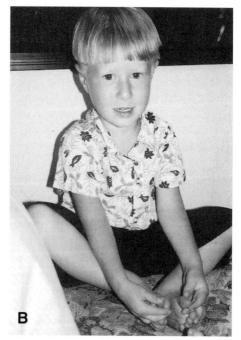

FIGURE 3–10 ■ Joe Polk. **A,** 3 days old; **B,** age 4.

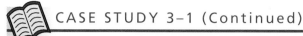

CASE STUDY 3–1 (Continued)

sue whenever possible. Mary observed that Joe's tissue softened after massage and that he also seemed mentally relaxed and far more bonded to his mother. She also frequently worked with Joe in a bathtub, doing range-of-motion exercises while he floated in the warm water. Joe's first set of casts to correct his clubfeet were put on when he was 3 days old, and a new cast was put on every week for many weeks. Mary knew that although the casting was necessary, Joe would not be receiving any sensory stimulation or movement when his feet were in the casts. She was so concerned about the effects of immobilization on Joe's feet that she purchased a cast cutter, and each week, she removed his casts the night before they were to be recast; this allowed her to bathe his legs and do massage and range-of-motion exercises on his feet and ankles before the casts were redone the next day. Joe also received a great deal of craniosacral therapy when he was 4 to 6 months old, which focused on dural tube mobilization to free his spinal cord, balance of his reticular system, and release of specific cranial restrictions. During some sessions, he released a great deal of anger and frustration, with intense screaming. His joint mobility continued to increase slowly but steadily. Joe continues to receive regular massage from his mother today at age 3, but not the intensive type of therapy he received in his first year.

Response

During his therapies, Joe gained range of motion in all of his joints. At age 4, Joe now looks completely normal. He no longer needs orthopedic shoes, his feet have no deformities, and his ankle range of motion is normal. He can dress and feed himself, dive off a diving board and swim underwater, ride a tricycle, climb a ladder, and use his hands to color and cut with scissors. He has slightly limited range of motion in his elbow joints and limited extension in one wrist, but as he continues to be highly active, his joint range of motion is expected to improve even more, and his doctors no longer feel further surgery will be necessary (Polk M, personal communication, September 2002).

Discussion Questions

1. What tissue was affected by Joe's arthrogryposis?
2. What symptoms did Joe have as a result of his arthrogryposis?
3. What therapeutic modalities were used with Joe, including massage therapy?
4. How did Joe show that the arthrogryposis had affected him psychologically, as well as physically?

Head and Neck

Movements are shown in Figure 3–11.

1. Place the fingers at the base of the child's skull, with the thumbs at the side of the head and slightly above the ears. Slowly and gently push the head forward until resistance is felt or the chin touches the chest. Slowly lower the head to its resting position. This flexes the neck (see Figure 3–11A).
2. Repeat Step 1, but as you bring the head back to the resting position, let it gently fall back on your fingers so that the child's chin is pointing toward the ceiling. This extends the neck (see Figure 3–11B).
3. Place one hand behind the child's head and the other hand under the chin. Elevate and support the head at a 45° angle to the child's body. Slowly turn the head to one side until a slight resistance is felt. Turn the head to the other side until a slight resistance is felt. Avoid flexing or extending the neck as you turn the child's head. This rotates the cervical spine (see Figure 3–11C).
4. With the palms on either side of the face, move the head to one side until resistance is encoun-

tered or until the ear touches the top of the shoulder. Repeat on the other side. This laterally flexes the cervical spine (see Figure 3–11D).

Upper Extremity—Shoulder, Elbow, Wrist, and Hand

Movements are shown in Figure 3–12.

Shoulder and Elbow

Grasp the arm with one hand beneath the elbow and one hand beneath the wrist, unless otherwise indicated.

1. Move the arm up to the ceiling and toward the head. This flexes, externally rotates, and extends the shoulder (see Figure 3–12A).
2. Move the arm away from the body and toward the child's head until the hand is touching the top of the head. This abducts and externally rotates the shoulder (see Figure 3–12B).
3. Move the arm across midline until the hand touches the child's other shoulder. This adducts the shoulder (see Figure 3–12C).
4. Place the arm out to the side at shoulder level (90° abduction) and bend the elbow so that the hand is pointing straight up. Move the forearm

POINT OF INTEREST BOX 3–1
How to Determine When a Joint Has Reached the End of Its Normal Range of Motion

When performing passive range-of-motion exercises, it is important to know when you have reached the end of a joint's normal range of motion. If you are not aware of how the joint feels at that point, you might force it too far and cause an injury. There is a characteristic quality to the resistance or limitation encountered at the end of the normal range of motion, known as the end-feel. Once you learn what the end-feel is like, you will know when to stop when the joint has reached its maximum range. To learn how to identify end-feel, when you reach the end of what feels like unrestricted motion, apply a gentle overpressure and notice how the joint feels at that end point.[1] When the joint has moved as far as it normally can, you will feel one of the following end-feels:

1. Bony end-feel. When two bones come together, it stops further motion at a joint. The resistance felt is hard and abrupt and motion comes to a full stop. Full elbow extension has this type of end-feel.
2. Capsular end-feel. The joint capsule and its surrounding soft tissue (but not muscles) limit the range of motion at the joint. The quality of the resistance felt is firm but not hard; there is a slight "give" to the movement, similar to when stretching a piece of leather. Full medial rotation of the hip has this end-feel.
3. Muscular end-feel. The length of the muscles limits the range of motion at a joint. The quality of the resistance felt is firm, although not as firm as the capsular end-feel, and somewhat springy. When the child is in a supine position with the leg lifted in the air and the knee is flexed and then extended, this is the muscular end-feel; the limitation in knee extension is from the muscles at the back of the knee.
4. Soft-tissue end-feel. Soft tissue limits the range of motion. The quality of the resistance is mushy or soft. When the child is supine and the knee is fully flexed and the posterior thigh stops the calf, the knee can flex no further. This is the soft-tissue end-feel.[1] The child's response to passive movement provides information about non-contractile elements such as ligaments and fasciae.

[1]Reese N, Bandy W: *Joint Range of Motion and Muscle Length Testing.* Philadelphia: W.B. Saunders, 2002, p 27-29, 394

down until the palm touches the therapy table. This rotates the shoulder externally (see Figure 3–12D).
5. Move the forearm back until the back of the hand touches the therapy table, close to the child's head. This rotates the shoulder internally (see Figure 3–12E).
6. Bend the elbow until the fingers touch the chin, and then straighten the arm out. This flexes and extends the elbow (see Figure 3–12F).
7. Grasp the child's arm, as for a handshake, and turn the palm up and down; make sure that only the forearm moves and not the shoulder. This pronates and supinates the forearm (see Figure 3–12G).

Wrist and Hand Movements

Flex the child's arm at the elbow until the forearm is at a right angle to the therapy table. Support the wrist joint with one hand and, with the other hand, manipulate the joint and the fingers.

1. Bend the wrist backward and, at the same time, flex the fingers so that they touch the palm. This hyperextends the wrist and flexes the fingers. Now, bend the wrist backward and extend the fingers. This hyperextends the wrist and the fingers (Figure 3–12H).
2. Bend the wrist forward and extend the fingers. This flexes the wrist and extends the fingers (Figure 3–12I).

Lower Extremity—Hip, Knee, Ankle, and Foot
Movements are shown in Figure 3–13.

Hip and Knee

1. Lift the leg by grasping the child's foot with one hand and the knee with the other hand. Bend the knee and flex it toward the chest until resistance is felt. This flexes the hip and the knee (see Figure 3–13A).
2. Support the child's knee underneath with one hand and support the ankle with the other hand; let the knee fall toward the outside as far as the child's tissue will allow. Now move the foot up toward the ceiling and then down in the opposite direction. This rotates the hip externally and internally. Note that careful draping is necessary to prevent the child's genital area from being exposed; even with careful draping, the child may feel exposed or vulnerable with the hip in this position. Explain what you are going to do before you attempt this hip rotation, and carefully check that the child is comfortable. If you have any doubt, omit this joint movement and Step 3 (see Figure 3–13B).
3. Continue to support the leg in the same way. Flex the hip by repeating Step 1 above, then

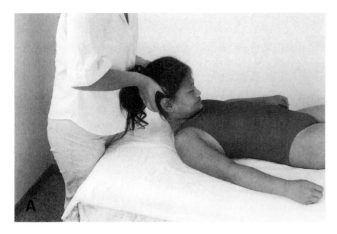
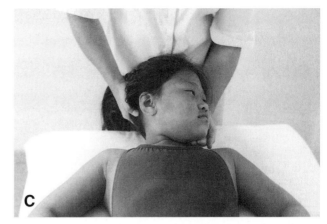
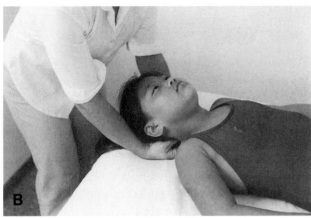
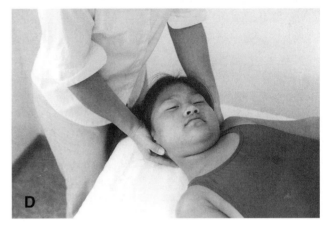

FIGURE 3–11 ■ **A-D,** Passive Range-of-Motion Exercises for the Head and Neck.

bring the thigh medially across the body toward the other side, down toward the outside, and laterally. This flexes, adducts, and abducts the hip (see Figure 3–13C).
4. With the child lying prone, place one hand on the hip to stabilize it and, with the other hand, lift the leg at the knee. Move the leg backward from the hip joint, then medially, then back toward the table, then laterally. This extends the hip (see Figure 3–13D).
5. With the child lying prone, lift the ankle and bring it toward the buttock until you feel resistance. Straighten the lower leg as you lay it back in the original position. This flexes and extends the knee (see Figure 3–13E).

Ankle and Foot
1. Grasp the foot with one hand and the ankle with your other hand. Make the entire foot rotate at the ankle. Rotate clockwise and counterclockwise. The ankle is a hinge joint and will not make a true circular movement; however, in trying to rotate it, you will be dorsiflexing, inverting, plantar flexing, and everting the

foot. This may be done with the child either prone or supine (see Figure 3–13F).
2. Grasp the top part of the toes of one foot using the thumbs and fingers. Rotate clockwise and counterclockwise (Figure 3–13G).

Adapted from: Kozier B, Erb G, Berman A, Snyder S: *Fundamentals of Nursing.* Upper Saddle River, NJ: Prentice-Hall, 2000.[3]

SENSORY STIMULATION OF THE SKIN

The various nerves in the skin that sense light pressure, deep pressure, and temperature change are stimulated by new and varied types of touch on the skin (see Figure 3–14).

These can be provided through the use of massage oils or lotions, textured massage tools, coarse towels, fake fur, different types of hairbrushes, hot packs, ice massage, ice packs, different temperatures of water, soap lather, and Epsom salts. By exposing the child to them as part of the massage experience, you not only decrease his fear of touch, you can also enrich the sensory experience of the child, reinforce body boundaries, and help build a more complete and accurate body image.

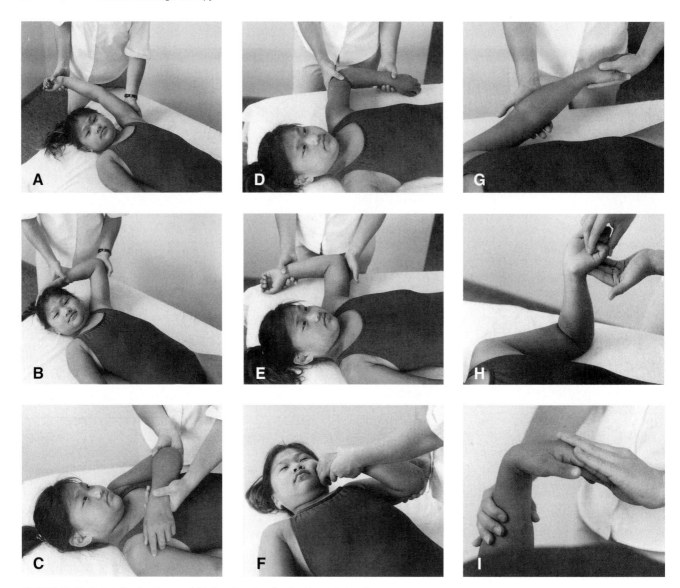

FIGURE 3–12 ■ A-I, Passive Range-of-Motion Exercises for the Upper Extremity.

BALL MASSAGE

Ball massage is a specific technique that combines continuous motion and compression of tissue; it can be done from one end to the other of the extremities, torso, abdomen, or back (see Figure 3–15). Its effect can be superficial or deep, and fast or slow, and stimulating or soothing, depending on the type, size, texture, and density of the ball and on how it is moved. By varying the texture and weight of the ball and the amount of pressure against the child's body, ball massage can give additional feedback about the skin, muscle and other soft tissue, and bone and about how the different layers of tissue relate to each other. Especially when used with deep pressure, ball massage releases tension in the child's muscles and stimulates the skin. As discussed in Chapter 2, keep a variety of appealing balls on hand for the child to choose from, including rubber balls; tennis balls; balls that are large, small, or spiked; and balls that make noise (such as balls with a bell inside or ones that squeak). Do not use hard wooden balls. Let the child pick a ball and then be playful with it. Children will enjoy a ball that has a novel color or texture, a ball that makes noise, or a ball that you roll on their body in rhythm to a rhyme or song; for example, a ball may be rolled slowly straight down the back in one smooth motion or it may be rolled gradually down the back, moving in tiny circles all the way. No exact directions are given for ball massage, but remember to thoroughly cover any area that is being massaged.

RELAXATION TECHNIQUES

Basic Relaxation Sequence

Each time you begin to massage a new part of a child's body, practice this simple relaxation sequence.

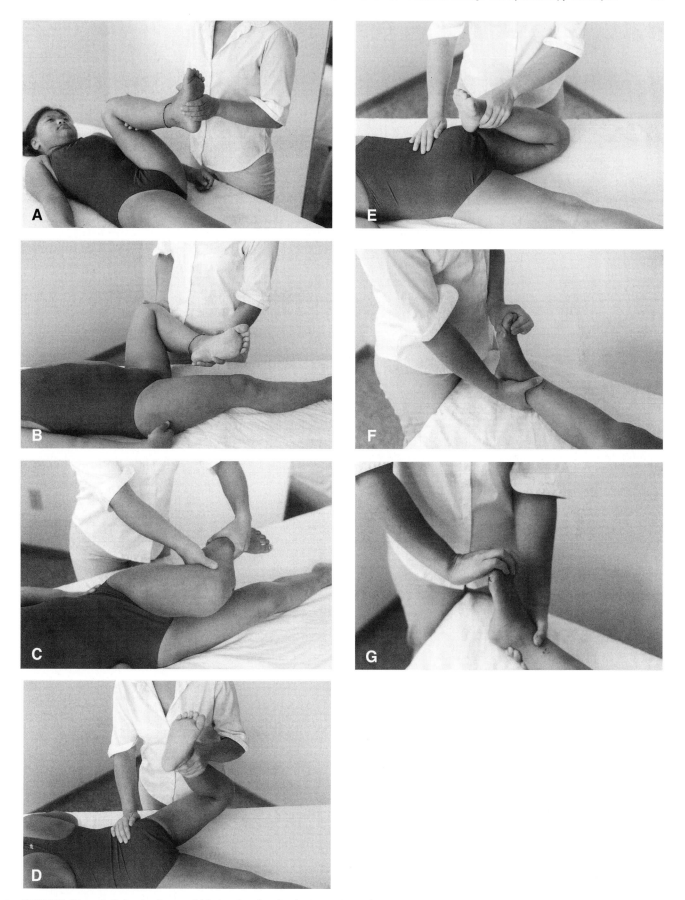

FIGURE 3–13 ■ **A-G,** Passive Range-of-Motion Exercises for the Lower Extremity.

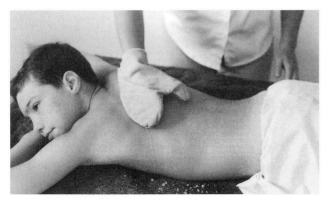

FIGURE 3–14 ■ Washing the back provides a variety of different skin sensations, including those of temperature, texture, and pressure.

It is simple, takes a short time, and yields profound results, greatly enhancing the relaxing effect of the massage and helping the child to learn to consciously relax.

Gently lay your hands on the part of the body you will be massaging. For massage of the head and shoulders, lay your palms gently on either side of the head (Figure 3–1). For massage of the arm, rest the child's hand gently between your palms. Both you and the child should take a few deep, comfortable breaths. As you exhale, consciously relax. Drop your shoulders, allow your face to soften, and relax your hands. If you feel tension anywhere in your body, relax that area as you exhale. Use the following suggestions to help the child relax while he or she is exhaling:

- Feel your stomach get nice and soft.
- Let your shoulders get heavy and melt into the table.
- Let your muscles melt like butter in the hot sun.
- Pretend you are as loose as a Raggedy Ann doll (you could use a doll to show the child what you mean).
- Let your hands hang loose.
- Let your whole body relax and sink into the table.

Use positive phrases, such as "relax more and more," rather than negative ones, such as "don't tense up." If you see the child holding tension, gently remind him to relax. Be sure to give the child lots of positive reinforcement whenever you see even small signs of relaxation.

Advanced Relaxation Sequence

This advanced relaxation technique is a method called "progressive relaxation," which was invented by physiologist Edmund Jacobson in the early 1900s. It consists of systematic tensing and releasing of various muscle groups throughout the body, while, at the same time, paying close attention to the sensations this creates. This method can teach a child how to relax while simultaneously increasing body awareness. It has been used for decades with children for medical and emotional problems, including general tension, insomnia, test anxiety, hyperactivity, tactile defensiveness, migraine headaches, depression, and phobias (Anneberg L: *A study of the different relaxation techniques in tactile deficient and tactile defensive children.* Master's thesis, Lawrence, KS: University of Kansas, 1973).[4-11]

The author has adapted Jacobson's method for use during pediatric massage. In this modified version, you will ask the child to tense and relax different muscle groups against your hands while you offer mild resistance. Your hand placement helps the child understand precisely where to contract the muscles. Suggest that the child tense the muscles in an exaggerated way, so that he or she can notice the contrast between how the muscle feels when it is tense and how it feels when it is relaxed. Because all the child needs to do is follow a simple instruction, such as "push up against my hands," the method can be used with even very young children. The entire sequence should be done at the beginning of a massage session and should take no more than 5 minutes. It is ideal to use with a child who seems to be lacking body awareness or with a child who is very tense upon arriving for a session. It may be used with a child who is concerned about modesty as well, as it can be done with the child fully clothed. Parents may be taught to do this sequence with their child before bed if he or she has insomnia.

1. Ask the child to lay supine on the floor or treatment table.
2. Place your hands gently on the area you will be asking the child to tense. Checklist Box 3-1

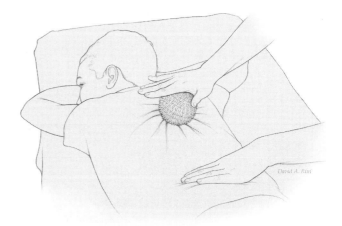

FIGURE 3–15 ■ Ball Massage.

gives a sample sequence. Then ask the child to push against your hands and offer mild resistance (push back gently).

3. Remind the child to tense only the specific area you have mentioned. Observe the child to see if other parts of the body are being tensed. If so, ask the child to relax everywhere except the area that is supposed to be tensed; for example, if you are asking a child to take a deep breath and tighten his chest, and you observe that he is clenching his hands, remind him to relax them.

4. Remind the child to tense hard.

5. Hold each contraction for 2 seconds for a small child and up to 5 seconds for a teenager. Remind the child to notice how tight the area feels. Then, instruct the child to relax and enjoy the pleasant feeling as the muscles let go. When you see him or her following the instructions, give lots of positive reinforcement. After a pause of about 10 seconds, go to the next area of the body. The pause is important; by allow-

ing the child a "rest time," the subtle changes that occur as the muscles relax can be felt. Otherwise, with too many contractions in too short of a time, the child may focus on the contractions alone.

ADAPTING MASSAGE TO THE INDIVIDUAL CHILD

Because every child is a unique individual, you may need to alter your massage treatment for each individual child, rather than try to do each massage as outlined here. Children and their parents can generally tell you what best suits them. Here are some general guidelines:

Attention Span

Children are truly individuals when it comes to how long they will lie quietly. Younger children usually have a shorter attention span, although this is not always true. Some toddlers will lie still for a full-body

---

✔️ **CHECKLIST BOX 3–1**
ADVANCED RELAXATION SEQUENCE (INSTRUCTIONS FOR THE CHILD ARE IN QUOTATIONS)

Tensing the Legs

❏ Hands on top of the lower legs: "Push up against my hands. Now let go all at once."
❏ Hands underneath the lower legs: "Push down against my hands. Now let go all at once."
❏ Hands on the outside of the lower legs: "Push out against my hands. Now let go all at once."
❏ Hands on the inside of the knees: "Push in against my hands. Now let go all at once."

Tensing Muscles Around the Pelvis

❏ Hands on top of the iliac crests: "Push up against my hands. Now let go all at once."

Tensing the Abdomen

❏ Hands on top of the abdomen: "Push my hands away with your tummy. Now let go all at once."

Tensing the Chest

❏ Hands on top of the chest: "Take a deep breath, hold it, and push up against my hands. Now let go all at once."

Tensing the Arm and Shoulder Muscles

❏ Hands on the top of each forearm: "Push up against my hands. Now let go all at once."
❏ Hands underneath each forearm: "Push down against my hands. Now let go all at once."
❏ Hands on the outside of each forearm: "Push out against my hands. Now let go all at once."
❏ Hands on the inside of each forearm: "Push in against my hands. Now let go all at once."

Tensing the Shoulders

❏ Stand at the child's head, and push down on both upper trapezius muscles: "Push up against my hands. Now let go all at once."

Tensing the Neck Muscles

❏ Slip both palms underneath the head: "Now lift your head up just a tiny bit off the table. Keep holding up your head and feel how heavy it is." When the child's head is held up off the table, slip a small pillow underneath her head. "Now let go all at once." She will drop her head on the pillow, and it will feel as if she is resting on a cloud.

Tensing the Muscles of the Face

❏ Slip both hands underneath the head, and hold gently: "Make a tight face. Wrinkle up your forehead, close your eyes tight, wrinkle your nose, stick out your tongue, and pucker your lips. Feel how tight a face you can make. Now let go all at once."

Tensing the Entire Body

❏ Continue to hold both hands underneath the head: "Tighten up every thing we've tightened before."
❏ Check to see that the child has tightened up from the feet to the head, including the face. Gently remind the child to tense any parts of the body that you see are still relaxed. When everything is gently tensed, ask the child to let go all at once. Now, as the child rests, ask him or her to say what feels different now.

massage, and some older children will be able to relax for only 5 minutes.

For those children who cannot seem to lie still, you can adapt your usual way of giving a massage. Here are some ideas that may be good solutions:

- Follow the child around and do massage as he or she plays.
- Ask the parent to distract children by playing with them while you continue to do the massage.
- Tell a story or sing during the massage. This may be successful with a small child.
- Give the child a toy or book to play with or look at.
- Change strokes frequently or use many different massage tools and different techniques for variety.
- Use warmth, such as microwave hot packs, steam packs, or warmed linens. One resourceful mother found that if she put a hot towel, fresh from the dryer, under her daughter, the girl would lie still much longer. Warm socks and put them on the child after a foot massage, or warm a T-shirt and have the child put it on after the upper body has been massaged.
- Use the advanced relaxation sequence during the massage session when the child becomes tired of laying still.

Amount of Pressure

This can vary from day to day, but most children usually prefer a certain type of pressure. Their preferences range from extremely light to very firm. Some children may ask for firmer pressure over very tight areas or lighter pressure over sore areas. You should always monitor nonverbal signals that indicate you are using too much pressure (such as flinching or grimacing), and check with the child often. Use phrases such as "Is this too hard?" or "Does it feel better if I go softer or lighter?"

Best Area to Massage

When in doubt, massage the back. Avoid any areas that the child does not like to have massaged or that cause discomfort. After some experience with the basic, full-body massage, children may begin to request massage of certain areas, for example, the back, for relaxation, insomnia, and shoulder tension; the stomach, for tension stomachaches; the face, for relaxation; the legs, for insomnia or growing pains; the neck, for tension headaches; and the feet, for fatigue or discomfort following vigorous exercise.

Which Strokes to Use

Use more of the strokes the child enjoys and use fewer or none of the strokes he or she doesn't enjoy. When in doubt, use superficial effleurage strokes,

which are generally well accepted. One mother found that her 11-year-old son would not tolerate anything but superficial effleurage and would giggle and flinch when she did anything else. So, every night, she used only superficial effleurage strokes and found that her son was able to relax and that she enjoyed giving him his massage. As he continued to benefit from his nightly massage, possibly, he would be able to enjoy other strokes in the future.

The Sequence of Strokes

It may be better to change the sequence of strokes for an individual child. For example, a child who comes in with a tension stomachache will be more relaxed for the rest of the massage if his or her abdomen is massaged at the beginning of the session. Or, you may wish to begin the massage in a different sequence; for example, if there is a reason to massage the back toward the end of the session, rather than the beginning.

FULL-BODY MASSAGE SEQUENCE

Before beginning a massage, children should be left alone with their parents to undress in private. (Teenagers may prefer to undress without parents present.) Let them know they should leave their underpants on and make sure that they know they will be carefully draped during their session. If there is any concern about disrobing, their wishes should be honored. While they are disrobing and getting under the drapes on the treatment table, you have the opportunity to wash your hands and get any supplies you need, from massage oil to toys. Now begin with the massage of the back.

BACK MASSAGE

Have the child lie face down. Place a small, rolled towel or pillow underneath the ankles. Sit on the side of the therapy table near her waistline. For a larger child, such as a teenager, you may stand at the head of the table, rather than sit, and do the back effleurage in reverse. Uncover the child's back and move her underwear down so that the posterior iliac crests are exposed but the gluteal cleft is still covered. (The following sequence is summarized in Checklist Box 3-2.)

1. Perform the basic relaxation sequence (see page 70) and passive touch on the lower back.
2. Apply oil or lotion.
3. Perform back effleurage (Figure 3–2). Begin with your hands just above the sacrum, parallel on either side of the spine, and with your fin-

gertips pointing toward the head. Glide toward the head, moving up the middle of the back, in between the scapulae and up to the base of the neck. Now move your hands away from each other and glide along the top of the upper trapezius to the points of the shoulders, down the sides of the torso and hips to the bottom of the buttocks, and then return to the starting position, with your hands just above the sacrum. Each hand is actually describing a large oval shape. Repeat 10 times. Begin with superficial pressure. Pressure can be increased as the child's tissue is warmed and relaxed.

4. Rake the back (see Figure 3–16). Beginning at the top of the shoulders and using medium pressure, rake downward (toward the feet). On a small child, each raking stroke should be about 1 or 2 inches long; on a teenager, up to 5 or 6 inches long. Gradually move down the back from the shoulders to the top of the sacrum. Repeat the entire stroke three times.

5. Perform back effleurage. Repeat three times.

6. Knead the upper trapezius (see Figure 3–17) Knead the upper trapezius from the base of the neck to the tip of the shoulder. Use medium pressure. Knead each side for 30 seconds or longer.

7. Perform back effleurage. Repeat three times.

8. Thumbstroke between the scapulae (see Figure 3–18). The thoracic spinal erectors, the rhomboids and the middle trapezius muscles are located between the scapulae. Thumbstroking will warm and relax all these muscles. With the

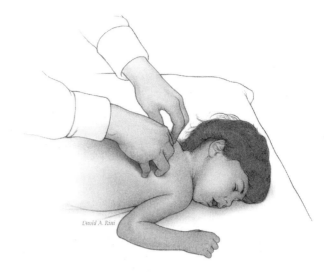

FIGURE 3–16 ■ Raking the Back.

thumbs, compress the tissue as you stroke toward the head. Press firmly, but do not cause pain; if the area hurts, lighten the pressure. Do for 1 minute or longer. Do not massage the spine.

9. Perform back effleurage. Repeat three times.

10. Thumbstroke the lower back (see Figure 3–19). Beginning at the top of the sacrum, use both thumbs to outline each posterior iliac crest, one at a time. Use medium to firm pressure. Push away from yourself, first with the flat of one thumb and then with the other. Let these small pushes or strokes overlap slightly and gradually slide out along the bone, from the sacrum to the lateral edge of the iliac crest. Imagine that

CHECKLIST BOX 3–2
BACK MASSAGE

1. Basic relaxation sequence and passive touch.
2. Apply oil or lotion.
3. Back effleurage, 10 times.
4. Rake the back three times.
5. Back effleurage, three times.
6. Knead the upper trapezius, 1 minute.
7. Back effleurage, three times.
8. Thumbstroke between the scapula, 1 minute.
9. Back effleurage, three times.
10. Thumbstroke the lower back, 1 minute.
11. Back effleurage, three times.
12. Knead the buttocks.
13. Back effleurage, 10 times.
14. Skin stimulation stroke.
15. Ball rolling.
16. Basic relaxation sequence.

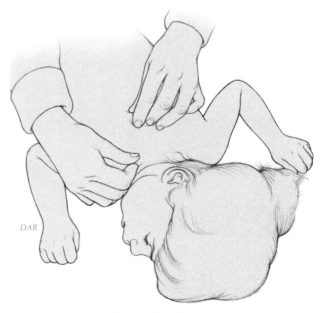

FIGURE 3–17 ■ Kneading the Upper Trapezius.

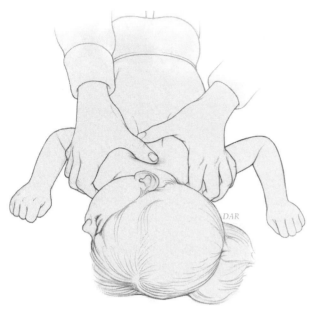

FIGURE 3–18 ■ Thumbstroking Between the Scapulae.

you can define its shape with the thumbs. Do one entire side and repeat on the other. Do once, slowly and thoroughly, taking approximately 1 minute.

11. Perform back effleurage. Repeat three times.
12. Knead the buttocks (see Figure 3–20). Knead the buttocks through the underwear from the sacrum out to the side of the hip. Do one buttock, then the other. Use medium pressure. Do each buttock for 30 seconds or more.
13. Perform back effleurage. Do three times.
14. Perform a skin stimulation stroke. Choose one: cover the back with a pillowcase or sheet and massage the entire back with a textured massage tool or hairbrush; remove the sheet and do pincement or tapping on the entire back; gently rub massage oil off the entire back with a coarse washcloth or a piece of fake fur; or perform a salt glow of the entire back.
15. Perform ball rolling. Cover the back with a pillowcase or sheet, and roll any size ball (chosen by the child) up and down the length of the back for 1 minute. Do not press on her vertebrae. To increase awareness of the spine and release tension in the paravertebral muscles, a small, soft ball may be rolled in tiny circles on either side of the spine. Begin at T1 level, and slowly proceed down to about waist level. Use firm pressure adjusted to the child's tolerance.
16. End with the basic relaxation sequence.

LEG MASSAGE (BACK)

Sit at the foot of the table, near the outside of the child's foot. Small children may lay one entire leg

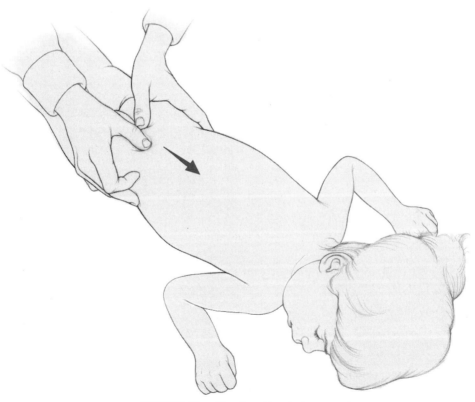

FIGURE 3–19 ■ Thumbstroking the Lower Back.

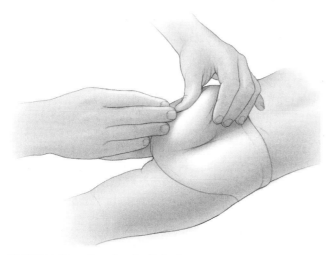

FIGURE 3–20 ■ Kneading the Buttocks.

CHECKLIST BOX 3–3
LEG MASSAGE (BACK)

1. Basic relaxation sequence and passive touch.
2. Apply oil or lotion.
3. Leg effleurage, 10 times.
4. Rake the back of the leg, 1 minute.
5. Leg effleurage, three times.
6. Thumbstroke the back of the leg, 1 minute.
7. Leg effleurage, three times.
8. Thumbstroke the sole of the foot, 1 minute.
9. Circle the anklebones six times.
10. Leg effleurage, 10 times.
11. Range-of-motion exercises for the hip and knee joints.
12. Skin stimulation stroke.
13. Ball rolling on the back of the leg and sole of the foot.
14. Basic relaxation sequence.

across your lap. For better body mechanics with children who are almost adult-size, stand to the outside of the leg you will be massaging; do not stoop or stretch to cover the entire area. As the child will be wearing underpants, a few strokes will be done over the underwear. Although this decreases some of the benefits from gliding effleurage strokes, it is important for the child to have the protective boundary that underwear provides. The following sequence is summarized in Checklist Box 3-3.

1. Perform the basic relaxation sequence (see page 70) and passive touch on the foot or calf.
2. Apply oil or lotion.

3. Perform leg effleurage (see Figure 3–21). Place the palms on either side of the ankle. With parallel fingertips pointing toward the head and hands, glide up to the top of the calf and continue up to the top of the thigh. This stroke mainly uses the fingertips on a small child and the entire hand (palm and fingertips) on a larger child. The inside hand covers the inside of the leg, and the outside hand covers the outside of the leg. Do not press on the back of the knee. When you reach the top of the leg, your outside hand will continue up to the top of the

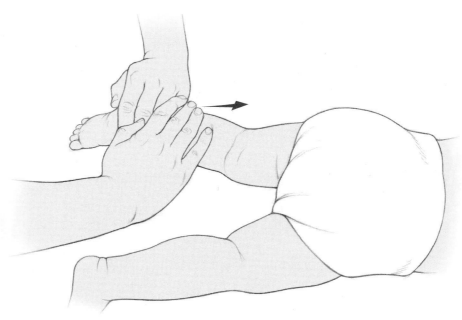

FIGURE 3–21 ■ Leg Effleurage.

buttock and turn and glide back down the outside of the leg, as the inside hand glides down the inside of the leg. Although your outside hand will have to glide a longer distance than your inside hand, coordinate the hands so that they are parallel on the way down. When you reach the foot, glide down and gently stroke over the sole of the foot with the fingertips. Begin with superficial pressure. As the child's tissue becomes warmed and relaxed, deeper pressure may be used. Perform 10 times.

4. Rake the back of the leg (see Figure 3–22). For a small child, move to a sitting position opposite the back of the knee. For a nearly adult-size child, move to a standing position opposite the back of the knee. Begin raking strokes at the top of the buttock, stroking toward the feet and gradually work down to the back of the knee. On a small child, each raking stroke should be 1 or 2 inches long; on a teenager, up to 5 or 6 inches long. Cover the muscles of the inner thigh, top of the thigh, and outside of the thigh. Do not press on the back of the knee. Return to the original position at the foot of the table and continue raking from the top of the calf to the ankle. Do the entire stroke—raking from buttock to ankle—once, using medium pressure.

5. Perform leg effleurage three times.

6. Thumbstroke the back of the leg (see Figure 3–23). Begin just above the ankle, thumbstroking the calf muscles and gradually moving up the calf. When you reach the top of the calf, change your position to sitting opposite the knee. Do not press on the back of the knee. Continue thumbstroking from just above the knee to the top of the thigh. Do the entire movement of thumbstroking from ankle to buttock once, using medium to firm pressure. Move back to sitting at the foot of the bed.

To perform a variation of this stroke, mentally divide the calf and thigh into three sections (inside, top, and outside), and thumbstroke each section separately.

7. Perform leg effleurage three times.

8. Thumbstroke the sole of the foot (see Figure 3–24). Begin at the base of the toes. Stroke away from you with many small pushes of the thumbs; work slowly and thoroughly up the sole of the foot to the heel. Imagine that the thumbs are dipped in ink and you want to completely ink the entire sole, with no areas left untouched. This is an area where firm pressure often feels good; ask the child what pressure feels best for her.

9. Circle the ankle bones (see Figure 3–25). Using the fingertips, slowly and gently circle around both ankle bones at the same time. Do six times.

10. Perform leg effleurage 10 times.

11. Perform passive range-of-motion exercises for the hip and knee. Extend the hip and flex and extend the knee (see page 66).

12. Skin stimulation stroke. Choose one:
    - Cover the back of the leg, including the buttock, with a pillowcase or sheet; massage it with a textured massage tool or a hairbrush.
    - Perform pincement or tapping on the entire back of the leg.
    - Gently rub the massage oil off of entire back of the leg with a coarse washcloth or a piece of fake fur.

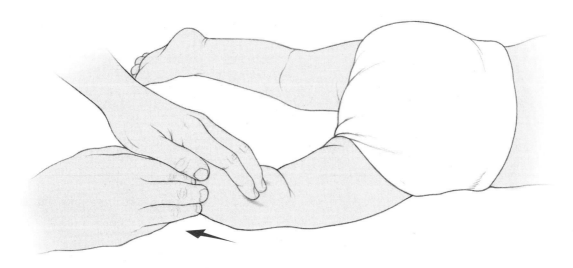

FIGURE 3–22 ■ Raking the Back of the Leg.

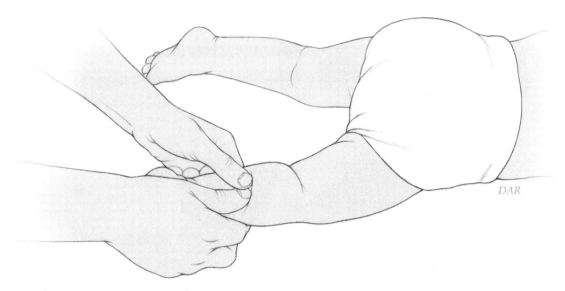

FIGURE 3–23 ■ Thumbstroking the Back of the Leg.

■ Do a salt glow of the entire back of the leg and the sole of the foot (see page 93).

13. Perform ball rolling. Cover the back of the leg with a pillowcase or sheet, have the child choose a ball, and roll the ball from the buttock to the tips of the toes and back. Massage the sole of the foot and each toe with the ball, moving in tiny circles. Press each toe into the massage surface with firm pressure.

14. End with the basic relaxation sequence. Now move to the other leg, and repeat the same series of strokes.

HEAD, NECK, AND SHOULDER MASSAGE

The child should lie on her back with a rolled towel or pillow under her knees. Use this position for the rest of the full body massage. Sit at the head of the table. With a small child, you may wish to sit cross-legged on the floor. (The following sequence is summarized in Checklist Box 3–4.)

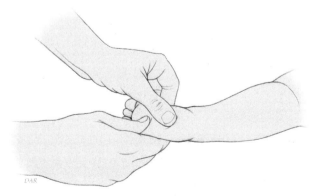

FIGURE 3–24 ■ Thumbstroking the Sole of the Foot.

1. Perform the basic relaxation sequence (see page 70) and passive touch.

2. Apply oil or lotion.

3. Perform shoulder and neck effleurage (see Figures 3–26 and 3–27). Use medium pressure. Begin the stroke at the medial ends of the clavicle. Place your hands palm down with the fingertips pointing toward each other. Your hands will be stroking along the clavicle, with your thumb above and your four fingers below the bone. Your hands move away from each other as they trace each collarbone from the medial ends of the clavicle out to the lateral ends and to the tips of the shoulders. When your hands reach the tips of the shoulders, slowly rotate

> **CHECKLIST BOX 3–4**
> *HEAD, NECK, AND SHOULDER MASSAGE*
>
> 1. Basic relaxation sequence and passive touch.
> 2. Apply oil or lotion.
> 3. Shoulder and neck effleurage, 10 times.
> 4. Diagonal neck stroke, 10 times.
> 5. Shoulder and neck effleurage, three times.
> 6. Scalp petrissage, 1 minute.
> 7. Shoulder and neck effleurage, three times.
> 8. Forehead and eye circles, six times.
> 9. Face effleurage, six times.
> 10. Cheek petrissage, 30 seconds.
> 11. Shoulder and neck effleurage, 10 times.
> 12. Neck range-of-motion exercises.
> 13. Skin stimulation stroke.
> 14. Basic relaxation sequence.

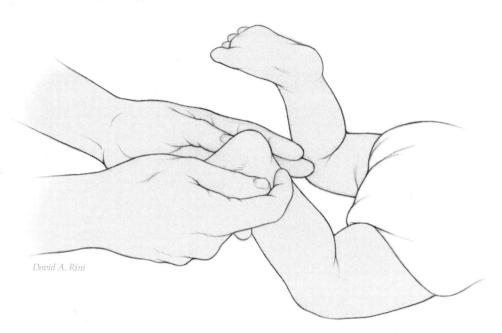

David A. Rini

FIGURE 3–25 ■ Circle the Ankle Bones.

them so that the fingertips are underneath the shoulders. Glide along the top of the upper trapezius back to the neck, up the back of the neck, under the head and off. Perform 10 times.

4. Perform diagonal neck stroke (see Figure 3–28). To begin, turn the left hand palm up. Slide it under the neck to the right shoulder. Now pull this hand (the left) diagonally from the right shoulder across the neck and finish below the left ear. Switch hands and do the same stroke; the right hand will move diagonally from the left shoulder across the neck and finish below the right ear. Imagine that you are drawing an X on the back of the neck with the fingertips. This diagonal stroke across the neck allows you to combine cross-fiber stroking with a gentle stretching along the many layers of muscle fibers in this area. Curl the fingers as you slide and use medium pressure with the fingertips. Encourage the child to relax her neck and allow the stroke to move her head from side to side. If she is not relaxing her neck muscles, her head will remain in the same position during the stroke. Perform 10 times.

5. Perform shoulder and neck effleurage three times.

6. Perform scalp petrissage (see Figure 3–29). Slip your hands under the child's head, then cradle it by letting the back of her head rest on your palms. Begin at the base of her scalp and move your fingertips in slow, small circles. Feel the shapes of the bones underneath the scalp, and

notice the mobility and level of tension in the tissue of the scalp. Tension in the face, eyes, or neck (such as in the posterior cervical and sternocleidomastoid muscles) may initiate trigger points in the scalp muscles, and injuries to the head may also cause tension in the tissue of the scalp.[12] Gradually perform petrissage up the back of the head. When your hands begin to be uncomfortable in this position, flip them around so that your palms are down and continue petrissage up to the forehead. The temples and the area above the ears should be massaged, as well as the sides of the head. Use light to medium pressure, depending upon the child's comfort level. Massage the scalp for 1 minute.

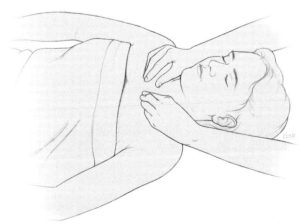

FIGURE 3–26 ■ Shoulder and Neck Effleurage. Your hands are in the starting position.

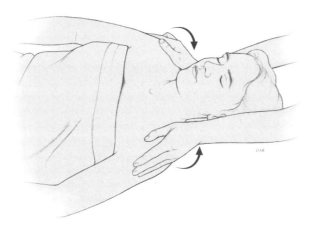

FIGURE 3–27 ■ Shoulder and Neck Effleurage. Your hands have reached the tips of the shoulders and are ready to rotate around them and glide up the upper trapezius to the neck.

7. Perform shoulder and neck effleurage three times.
8. Circle the forehead and eyes (see Figures 3–30 and 3–31). Place both hands palm down on the forehead with your fingertips pointing toward each other. (For a small child, you may have room for only the fingertips.) Slowly and gently rake from the middle of the forehead out to the temples. Make small circles with the fingertips on both temples simultaneously; then, using the index fingers, glide smoothly under the eyes up the sides of the nose and back to the forehead. Use light pressure when gliding in one smooth, flowing stroke. Repeat six times.
9. Perform face effleurage (see Figures 3–32 and 3–33). Use light pressure. Begin with the thumbs touching under the nose, index fingers touching below the lower lip, and the last three fingers curled below the tip of the chin. Stroke from the center of the face out toward the side of the face. The fingers will simultaneously outline the cheekbones, lips, and jawbone. When the fingertips reach the sides of the face, rotate your hands and let the fingertips slide up in front of the ear, over the temples, and up to the middle of the forehead. Glide the index fingers down the bridge of the nose to the chin, and begin again. With practice, this stroke can be done smoothly and continuously and has a very calming effect. Repeat six times.
10. Perform cheek petrissage. Using the fingertips, make small circles under the cheekbones (zygomatic arches) and on the cheeks. You are massaging the masseter muscle, one of the most common muscles in the entire body to harbor trigger points. Even infants may carry considerable tension in this area because of almost constant suck-

ing, chewing, and mouthing of objects. Dental pain or injury can initiate tension in the masseter, even in small children. By adulthood, unfortunately, many adults have substantial knots in this muscle. Perform petrissage gently, slowly, and thoroughly. Continue for 30 seconds or more.
11. Perform shoulder and neck effleurage 10 times.
12. Perform passive range-of-motion exercises for the neck (these include flexion, extension, rotation, and lateral flexion of the cervical spine; see page 67).
13. Perform a skin stimulation stroke. Choose one:
    ■ Gentle tapping of the entire face with the fingertips, taking care to avoid the eyes.
    ■ Gently wipe massage oil off the face with a washcloth. The cloth may be wrung out in warm water on a cool day or in cold water on a hot day.
14. End with the basic relaxation sequence.

CHEST AND ABDOMEN MASSAGE

Stand at the head of the therapy table. The following sequence is summarized in Checklist Box 3–5.

1. Perform the basic relaxation sequence (see page 70) and passive touch on the top of the shoulders.
2. Apply oil or lotion.
3. Perform chest and abdomen effleurage (see Figure 3–34). Place your hands on the chest, just below where the collarbones meet. Point the fingertips toward the feet. With hands parallel, glide down the center of the chest to the lower part of the abdomen. Here, move your

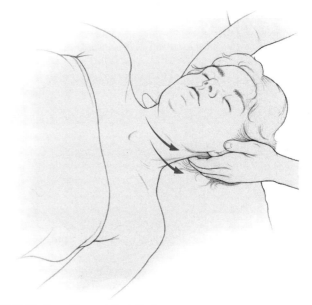

FIGURE 3–28 ■ Diagonal Neck Stroke.

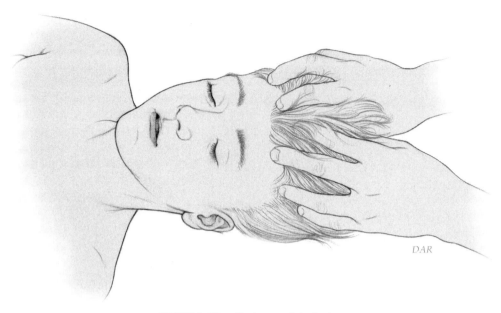

FIGURE 3–29 ■ Petrissage of the Scalp.

hands away from each other to the side and glide over the anterior iliac crests, up the lateral aspect of the hips and torso, onto the upper chest, and back to the starting position. Use gentle pressure, gradually increasing the pressure as the child's tissue becomes warmer and more relaxed. Repeat 10 times.

Be careful to preserve the child's modesty and respect his right to refuse chest massage. Modesty is not usually a concern for very small children but, with older children, you should

always obtain their permission before the chest area is massaged. Although this is not usually a concern for boys, it is still wise to ask their permission first. The breasts and nipples should never be massaged unless you, the child, and the child's parent have agreed that there is a specific therapeutic purpose for doing so.

■ Prepare the child before you remove the drape covering the torso and abdomen. For example, you might say, "I'm going to uncover your chest and stomach now. Is that okay

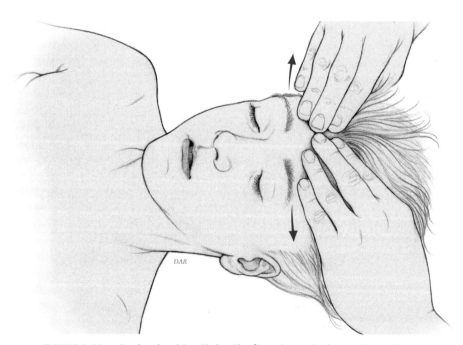

FIGURE 3–30 ■ Forehead and Eye Circles. The fingertips are in the starting position.

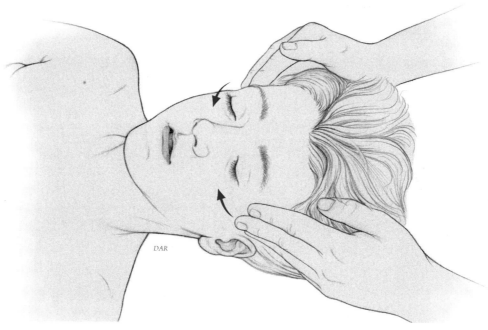

FIGURE 3–31 ■ Forehead and Eye Circles. The fingertips have reached the temples and are ready to glide under the eyes.

with you? And how do you feel about me massaging your chest?" If the child indicates any concerns, drape the breast area and massage only the abdomen.

- A powerful way to help the child experience the connectedness of his upper and lower body is to combine this stroke with the last part of the shoulder and neck effleurage stroke. Instead of returning to the starting position on the chest, as your hands move up the sides of the hips and torso, let them glide over the tips of the shoulder, along the upper trapezius, under the back of the neck, under the head, and off.

4. Perform chest friction (see Figure 3–35). Place your hands as you would for the beginning of the chest and abdomen effleurage. Then glide just a few inches down the center of the chest (over the sternum) with your right hand. Return the right hand to the starting position and glide a few inches over the sternum with your left hand; return the left hand to the

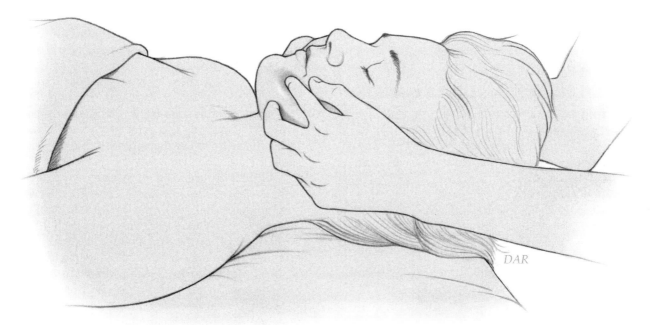

FIGURE 3–32 ■ Face Effleurage. The fingers are simultaneously outlining the cheekbone, lips, and jawbone.

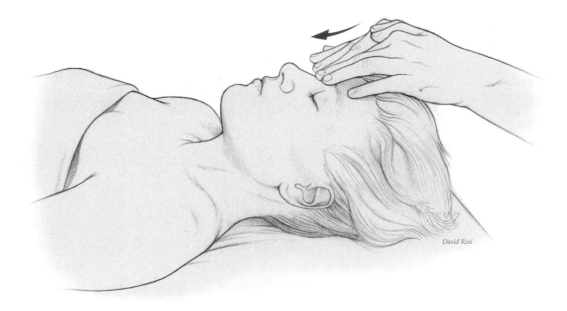

David Rini

FIGURE 3–33 ■ Face Effleurage. The fingers have come up the side of the face to the middle of the forehead, and are ready to glide down the center of the face to the chin.

starting position and glide a few inches with your right hand. If you are working with a girl, be careful that the stroke stays over the sternum and that the breast area is not massaged. Continue alternating your hands, moving briskly. The size of the child's chest will determine how far each stroke can go; try to cover the area from the sternal notch to the bottom of the sternum, but do not press on the xyphoid process. Keep your hands soft so that they glide smoothly over the ribs; use gentle pressure. Continue for about 30 seconds. As with any friction stroke, your hands and the

child's tissue will soon feel dramatically warmer.

5. Perform chest and abdomen effleurage three times. Now move from the head of the table to stand on the right side of the table beside the right hipbone.

6. Perform abdominal effleurage (see Figure 3–36). The abdomen is often an especially vulnerable area. Physically, the internal organs of the abdomen lack bony protection, as compared with the heart, lungs, or pelvic organs, which are surrounded by bone. This may be the cause of the extra vulnerability many adults and children feel in this area. Be especially gentle when you first touch the abdomen. If the child has any history of abuse or simply seems unhappy about this area being massaged, do not proceed without specific consent. Begin by slowly making contact using the palm of your right hand (the hand closest to the abdomen). Rest it gently on the abdomen for a few moments to help the child become accustomed to touch. Make clockwise circles with your palm, covering the entire abdomen. After a few circles, include your left hand; the left makes clockwise half-circles on the top half of the abdomen, while your right hand makes the bottom half of its circle. Then take your left hand off the abdomen until your right hand completes the top half of its circle and returns to the bottom half of its circle. Use gentle pressure. Repeat 10 times. If the child is ticklish, you may try covering the abdominal

---

✔️ **CHECKLIST BOX 3–5**
CHEST AND STOMACH MASSAGE

---

1. Basic relaxation sequence and passive touch on the tops of the shoulders.
2. Apply oil or lotion.
3. Chest and abdomen effleurage, 10 times.
4. Chest friction, 30 seconds.
5. Chest and abdomen effleurage, three times.
6. Abdominal effleurage, 10 times.
7. Knead the abdomen, 1 minute.
8. Chest and abdomen effleurage, 10 times.
9. Skin stimulation stroke.
10. Basic relaxation sequence.

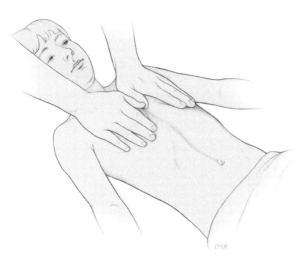

FIGURE 3–34 ■ Chest and Abdomen Effleurage.

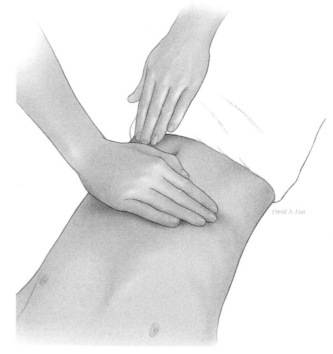

FIGURE 3–36 ■ Abdominal Effleurage.

area with a sheet and gently stroking through it; this may decrease the amount of skin stimulation enough to stop the ticklishness.

- For a small child, you may not be able to fit your entire palm on the abdomen and may need to glide more with your fingertips. Even so, remember that this effleurage stroke should be performed as smoothly as possible; do not poke or use direct pressure on the abdomen. Also, do not touch or put any pressure on the xyphoid process.

7. Knead the abdomen (see Figure 3–37). Reach across the abdomen and begin above the left iliac crest, kneading the abdomen. Knead across the abdomen, ending above the right iliac crest. Continue for about 1 minute. Many children are not fleshy in this area and knead-

ing can be a challenge—there is just not a great deal of tissue to grasp.

8. Perform chest and abdomen effleurage. Return to the original position, standing at the head of the table, and repeat the chest and abdomen effleurage 10 times.

9. Skin stimulation stroke. Choose one:
   - Cover the chest and abdomen with a pillowcase or sheet and massage gently with a textured massage tool or soft hairbrush. This

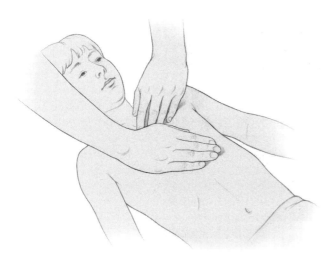

FIGURE 3–35 ■ Chest Friction.

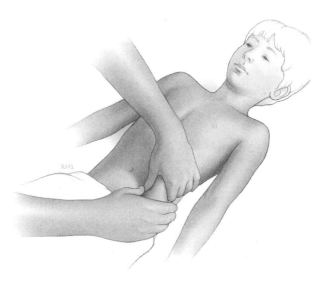

FIGURE 3–37 ■ Kneading the Abdomen.

may cause tickles, which some children will enjoy and some will not. Ask, "Do you want me to stop?" If the child cannot tell you, err on the side of caution and skip this stroke.

- Wipe massage oil or lotion off with a washcloth.
- Use a prewarmed towel that is large enough to cover the entire torso and abdomen. Cover the entire area with the towel and perform one or two effleurages over the towel to bring it in contact with the child's skin. Then leave the towel there and cover it with a drape to keep in the heat.

10. End with the basic relaxation sequence.

ARM MASSAGE

Stand opposite the arm, at about the level of the child's hand. The following sequence is summarized in Checklist Box 3–6.

1. Perform the basic relaxation sequence (see page 70) and passive touch on the hand or forearm.
2. Apply oil or lotion.
3. Perform arm effleurage (see Figure 3–38). This stroke is similar to the leg effleurage stroke on both the front and the back of the legs. Begin by placing your inside hand palm-to-palm with the child's hand. Place your outside hand palm down on the back of the child's hand. With your fingertips pointing toward the shoulder, glide up the arm with both hands. Keep your hands parallel. When your inside hand reaches the armpit, it will simply glide back down the inside of the arm again. Your outside hand will glide up and over the top of the shoulder, crossing the anterior deltoid, the lateral end of the collarbone, the posterior deltoid and then, finally, glide back down the outside of the arm. Synchronize your hands by slowing down your inside hand as it leaves the armpit until your outside hand has circled the shoulder and comes back down parallel to the inside hand. Then both hands continue at the same time, gliding all the way down the arm and hand and gently stroking out to the fingertips. If the child is ticklish, avoid the ticklish area. Very light stroking generally makes the tickling worse. Begin with superficial pressure and, as the child's tissue becomes warmer and more relaxed, you may use medium pressure. Repeat 10 times.

4. Thumbstroke the inside of the arm (see Figure 3–39). Begin at the wrist and work up to the armpit, skipping over the antecubital area. Stay away from any ticklish areas. Use medium pressure. Do the entire inside arm once, slowly and thoroughly. This should take about 1 minute.

5. Perform arm effleurage three times.

6. Rake the outside of the arm (see Figure 3–40). Start at the top of the shoulder and work down the outside of the upper arm and the top of the forearm to the wrist. Do once, slowly and thoroughly, using medium pressure. This will require about 1 minute.

7. Perform arm effleurage three times.

8. Perform friction on the hand. Begin by rubbing your hands together as if you were warming them. Then make a "hand sandwich" with your inside palm against the child's palm and your outside palm on top of the back of the child's hand. Now rub briskly, just as you did to warm your hands. Continue for 15 seconds or more.

9. Thumbstroke the back of the hand (see Figure 3–41). Beginning at the base of the fingers, thumbstroke the entire back of the hand up to the wrist. Use medium pressure. Continue for 30 seconds or more.

10. Thumbstroke the palm (see Figure 3–42). Thumbstroke the entire palm, pushing from the base of the fingers toward the wrist and smoothing out all the creases. Continue for 30 seconds or more.

11. Stretch the fingers (see Figure 3–43). Use the thumb on top and index finger underneath as you massage each finger. Beginning at the base of the child's finger, slide out to the fin-

---

☑ CHECKLIST BOX 3–6
ARM MASSAGE

1. Basic relaxation sequence and passive touch.
2. Apply oil or lotion.
3. Arm effleurage, 10 times.
4. Thumbstroke the inside of the arm, 1 minute.
5. Arm effleurage, three times.
6. Rake the outside of the arm, 1 minute.
7. Arm effleurage, three times.
8. Hand friction, 15 seconds or more.
9. Thumbstroke the back of the hand, 30 seconds.
10. Thumbstroke the palm, 30 seconds.
11. Stretch the fingers, three times for each finger.
12. Arm effleurage, 10 times.
13. Range-of-motion exercises for the shoulder, elbow, wrist, and finger joints.
14. Skin stimulation stroke.
15. Ball rolling.
16. Basic relaxation sequence.

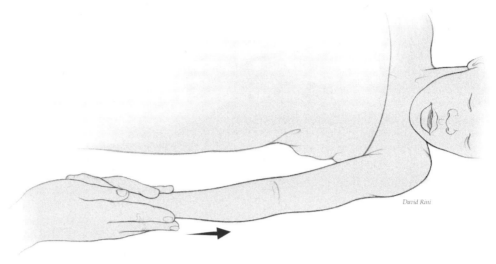

FIGURE 3–38 ■ Arm Effleurage.

gertip, gently pulling at the same time. Gently pinch the end of each finger as you slide off, so that the fingertip receives a tiny bit of extra stimulation. Do each finger three times.

12. Perform arm effleurage 10 times.
13. Perform range-of-motion exercises for the entire upper extremity:
    ■ Perform range-of-motion exercise for the shoulder joint, including flexion, extension, abduction, adduction, and internal and external rotation of the shoulder (see page 65).
    ■ Perform range-of-motion exercise for the elbow joint, including flexion and extension of the elbow and pronation and supination of the forearm (see page 65).
    ■ Perform range-of-motion exercise for the wrist joint, including hyperextension and flexion of the wrist (see page 66).
    ■ Perform range-of-motion exercises for the fingers, including extension and flexion (see page 66).
14. Skin stimulation stroke. Choose one:
    ■ Cover the arm with a sheet and massage it with a textured massage tool or brush.
    ■ Do pincement or tapping of the entire arm.
    ■ Wipe off massage oil or lotion with a washcloth or piece of fake fur.
    ■ Perform a salt glow of the entire arm.
15. Perform ball rolling of the entire arm. Move the ball up and down the length of the arm, then massage the back of the hand and each finger with the ball, moving in tiny circles. Press each finger into the massage surface with firm pressure.
16. End with the basic relaxation sequence. Now move to the other arm, and repeat this series.

LEG MASSAGE (FRONT)

Sit at the foot of the table, near the lateral side of the child's foot. Small children may lay one leg across your lap. For better body mechanics, stand to the outside of the leg of when working with adult-size children; do not stoop or stretch to cover the entire area. The following sequence is summarized in Checklist Box 3–7.

1. Perform the basic relaxation sequence (see page 70) and passive touch on the top of the foot or lower leg.
2. Apply oil or lotion.
3. Leg effleurage (see Figures 3–44 and 3–45). This stroke is similar to the leg effleurage for the back of the leg (see page 75). Use medium pressure.

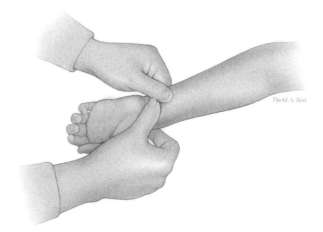

FIGURE 3–39 ■ Thumbstroking the Inside of the Arm.

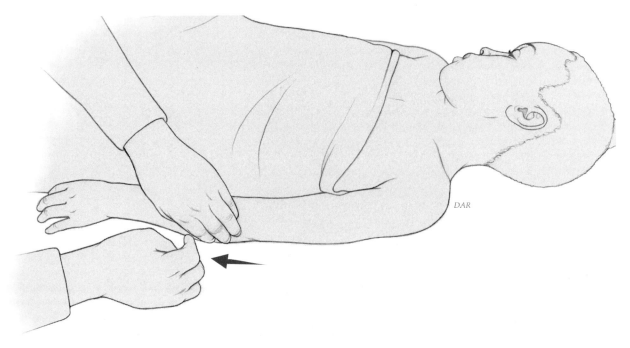

FIGURE 3–40 ■ Raking the Outside of the Arm.

Place both palms on the ankle. With your fingertips pointing toward the head and with your hands parallel, glide up to the top of the leg. Your inside hand will cover the inside of the leg, and your outside hand will cover the outside (lateral aspect) of the leg. Keep your hands directly across from each other. When your inside hand reaches the top of the leg, it will sim-

ply glide back down the inside of the leg again. The outside hand will glide up the outer half of the leg, trace the anterior iliac crest from its medial edge to its lateral edge, and then glide back down the outside of the leg. Synchronize your hands by slowing down the inside hand as it leaves the top of the leg until the outside hand has traced the iliac crest and come back down

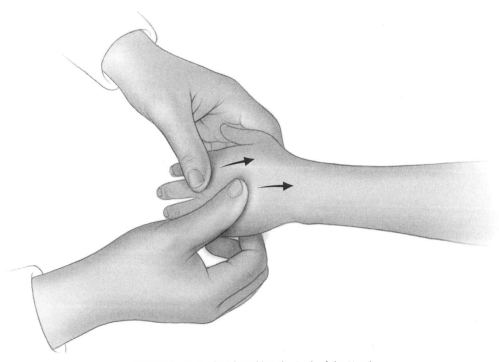

FIGURE 3–41 ■ Thumbstroking the Back of the Hand.

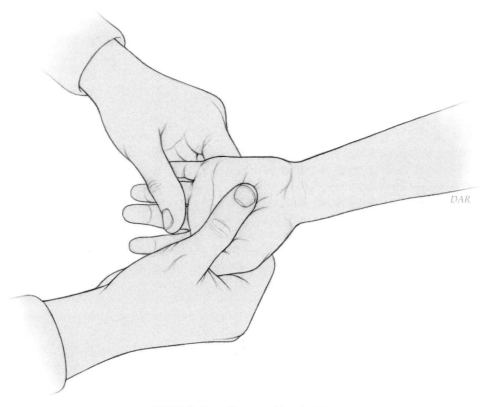

FIGURE 3–42 ■ Thumbstroking the Palm.

parallel to the inside hand. Both hands then glide all the way down the leg and foot at the same time, gently stroking over the top of the foot and out to the tips of the toes. Use superficial pressure at first. As the child's tissue becomes warmed and relaxed, you may use medium pressure. Repeat 10 times.

4. Rake the front of the leg (see Figure 3–46). Begin at the top of the leg. Move towards the feet; rake the entire thigh and around the patel-

la. Continuing toward the foot, rake the muscles on the medial side of the tibia from knee to ankle, then the muscles on the lateral side of the tibia from knee to ankle. Do the entire leg once, slowly and thoroughly. Use medium pressure. The entire stroke should take about 1 minute.

CHECKLIST BOX 3–7
LEG MASSAGE (FRONT)

1. Basic relaxation sequence and passive touch.
2. Apply oil or lotion.
3. Leg effleurage, 10 times.
4. Rake the front of the leg, 1 minute.
5. Circle the sides of the knees.
6. Tap directly on the patella.
7. Leg effleurage, three times.
8. Foot friction, 15 seconds or more.
9. Thumbstroke the top of the foot, 30 seconds.
10. Stretch and stroke the toes, three times for each toe.
11. Leg effleurage, 10 times.
12. Range-of-motion exercises of the hip, knee, ankle, and toe joints (see page 66–67).
13. Skin stimulation stroke.
14. Ball rolling.
15. Basic relaxation sequence.

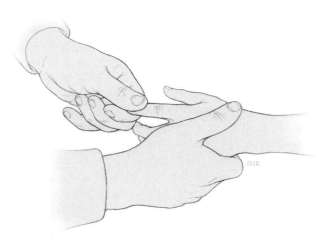

FIGURE 3–43 ■ Stretching the Fingers.

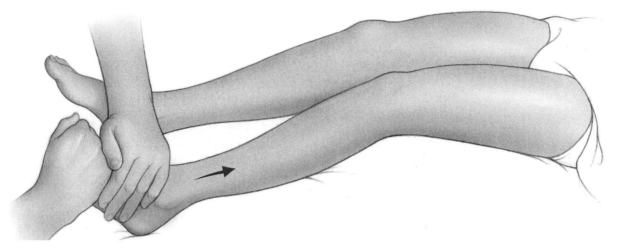

FIGURE 3–44 ■ Leg Effleurage. Starting position.

5. Circle the sides of the knees. Use the palm and fingertips of both hands at once, making wide circles on either side of the knee; this is similar to a tiny effleurage stroke. Repeat six times.
6. Tap directly on the patella with the fingers of both hands. Continue for 10 seconds.
7. Perform leg effleurage three times.
8. Perform friction on the foot (see Figure 3–47). Begin by rubbing your palms together as if you were warming them. Make a "foot sandwich" by placing your outside hand palm down on the top of the foot and your inside hand palm

up on the bottom of the foot. Now rub briskly, just as you did to warm your hands. Continue for 15 seconds or longer.
9. Thumbstroke the top of the foot (see Figure 3–48). Beginning at the base of the toes, thumbstroke the entire top of the foot up to the ankle. Imagine that your thumbs are dipped in ink and you want to completely ink the top of the foot. Using medium pressure, thumbstroke for 30 seconds or longer.
10. Stretch and stroke the toes (see Figure 3–49). Hold the foot steady by putting your outside

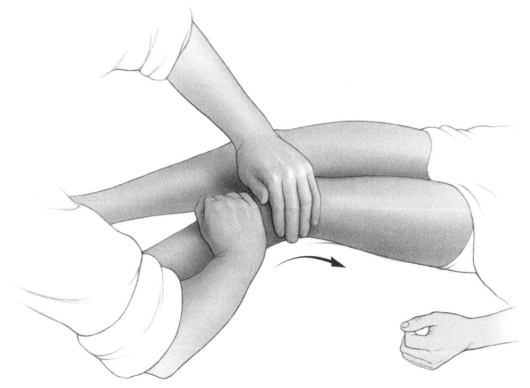

FIGURE 3–45 ■ Leg Effleurage. Your hands have glided over the knee and will continue to the top of the leg before returning to the starting position.

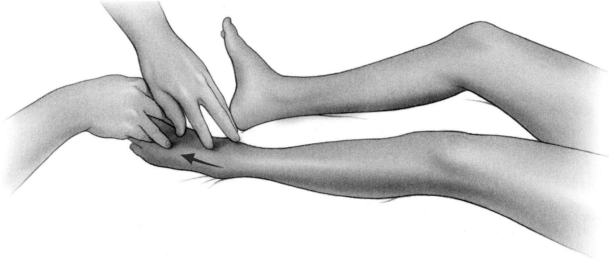

FIGURE 3–46 ■ Raking the Front of the Leg.

hand palm down on top of the ankle. With your inside hand, stretch and stroke one toe at a time. Beginning with the great toe, grasp each toe and gently rotate it in a circle three times, then rotate it in the opposite direction three times. To stroke, put your index finger beneath each toe and your thumb on top; gently pull as you slide from the base to the tip and off. Gently pinch the end of each toe as you slide off, so that the tip receives a tiny bit of extra stimulation. Stroke each toe three times. If the child is ticklish, skip this stroke and go back to foot friction instead.

11. Perform leg effleurage 10 times.
12. Perform range-of-motion exercises for the entire lower extremity:
    ■ Perform range-of-motion exercises of the hip joint, including flexion, extension, internal and external rotation, adduction, and abduction (see pages 66–67).
    ■ Perform range-of-motion exercises of the knee joint, including flexion and extension (see pages 66–67).
    ■ Perform ankle rotation (see page 67).
    ■ Perform toe rotation (see page 67).
13. Perform a skin stimulation stroke. Choose one:
    ■ Cover the entire leg and foot with a sheet, and massage with a textured massage tool or brush.
    ■ Do pincement or tapping of the entire leg and foot, including the kneecap.
    ■ Wipe massage oil or lotion off with a washcloth or piece of fake fur.
    ■ Perform a salt glow of the entire leg.
14. Perform ball rolling of the entire leg.
15. End with the basic relaxation sequence. Now move to the other leg and repeat.

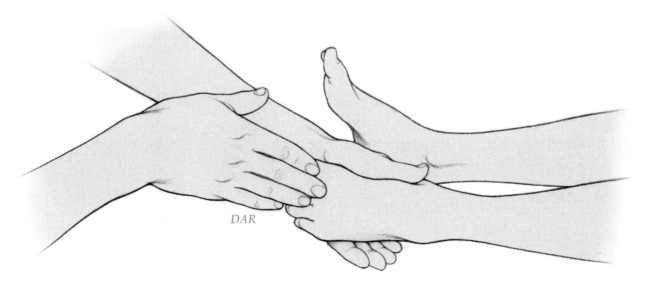

FIGURE 3–47 ■ Foot Friction.

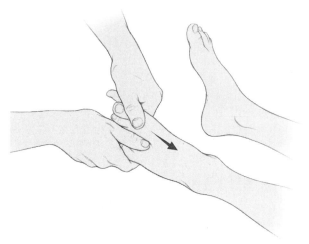

FIGURE 3–48 ■ Thumbstroking the Top of the Foot.

PRESSURE POINT MASSAGE

Many of the basic whole-body massage strokes you have learned so far are smooth and gliding and sweep over large areas. Except during passive touch, your hands are always in motion. The pressure point massage you will learn next is a different approach. As shown in Figure 3–50, individual fingers put slow, steady pressure on small, specific areas. Pressure point massage is an effective way to release deep tension, as long as great care is taken to apply the proper amount of pressure. Too little pressure will not release deep tension; too much pressure will be painful for the child. In Chapters 4, 5, and 6, you will learn how to use pressure points in combination with the basic Swedish massage strokes to treat common injuries and discomforts.

For each new pressure point, place the thumb or fingers on the specified spot. Use the flat of the finger, not the tip. Slowly increase your pressure until the child says the point is just beginning to hurt. Let up a little bit so that the point does not hurt. Hold each point for about 10 seconds, then slowly decrease the pressure and take your finger away. If you have difficulty locating a spot, the child can tell you where he or she is especially sensitive or tense.

HYDROTHERAPY AS AN ADJUNCT TO PEDIATRIC MASSAGE

BENEFITS AND TECHNIQUES OF HYDROTHERAPY

The therapeutic application of water, ice, or steam to the body is known as hydrotherapy. Because hydrotherapy, like therapeutic massage, can relax muscles, increase circulation, decrease muscle spasm,

relieve musculoskeletal pain, and help a child feel nurtured, it reinforces the effects of massage. Using hydrotherapy before massage allows you to work more effectively and can greatly increase a child's comfort and relaxation.

In the United States, hydrotherapy is not always within the scope of a massage therapist's practice. Statutes vary from state to state; in the state of Oregon, for example, the practice of massage includes "external use of hot, cold, and topical preparations such as lubricants." Therapists should investigate the regulations in their own state before treating children with the hydrotherapy treatments described in this book.

During hydrotherapy treatments, water may be applied externally to the entire body or to specific areas. Baths may be of varying temperatures. Sprays, frictions, hot or cold packs, hot or cold compresses, showers, saunas, or steam baths are external treatments, as well. Water may be also applied internally, in the form of steam inhalation, nasal rinses, gargles, douches, and drinking of water.

The most common forms of hydrotherapy used by massage practitioners today are the application of moist heat or ice. The application of moist heat to a specific area before massage increases blood flow, relaxes the tissue, and decreases pain. This allows you to work on deeper tissues with less discomfort for the child. A local ice application before massage increases local circulation and decreases pain and muscle spasm. This allows you to massage an area that is less sensitive and has more blood flow. These hydrotherapy applications not only have the direct physiologic effects mentioned above, they also involve careful personal attention and touch, which adds another nurturing element to a massage session. Before using any hydrotherapy application with children, always explain what the application is and why you are using it. Make sure they are comfortable during the application, and never allow them to become chilled.

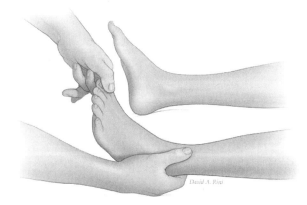

FIGURE 3–49 ■ Stretch and Stroke the Toes.

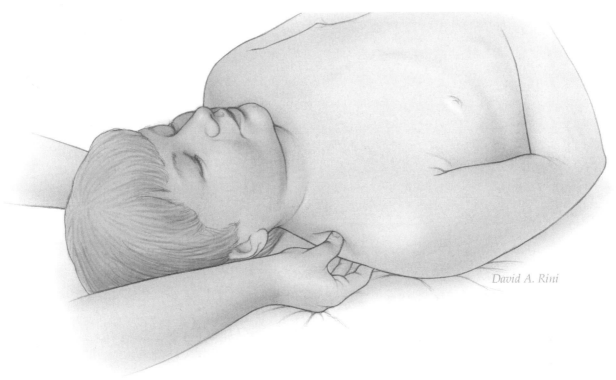

FIGURE 3–50 ■ Pressure Point Massage.

Children have a greater proportion of skin surface area and can become chilled more easily than an adult. Observe them carefully and, if they appear to be having a bad reaction to a treatment, stop the treatment immediately.

Effects of Cold Applications and Treatments

The primary effect of a local application of cold is the contraction of the small blood vessels of the skin. There is an immediate reduction in blood flow as capillary blood pressure falls 6–11 mm of mercury and the skin pales. Blood is driven to the interior of the body as the blood vessels of the skin contract and the internal blood vessels dilate. This constriction of the capillaries of the skin lasts 5 to 8 minutes after the cold application is removed, when the capillaries then dilate. The final result is a capillary diameter, which is actually larger than before the cold was applied. This is the secondary effect of a cold application.

The contraction of the blood vessels in the skin and the shunting of blood into the interior is a reflex reaction to cold on the skin, and it takes place even before the tissue is significantly chilled. This is the body's attempt to maintain a core temperature of 98.6° F; by shunting warm blood back into the interior of the body, the brain and other vital organs are kept warm and heat loss through the skin is reduced. When the cold is removed, this pattern is reversed; the small blood vessels of the skin dilate and the internal blood vessels contract. An increased amount of blood flows to the capillaries, and the skin flushes as blood is drawn to the surface.[13]

During the cold application, the decrease in surface blood flow, in turn, decreases inflammation. This makes cold therapy appropriate for acute sprains, bruises, muscle strains, acute bursitis, and acute joint inflammation.

Ice Massage

Ice massage is the application of ice to the skin, using an ice cube or ice chunk. After an injury (such as a severe bruise or joint sprain) or for a severe muscle spasm, ice massage can decrease local swelling and inflammation and relieve muscle spasm. Make a chunk of ice by filling a paper cup with water and freezing it. Hold the cup of ice in one hand and gently rub the ice in a circular motion over the particular body area, including a few inches above and below the area as well (see Figure 3–51). Perform ice massage for about 5 minutes.[14] After an injury, ice massage can be done as often as once an hour to relieve pain and to increase circulation.

Many children dislike ice applications unless a few simple precautions are followed. First, make sure the child is warm and that rivulets of water are not going to trickle down in a sensitive area. Drape towels around the area to be iced, if necessary. Second, warn the child before the ice first touches the skin. Finally, if the child complains about the cold after a few min-

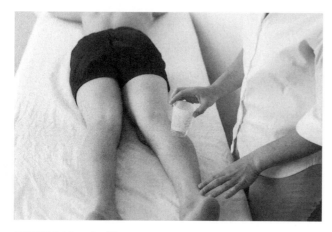

FIGURE 3–51 ■ Ice Massage.

utes, stop using the ice for a short time, then try again. Ice massage feels more intense than an ice pack and, for some children, it is also more difficult to tolerate.

Ice Pack Application

Commercial ice packs or ice bags are easy to obtain or you may use homemade ice packs (a plastic bag filled with crushed ice or ice cubes). Place a thin layer of cloth, such as a pillowcase, on the skin and lay the ice pack on top. Ice packs should be applied for no longer than 15 minutes; after an injury, they may be used in intervals of 15 minutes on and then 15 minutes off. Repeat as needed. The rest period avoids any cold damage to the child's tissue, such as frostbite.

Many children are reluctant to have ice on their body, so be sure to warn them before the ice is applied and tell them a special effort will be made to keep the rest of their body warm.

Heating Compress

A heating compress is a mild, prolonged application of moist heat that, despite its name, begins with cold water. It is generally applied for several hours or overnight. Typically, a cotton cloth dipped in cold water is applied to one area of the body and then covered with wool or other insulating material. The child should always be thoroughly warm before the compress is applied. Heating compresses are used to relax muscles and to relieve the discomfort of sore throats, rheumatic joints, or chest colds, and can relieve congestion in certain areas. The cold socks treatment (see page 121), which is used to decongest the head of a child who has a cold, is a type of heating compress.

Heat Application and Treatment

The primary effect of local heat application is dilation of the blood vessels of the skin. This increases the loss of heat from the skin and helps the body maintain its core temperature of 98.6° F, protecting the brain and other internal organs from overheating.

The peripheral blood vessels dilate as a reflex reaction, even before the area is significantly heated. As blood rushes to the area, the skin turns pink, local tissue metabolism increases, and more white blood cells move to the area. The tissue under the hot application begins to sweat, the muscles relax, and pain is reduced.

You can take advantage of the body's reaction to heat in many therapeutic ways. The primary effect of heat, the dilation of blood vessels, will shift blood from somewhere else in the body to fill the dilated vessels. When congestion may be causing symptoms, such as migraine and sinus headaches, a hot foot or hand bath can help draw congestion from that area (see Migraine Headaches, page 135-136). Hot applications in local areas relieve muscle tightness and pain. Heat, like touch, is experienced by children as comforting and nurturing. When a child is tense or nervous about receiving a massage, the addition of heat through warmed linens, rice-filled, microwaveable bags, or moist heat packs can help them feel more relaxed. Do not apply heat in the acute stages of injuries such as bruises, sprains, and dislocations.

Hot Footbaths

The hot footbath is a local heat treatment. The child sits in a chair wrapped in a sheet or blanket, with both feet in a container of water (110° F) for about 20 minutes; he receives a cold compress to the forehead at the same time. However, a hot footbath can also be given with the child laying supine on a treatment table with the feet in the container of water (see Figure 3–52). The water temperature must remain at 110° F during the entire treatment, and the cold compress should be changed every 3 minutes. At the end of the treatment, cold water is poured briefly over the child's feet, they are dried, and the child then rests for 10 to 15 minutes. This technique is contraindicated for those with insulin-dependant diabetes or loss of feeling in the legs.[13]

Hot Packs or Hot Moist Towel Application

The application of moist heat relaxes muscles, relieves pain, and helps the child feel comforted and nurtured. It can also keep a child warm during a massage. Moist heat is used because it penetrates more deeply than dry heat.

- Hot moist heating pads or Hydrocollator packs: Put one or two dry towels on the area of the child's body that is going to be treated. Then apply a moist heating pad or Hydrocollator pack, and cover with another dry towel. The dry towel against the child's skin protects against burns and the dry towel on top of the hot pack keeps in the heat. Check with the child to make sure the hot application is not too hot and check it frequently. Add more towels underneath the hot pack if it is too hot. Cover the

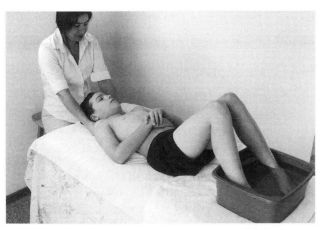

FIGURE 3–52 ■ Hot Footbath. Normally the child would be covered by a sheet or blanket, but it has been removed for clarity's sake.

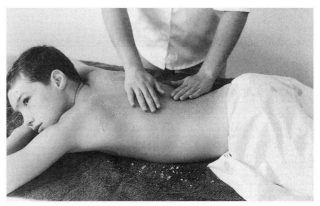

FIGURE 3–53 ■ Salt Glow Massage. A massage performed using salt; the skin becomes pink as a result of increased circulation in the skin.

child with a sheet. Hot packs should be left on for 15 minutes unless otherwise noted.

- Hot moist towels: They can be applied directly to the child's skin, as they are generally not as hot as heating pads or Hydrocollator packs. Wring them out in hot water, apply to the child's skin, and cover with a dry towel. Check with the child to make sure that the hot towels are not too hot and check his or her skin frequently.

Salt Glow

A salt glow, or salt rub, is both stimulating and relaxing to the skin and the underlying muscles. It also increases local blood flow. Many children enjoy it as a combination of a back massage and a "back scratch." It is excellent for any child who is immobilized because of illness or injury and cannot increase his or her own circulation through exercise. During a salt glow, three types of skin stimulation are combined: the temperature of the water; the actual friction with the salt; and the washing and drying of the skin. While it is possible to do a salt glow of the entire body, you would need to use a bathtub and have the child completely undressed. Instead, it is more practical for you to do salt glows on smaller areas, such as the back, the legs and feet, or the arms and hands. A salt glow of the back is shown in Figures 3–53 and 3–54. For a child who is sensitive or tactile defensive, you may do a salt rub of a very small area, such as the hands. You will need the following equipment:

- two bowls of warm water at 110° F
- one towel
- two washcloths or terrycloth mitts
- about one-quarter cup Epsom salts, moistened with just enough water so that it clumps together but does not dissolve the salt

To perform a salt glow on one part of the body, begin with the child lying on a towel on the therapy table or on the floor. Explain that he will feel warm water on the area. Gently wash the back, arm, or leg with warm water. Now tell the child that he will feel the salt on the body part. Take about one tablespoon of the moistened salt in your hands, and spread it on the back or arm or leg. More salt may be needed, depending on the size of the area. Use a brisk upward movement with one hand while making a brisk downward movement with the other hand; as you alternate hands, you will be giving a friction-type massage. Move from one end of the area to the other and back again, using gentle pressure and always moving briskly. Continue for 1 to 3 minutes, depending on the size of the child and the child's reaction. The skin will quickly become pink. Ask the child to tell you when the salt starts too feel "too scratchy." Often the child will enjoy the abrasive and stimulating nature of the salt for a time and then will start to feel that it is too abrasive. Should the child complain that the salt glow is uncomfortable, stop immediately. To complete the salt glow, gently wash the salt off with the wet washcloth or terrycloth glove, and dry the child with the other one. An additional sensory stimulation technique that may be added at this point is to wash the salt off

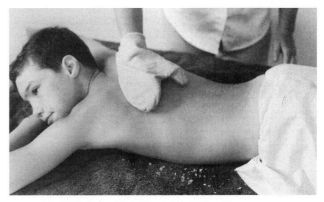

FIGURE 3–54 ■ The salt glow is completed by gently washing off the salt with water.

with water, then use a small amount of liquid soap and wash the back with soap lather, rinse it off with clean water, and dry the back. This gives the child a dramatic contrast between the scratchy feeling of the salt and the creamy feeling of the soap lather.

The towel that was underneath the child will have salt crystals on it and should be removed before proceeding with the massage. Ask the child to roll first to one side and then to the other as you fold the towel over the crystals and remove it.

The salt glow is contraindicated if the involved area has a cut, rash, or any open skin. It is also contraindicated in any child who shows extreme fearfulness.

Contrast Treatments

Contrast treatments are applications of heat alternated with applications of cold. They produce a greater increase in the local circulation than either a hot or a cold application alone. Alternating hot and cold applications causes the blood vessels to alternately dilate and contract, increasing the circulation to an area by 70–100%. Contrast treatments are excellent for reducing swelling in sprains and other traumatic injuries and can dramatically relieve pain.[13]

In contrast treatments, one cycle of hot followed by cold is called one *change*. The number of changes may be different for different conditions, as may be the amount of time the hot or cold is continued. A standard contrast treatment, however, consists of three changes of 3 minutes of heat followed by 30 seconds to 1 minute of cold. Different forms of heat, such as hot water, Hydrocollator packs, moist heating pads, or hot compresses may be used. Different forms of cold such as cold water, cold compresses, or ice massage may be used. Figure 3–55 shows a contrast treatment for the chest, and Figure 3–56 shows a contrast treatment for the eyes.

Hydrotherapy Safety Precautions

Hydrotherapy is safe, but you should always follow these precautions, using common sense:

1. Because some hydrotherapy treatments involve immersing a part of the child's body in water, it is possible that some water might be spilled on the floor. Mop up any spills immediately so that there is no chance of anyone slipping.
2. Children should be monitored even more carefully than adults for their reaction to the hydrotherapy applications. Their skin is thinner, and they may be burned more quickly by hot applications. Use plenty of towels under hot packs so that children do not get burned. Ask the child frequently how the hot pack feels on his skin and, occasionally, lift up the hot pack and check it. Add more towels on the child's skin if necessary.
3. Although highly unlikely that a child's skin might be frost-damaged from ice therapy, it is possible. Watch the clock when timing ice treatments—don't leave ice on for more time than called for.
4. Pay close attention to your pediatric patient. If you see a child reacting in an unusual way, immediately ask him or her about it. Terminate the treatment if the child seems to be uncomfortable.
5. Always check water temperature with both a water thermometer and your hand.
6. Exercise caution when handling hot packs, so your hands are not burned. Use metal tongs or rubber or leather gloves while handling hot packs of any type.

In this chapter, you have learned how to perform a full-body Swedish massage that is suitable for all chil-

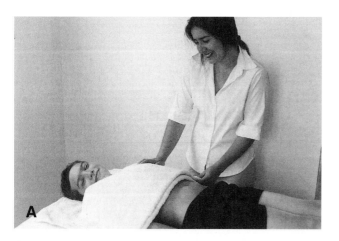

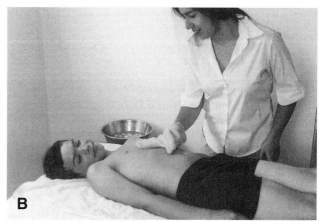

FIGURE 3–55 ■ Contrast Treatment of the Chest. **A,** The boy has just had a hot pack applied to his chest. **B,** The therapist is rubbing his chest with cold water.

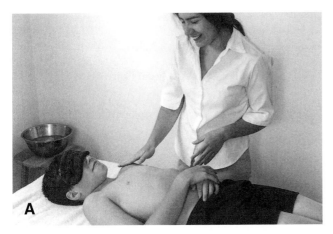 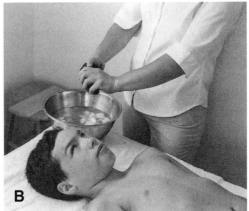

FIGURE 3–56 ■ Contrast Treatment for the Eyes. **A,** The boy has just had a hot cloth applied over his eyes. **B,** A cloth is being wrung out in cold water for the cold application over his eyes.

dren. It incorporates the classic Swedish techniques of passive touch, effleurage, petrissage, tapotement, friction, and range-of-motion exercises. It also includes sensory stimulation and relaxation techniques. Once you have thoroughly learned these techniques, you may enrich them by including techniques from other forms of massage and bodywork. However, the basic techniques presented in this chapter contain enough variation and possibility for creativity to keep your work both effective and interesting for years to come. In Chapters 4, 5, and 6, you will learn adaptations of the basic techniques for specific situations. This will enable you to treat children with injuries, minor discomforts, special needs and chronic conditions.

REVIEW QUESTIONS

1. Explain the benefits of using Swedish massage, passive range-of-motion exercises, skin stimulation techniques, ball massage, and pressure point massage with children.

2. Discuss some reasons for using relaxation techniques prior to and during the massage.

3. Give three examples of how a hands-on therapist can alter the strokes and structure of a massage session to reflect the child's unique needs and preferences.

4. Explain how the massage techniques in Chapter 3 can be adapted for these individual children:
   a. A 3-year-old child with stranger anxiety.
   b. An active middle school boy whose body has many bruises and scrapes in various stages of healing.
   c. An athletic teenage girl who has deep concerns about her weight, despite the fact that she is actually at her ideal weight.

   d. A teenage boy who has been experiencing a great deal of stress. He has been referred by his physician for help with severe headaches. He would rather "die" than remove an article of clothing in front of his mother, let alone in front of a strange therapist.

5. Discuss the body's reactions to local application of heat. Why does the body react to the hot application in these ways? List three examples of situations when local heat application is indicated.

6. Discuss the body's reactions to local application of cold. Why does the body react to the cold application in these ways? List three examples of situations when a local cold application is indicated.

REFERENCES

1. Boone DC, Azen SP: Normal range of motion in male subjects. *Journal of Bone and Joint Surgery*, 61-A:756, 1979
2. Upledger J: Mighty Joe Defies the Odds. *Massage Today*, June 2002, p 10
3. Kozier B, Erb G, Berman A, Snyder S: *Fundamentals of Nursing.* Upper Saddle River, NJ: Prentice-Hall, 2000, p 1003-1007
4. McBrien R: Using relaxation with first grade boys. *Elementary School Guidance and Counseling*, February 1978, p 146-152
5. Richter I, et al: Cognitive and relaxation treatment of pediatric migraine. *Pain*, 25:195-203, 1986
6. Bernstein D: *Progressive Relaxation Training: A Manual for the Helping Professions.* Champaign, IL: Research Press, 1973, p 8
7. Olness K: *Hypnosis and Hypnotherapy with Children.* New York: Guilford Press, 1996
8. Cautela J, Groden J: *Relaxation: A Comprehensive Manual for Adults, Children, and Children With Special Needs.* Champaign, IL: Research Press, 1978
9. Jacobson E: *You Must Relax.* New York: McGraw-Hill, 1934

10. Jacobson E: *Progressive Relaxation*. Chicago: University of Chicago Press, 1938

11. Platania A, et al: Relaxation therapy reduces anxiety in child/adolescent psychiatry patients. *Acta Paedopsychiatrica*, 55:115-120, 1992

12. Simons D, Travell J: *Myofascial Pain and Dysfunction: The Triggerpoint Manual*, vol. 1, ed. 2. Baltimore, MD: Lippincott Williams & Wilkins, 1999, p 430

13. Thrash A: *Home Remedies: Hydrotherapy, Massage, Charcoal and Other Simple Treatments*. Seale, AL: Thrash Publications, 1981, p 34-38

14. Packman H: *Ice Therapy: Understanding Its Application*, ed. 4. Whitestone, NY: self-published booklet, 1998

MASSAGE AND HYDROTHERAPY FOR PEDIATRIC INJURIES

4

■ **KEY POINTS**

After reading this chapter, the student will be able to:

1. Explain the most common causes of childhood injury and list strategies to prevent these injuries.
2. Give specific examples of injuries that children are more likely to have than adults and explain the reasons why.
3. Discuss, in detail, the impact of dislocations, fractures, and sprains on soft tissue in or near the sites of these injuries.
4. Understand the differences between acute injuries and their long-term effects and give examples.
5. Explain the rationale for using massage and hydrotherapy to treat each injury in this chapter.

It is a rare child who grows to adulthood without having many minor injuries and at least one major injury. Because they are not developmentally mature enough to assess danger or understand the consequences of their behavior, children are far more likely to be injured in accidents than are adults. Jumping from dangerous heights, riding bicycles unsafely, playing with fire, and darting out into traffic are just some of the risk-taking behaviors that put children in harm's way. Injuries are the leading cause of pediatric death and the second leading cause of hospitalization in the United States.[1] In 1999, 25% of American children sustained an injury that required medical attention. Of those children, nearly 120,000 were injured severely enough to become permanently disabled. One of 25 children received medical attention as a result of head injury alone. (These statistics do not include the number of children injured by violence or suicide attempts, which are considered intentional injuries, rather than by accidents). Any massage ther-

apist who works with children will most likely be treating both acute and chronic injuries.

PEDIATRIC INJURIES

PATTERNS OF PEDIATRIC INJURIES

Knowing about the causes of pediatric injuries can help you understand when children are most at risk of being injured and how many of their injuries are preventable.

■ Falls and motor vehicle accidents are the two most common causes of injuries, followed by drownings and fires. A concussion caused by a fall is a common reason for children to be hospitalized for trauma; however, a fall can also cause serious injury to other parts of the body. Motor vehicles are such a major source of injuries that orthopedic surgeon John Ogden calls the automobile "the principal crippler of children."[2] Children injured in car accidents may be involved as passengers, pedestrians, or bicyclists.

- 10–25% of all injuries in preschool children may be a result of child abuse.[2]
- 40% of emergency department visits for injuries occur between May and August when children are more likely to be playing outdoors without adult supervision. The majority of accidents occur in the evening hours for the same reason.
- 50% of nonfatal injuries are in or around the home. The typical bike crash occurs within one mile of home.[3]
- In all stages of childhood, boys receive far more injuries than girls, as a result of their engaging in more rough play and more dangerous activities.
- Poor children have higher levels of both nonfatal and fatal injuries.

REDUCING PEDIATRIC INJURIES

Because pediatric injuries are a major public health problem, information on how to prevent them should be common knowledge. Reducing unintentional childhood injury is possible through the following preventive measures:

- Use protective gear for activities such as biking, horseback riding, skateboarding, scootering, inline skating, and snowboarding. If a child hits his head during one of these activities, helmets can reduce the risk of brain injury by as much as 88%; however, only 15–25 % of children wear helmets when bicycling. In a nationwide study, 56% of children hospitalized for a bicycle-related injury had a traumatic brain injury; almost all were caused by automobile collisions.[3] Other examples of protective gear are knee and elbow pads and athletic mouth guards.
- Wear car seat belts.
- Provide adequate supervision during sports and at home. Responsibility for traffic safety should not be given to children; those younger than ages 11 to 12 are not developmentally mature enough to assess distance and speed and negotiate traffic safely.[4]
- Teach children about fire safety.
- Teach children how to act safely at home, at school, and in public. Traffic safety should be a priority because a large number of serious childhood injuries involve motor vehicles.

GENERAL APPROACHES TO PEDIATRIC INJURIES

When medical cautions/contraindications are followed, massage and hydrotherapy can be extremely

POINT OF INTEREST BOX 4–1
Pediatric Sports Injuries

The sports with the highest risk of injury to children are football, basketball, gymnastics, soccer, and baseball.[1] Injuries occur more frequently in contact sports; for example, 20–40% of high school football players are injured each year. Older children are more likely than younger children to be injured while playing contact sports, probably because sports are played more aggressively as children grow older. Injuries in young athletes cover a broad spectrum of damage to bone and soft tissue; the severity of the injury will depend on the skeletal and physiologic age of the child, the particular sport, and the severity of the trauma.[2] Teenagers have more lower-extremity trauma, with knee injuries being the most common, and younger athletes have more contusions, sprains, and simple fractures of their upper extremities. The joint most commonly sprained is the ankle.[1] Organized sports account for only about one-third of sports injuries, with the remainder occurring in physical education classes and in nonorganized sports, such as skateboarding.[1] Prevention of sports injuries should include:

1. The use of safety gear appropriate for each sport, including helmets, face guards, eye protection, proper footgear, padding, and other body protection.
2. Careful supervision of children while they are playing.
3. Following appropriate rules.
4. A preseason-conditioning program, which includes warm-up, stretching, running, weight training, and skill development. This type of program can prevent injuries, especially in collision and contact sports.[1]
5. Adequate rehabilitation of injuries. Inadequate rehabilitation probably accounts for one-fourth of sport-related injuries, due to residual problems from prior injuries.[1]

References

1. Morrissy R: *Lovell and Winter's Pediatric Orthopaedics*. Vol. 2. Baltimore, MD: Lippincott Williams & Wilkins, 2001, p 1289, 1290
2. Waters P, Millis M: Hip and pelvic injuries in the young athlete. *Clinics in Sports Medicine*, 7:525, 1988

important in relieving discomfort, promoting healing, preventing long-term soft tisssue dysfunction and pain, and helping with long-term symptoms from injuries such as spinal cord and traumatic head injuries.

AMPUTATIONS

"It is imperative, when massaging a person with an amputation or any other deformed condition, to approach them with pure love, respect, and willingness . . . approach this body with confidence. It's a survivor!"

—*Dianne Percoraro*[1]

An amputation is the removal of a limb or a part of a limb. Trauma is the major cause of amputation in childhood. Power lawn mowers are the primary cause of traumatic injuries resulting in amputation, followed by motor vehicle accidents, farm injuries, and gunshot wounds. In war-torn countries, land mines are a leading cause of amputation. Amputations of the upper extremity, more common than those of the lower extremity, are most often caused by machinery. Amputations may also follow tissue damage from tumors, burns, or gangrene. Boys suffer amputations twice as often as girls.[2]

APPROACH AND GOALS

Traumatic amputation is acutely stressful because it involves significant pain, stressful medical treatment, and a significant alteration of the child's body image. Long after the initial injury, the use of prostheses and changes in mobility and appearance may continue to cause the child significant stress. However, each child's situation is different; the long-term psychological effect of an amputation depends on where it is located, how different the child now looks from other children, and how much emotional support the child has.

The initial physical therapy goals for children with amputations are maintenance of range of motion and muscle strength. Massage helps maintain range of motion and also benefits the child in other ways. Locally, it softens stump adhesions and decreases edema in and around the stump and can increase range of motion in the joints proximal to the stump. When other muscles compensate for the missing body part, they can become overly tense or sore. For example, when one leg is amputated above the knee, there will be compensations and discomfort at the hip directly above the knee, the entire other leg, or in the back. Massage helps relieve discomfort and tension in the compensating muscles and prevents contractures from developing. Massage can help children accept the stump and have a positive, whole body image.

Use the basic massage techniques presented in Chapter 3, adjusting pressure to the child's tolerance level and causing no pain. A whole-body massage is ideal for any child with an amputation because

POINT OF INTEREST BOX 4–2
Massage in Thailand for Children With Amputated Limbs

Pamela Yeaton, a nurse and massage therapist, has worked in health care and health education in a number of third-world countries, including 3 years with the Peace Corps in Bangkok, Thailand. In Bangkok, she worked with the Foundation for the Welfare of the Crippled, treating children, training physical therapy aides, and supervising the therapy of more than 200 children. Crippled by polio, cerebral palsy, and accidents, children came from throughout the country. Those with amputations, most commonly from leg injuries from land mines, came to the Foundation about 6 months after the surgery. Children, as young as age 5, were taught to self-massage and stimulate their stumps and to help each other with range-of-motion exercise. Much of the information in this section is drawn from Ms. Yeaton's extensive experience (Yeaton P, personal communication, April 1992).

musculoskeletal compensations are likely to be found throughout the entire body. A child using crutches, for example, will have increased strain and tension in the muscles of the upper body. The following massage technique is effective for treating local discomfort and muscle tension:

- An ideal method of treating the stump is 10 minutes of massage on the stump in the morning before putting on the prosthesis and 10 minutes at night after removing it.
- A parent or other family member would be the ideal person to perform this daily therapy.
- Any touch may be difficult on a painful stump. Hydrotherapy is an excellent way to improve the child's tolerance for tactile stimulation; it can improve circulation to the stump and is an excellent beginning to the massage experience.

MASSAGE AND HYDROTHERAPY FOR AMPUTATIONS

CONTRAST TREATMENT OF THE STUMP

When performing a contrast treatment, use caution with the temperature of hot and cold applications. If the stump is sensitive, hot applications may need to be cooler and cold applications warmer. Ask the child to tell you what feels right. The contrast treatment may be extended to the entire extremity by using a larger hot pack or multiple hot packs.

Step 1. Apply a moist heating pad or Hydrocollator pack to the amputation stump for 3 minutes.

Step 2. Wring out a washcloth in ice water, and rub the stump for 30 seconds, or do ice massage for 1 minute.

Step 3. Repeat hot and cold twice (three changes total).

MASSAGE SEQUENCE FOR AMPUTATIONS

Step 1. Begin with the basic relaxation sequence, followed by visualization. Have the child visualize the missing limb and then breathe into it while exhaling. For example, if a hand has been amputated, she can visualize the hand while inhaling and, when exhaling, breathe all the way to the visualized fingertips.

Step 2. Apply oil or lotion to the entire extremity, but not on the stump. Cocoa butter or vitamin E oil on the incision, if newly healed, prevents cracking and drying of the scar tissue and relieves itching.

Step 3. Use the arm effleurage or leg effleurage strokes presented in Chapter 3 and give 2 to 3 minutes of warming superficial effleurage to the stump and the entire extremity.

Step 4. Specific Massage of the Amputation Stump

■ Start with gentle, but firm, pressure on and around the stump; hold this pressure to the count of 10. When the child can tolerate this pressure, the therapist can slowly work into gentle massage techniques. If pain continues to be a problem, consult the child's physical therapist, physician, or prosthetist.

■ Use gentle thumbstroking massage over the stump for about 2 minutes, depending on the child's tolerance.

Step 5. Passive range-of-motion exercises. Perform passive range-of-motion exercises on all joints of the extremity. If the child's hand has been amputated, for example, do the exercises on the wrist, elbow, and shoulder joints. The exercises should always be done on the other limb, as well. While passive range-of-motion exercises are helpful, when the joint has full range of motion, the child should learn to perform active range-of-motion exercises.

 Consult with the child's physician to obtain permission before massaging a child's amputation stump.

BIRTH TRAUMA

As labor begins, the fetal head is nearly half of the total body mass and the largest impediment to passage through the birth canal. The lower jaw is relatively undeveloped—a prominent, bony chin would make birth even more difficult. For the head and body of the fetus to leave the womb during the normal birth process, the mother's pelvis must become as wide as

possible, and the head of the fetus must become as narrow as possible. (To prepare for birth, the mother's pelvic ligaments began to soften months before delivery.) As labor begins, the vaginal wall muscles stretch and the cervix widens. As the mother's uterine muscles propel the fetus toward the birth canal, the head is compressed and the skull becomes longer and narrower as the cranial bones overlap each other. In 95% of all births, the baby's occiput faces toward the inside of the mother's pubic bone, with one cheekbone turned toward the mother's tailbone. The top of the baby's head, which is the narrowest part, comes through the birth canal first (see Figure 4–1). The occiput is still in four separate pieces and receives great pressure as it leads the way out of the birth canal. Normally its upper edges slide under the parietal bone. Either or both condyles of the occiput can be compressed, or one can shift forward and one shift backward.[1]

The normal birth described above causes a certain amount of stress to all infants, but does not cause actual physical injury. Complications that may lead to birth trauma or injury include:

1. Caesarean section. Before this surgery takes place, labor may have been prolonged for some reason, such as the mother's pelvis not being wide enough to accommodate the fetal head. Molding of the cranial bones may be exaggerat-

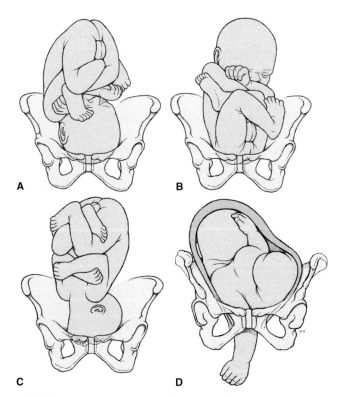

FIGURE 4–1 ■ Various Fetal Positions at Delivery. Reprinted with permission from *Stedman's Medical Dictionary*. Ed. 27. Baltimore, MD: Lippincott Williams & Wilkins, 2000, p 1441.

ed, such as when the frontal bone overlaps the parietal bone.[1]

2. High forceps delivery. The use of forceps to draw the fetal head out of the birth canal can cause compression of the temporal bones, the wings of the sphenoid bone, or the maxillary bones. Facial paralysis may result if the pressure applied to the sides of the head irritates the facial nerves. This condition often disappears spontaneously within a few weeks; however, the pressure may have long-term effects on the infant's soft tissue.

3. Induction of labor and prolonged or precipitous labor can traumatize the head of the fetus. A small percentage of infants acquire cephalohematomas (a collection of blood under the skin of the scalp, on the back or side of the head) caused by trauma to the blood vessels in the scalp during delivery. Rarely, this hemorrhage occurs together with damage to the brain. Overly intense or prolonged uterine contractions can also cause subdural hemorrhage or suboccipital strain.[2]

4. A breech delivery, in which the buttock presents first, occurs in about 3% of births. Problems delivering the fetus's head can result in muscular torticollis; dislocations or fractures of the clavicle, hip, or shoulder joint; and brachial plexus birth palsy. Minor spinal cord damage can occur during breech delivery, with traction applied to the trunk when manipulating the aftercoming head.[3] Because breech position in utero is now an indication for cesarean birth, breech deliveries are less frequent than in the past.

5. Severe trauma to the mother during pregnancy, such as a motor vehicle accident resulting in pelvic fracture.

6. Other problems with the delivery of the head, as sometimes occurs when twins lie on top of each other in utero, or in face-first or transverse presentations.

Every infant's cranial bones are molded to some extent to exit the birth canal. In a normal birth, the molding will correct in 5 to 6 days, partially via lusty crying and active sucking.[1] If the infant's position was abnormal during delivery, the position of the cranial bones may be affected. There may be compression or lateral strain of the cranial base, or a distortion of the occipital condyles may affect the way the occiput is positioned on top of the atlas (first cervical vertebrae). Birth trauma can have lasting effects, as shown in the following examples:

1. Birth trauma may initiate patterns of myofascial restriction, malalignment of bones, or

myofascial trigger points that continue to influence a person throughout life. For example, although a link between cephalohematoma at birth and the presence of head and neck trigger points has not been proven in an older child, the amount of force it requires to cause trauma to the blood vessels in the scalp is also enough to cause trigger points in the myofascia of the skull. Psychiatrist and former pediatrician, using age-regression hypnosis, David Cheek found a connection between a 50-year-old man's lifelong migraine headaches and the man's birth. When forceps were applied to the head during birth, one blade had pressed hard just above one eye orbit, and the other blade had compressed his occiput.[4] Trigger points in the temporalis, occipitalis, and posterior cervicals, all of which may be caused by birth trauma, are known to induce migraines.[5]

2. Brachial plexus birth palsy is a birth injury that causes paralysis of the arm muscles. Occurring in about one in 400 births, it is more common in large babies; babies who experienced prolonged or traumatic deliveries, especially when extraction techniques were used; babies born in a breech position; and babies born shoulder first. In these situations, the infant's shoulder is easily stretched and the nerves can be stretched, torn, or ruptured. The actual injury site is the upper trunk of the brachial plexus (less common) or the roots of cervical nerves C5 and C6 (most common). The nerve damage causes weakness in the deltoid, bicep, brachialis, supinator, supraspinatus, infraspinatus, and subscapularis muscles. Injuries that do not heal well are likely to cause permanent weakness, deformities, and contractures of the upper extremity.[6] Regular massage is an effective therapy for the symptoms of this condition. A patient of the author's was born in Germany in 1930 with brachial plexus birth palsy. As a child, he went weekly to a physical therapist who massaged and stretched his arm. His arm was straight and he had full use of it until his treatments stopped at age 11. His arm then became progressively flexed against his chest until, in his forties, it was permanently fixed in that position (Ze'ev O, personal communication, July 1991).

3. Ten percent of cerebral palsy cases are from birth injuries.[2]

4. Although no statistics are available, research generally supports the theory that there is a higher incidence of attention deficit disorder in children who had problems during delivery, such as a long or hard labor or forceps delivery.[7]

5. Clint Nelson, a cranial dentist and massage therapist, believes that cranial bones that are compressed into abnormal positions during delivery can cause other bones, such as the maxilla, to shift position, eventually ossify, and lead to malocclusion and bite problems (Nelson C, personal communication, July 2002).

APPROACH AND GOALS

Massage therapists should not treat newborns without special training. If you are working with children, however, be aware that, although they are young, children may have long-standing myofascial or skeletal restriction from birth events. Infant massage is an excellent therapy that can help infants relax and accept healthy touch. Gentle stretches, facial massage, and stroking can ease newborn discomfort from suboccipital strain.[8] Barry Gillespie, dentist, massage therapist, and teacher, teaches a newborn bodywork sequence that involves craniosacral, fascial, and muscle therapy. First the child's occiput, sacrum, and frontal bones are treated with craniosacral manipulation. Then the entire body is treated with myofascial release techniques. Finally, the sequence includes Swedish massage that begins at the legs and proceeds to the head. The average treatment lasts 15 to 20 minutes. If the child had an uncomplicated delivery with no major problems, she should not need further bodywork until about age 1, when children begin walking and, frequently, falling.[9]

BRUISES

A bruise is an area of discolored or black-and-blue tissue that is a result of injury (usually some kind of an impact). Capillaries beneath the skin break and blood leaks into the surrounding tissue. Bruises come in all sizes, from a tiny bruise on a toe to a bruise covering large parts of the child's body. Bruises usually are painful for at least the first 2 days after the injury. Bruises are common in children, especially active children.

APPROACH AND GOALS

Massage and hydrotherapy can soothe a bruised area, reduce muscle tightness caused by pain, and promote good circulation to help the bruise heal. If the child's bruise is part of a major injury, massage in a larger area may be indicated to reduce muscle tension and enhance healing. If a child has bruises from falling off a bicycle and also has a wrenched knee and sore back muscles, massage should be done both above and below the bruise. Massage could then be used to address the other sore areas.

MASSAGE AND HYDROTHERAPY FOR BRUISES

ICE APPLICATIONS

Ice should be applied as soon after an injury as possible. Apply an ice pack for 15 minutes and then remove it for 15 minutes; repeat this sequence several times. Bruises on small areas, such as fingers and toes, can be placed in a container of ice water (containing ice cubes). Heat should not be used for the first 24 hours. Ice massage can be performed around the bruise; use extra caution to not press on sore or sensitive areas.

CONTRAST TREATMENT

Step 1. Dip a washcloth or small bath towel in hot water, then wring it out. Mold the towel over the bruised area for 3 minutes. A moist heating pad or Hydrocollator pack may also be used.

Step 2. Replace the hot application with another washcloth or small bath towel, which has been wrung out in ice water, for 1 minute. An ice pack may also be used. Repeat twice.

MASSAGE SEQUENCE FOR BRUISES

Step 1. Basic relaxation sequence.

Step 2. Effleurage around the bruise. Begin by stroking gently around the bruise. It is critical that the child does not experience any pain. The combination of pain from the injury and pain from massage creates muscular guarding and fear of touch. Use your palms (or fingertips, if the area is small) and alternate your hands. Stroke toward the heart. Begin with gentle pressure and, as the circulation improves and the area becomes more relaxed, deeper pressure may be used, as long as the child is not experiencing pain. Continue for approximately 5 minutes.

 Do not apply massage or hydrotherapy to a bruised area unless the cause of the bruise is known. The child's physician should be consulted about bruises developing without obvious cause because this could be a sign of a serious health problem, such as leukemia or a blood clotting disorder.

BURNS

I am aware that I like touching friends more than I like being touched. That's related, I'm sure, to a severe childhood burn that meant I was constantly handled as my painful injury was treated and bandaged. . . . I care very much about touch, but I don't like being massaged.[1]

—*Helen Colton, family therapist*

Fire is the fourth leading cause of accidental death in the United States, and the leading cause of death for children ages 1 to 4. Approximately 100 children die in the United States each year from fires and burns and about 5,000 more are seriously injured. House fires and scaldings are the two leading causes of pediatric burn injuries. Young children have trouble escaping a house that is on fire and scaldings occur when children spill something hot or jump in a bathtub of very hot water. It takes only seconds for water at 125° F or higher to cause a severe burn to their tender skin.[2] Sadly, up to 10% of burns in children are a result of abuse by adults.[3] As children get older, they are generally more at risk of fire injuries because they engage in more high-risk behavior. Boys are at higher risk than girls, partly because they are more likely to play with fire.[2]

Because a severe burn destroys both the dermis and the epidermis, which does not grow back, skin grafts must be performed.[2] Contractures and scarring of skin may occur around joints. Major burns are painful, sometimes excruciatingly so, and the child may experience pain for extended periods. Children with serious burns may have multiple challenges, including the stress and pain of the original injury; painful medical procedures, such as debridement and dressing changes; painful scars; postoperative discomfort; and, possibly, physical disability. Children not only experience pain, but lack control over much of their care. Changes in their appearance or ability to function may cause even more stress. While it is important for children to reenter school as soon as possible, teasing and name-calling frequently occur. Insomnia, anxiety, and depression are common responses.

APPROACH AND GOALS

Massage can be soothing and healing for severely burned children. It helps improve their self-image, which suffers greatly from the disfiguring effect of burns. It helps them become more trusting of touch, which they may have learned to associate with pain. It gradually softens scar tissue fibers that restrict muscle and fascia, helping them feel less tight and increasing their range of motion. If the child's parents are taught to massage their children, it helps them become more comfortable with their child's changed body, as well. Emphasizing relaxation skills helps the children learn to have a measure of control over their response to pain. Pediatric psychiatrists Karen Olness and David Cohen use medical hypnosis to help children learn to control their pain responses and to facilitate their healing; they even use medical hypnosis for anesthesia during surgery.[4]

Three studies at the Touch Research Institute explored the use of massage therapy with adult and pediatric burn survivors. In the first study, simple pressure stroking given to adults before debridement decreased their depression and anger and lowered their pulse and cortisol levels, compared with those who were not stroked. They appeared less anxious and also reported less pain.[5] Adult burn patients in the second study were randomly assigned to a massage therapy group or a standard treatment control group at the beginning of the scar formation stage. The massage group received 30 minutes of massage with cocoa butter, twice a week for 5 weeks; the other group did not receive massage. The massage therapy group patients had more positive self-reports on their levels of anxiety, depression, pain, and itching immediately after the first and last therapy sessions and their ratings on these measures improved over the 5-week period.[6] Finally, the third study found that young children who were burn victims showed less distress during painful dressing changes after a 15-minute massage than children who did not receive the massage therapy.[7]

The author has treated children who were in excruciating pain from recent burns. They were receiving physical therapy to maintain range of motion that, although necessary, was excruciatingly painful. Swedish massage on the nonburned areas gave the children significant release from the extreme stress they experienced, not only from the injury itself, but also from the stress and pain of their rehabilitation. When the burns are healed, massage can release tension, soften scar tissue, and help the children feel that their bodies are more like normal. Whole-body massage is important in order to integrate burned areas into the child's body image. It is beneficial to regularly incorporate passive range-of-motion exercises into every massage treatment to prevent contractures and to teach the child to release tension around the joints.

Massage can also rehabilitate badly burned hands. If there is hypersensitivity (pain with any moderate stimulation), the area can be massaged using progressively more pressure as the hand becomes less sensitive. If there are scar tissue bands at the web spaces or on the palm, use circular fingertip massage applied perpendicular to the scar bands, using firm pressure. Also, stretch the skin to increase its surface area.

MASSAGE SEQUENCE FOR BURNS

MASSAGE SEQUENCE FOR ANY PART OF THE BODY, LASTING NO MORE THAN 10 MINUTES

Step 1. Basic relaxation sequence.
Step 2. Apply cocoa butter or vitamin E oil to help keep scar tissue soft.
Step 3. Perform superficial effleurage, moving slowly and gently. Move from distal to proximal (stroking

toward the heart). This allows any edema to be readily absorbed by muscle tissue, rather than lodging in areas that have little muscle tissue and, therefore, lack circulation. Repeat for about 5 minutes.

Step 4. Pick the skin up gently and roll it between your thumb and fingers, as in pincement, only slowly. Never cause pain! If the burned areas are massaged regularly, over time, the child's tolerance for pressure will increase. Repeat for 1 to 2 minutes.

Step 5. Use deeper pressure. Using the bones as a guide, glide over areas while pressing with your fingertips. For example, if you are massaging the forearm, use the thumb and fingers to stroke along the radius and ulna from elbow to wrist.

Step 6. Perform superficial effleurage for 1 minute.

Step 7. When the burned area is on a limb, perform passive range-of-motion exercises on the entire extremity.

 Massage should not be done too soon after a burn occurs. Check with the child's physician or physical therapist to find out when it is safe to begin. However, massage unburned parts of the body at any time to accustom the child to massage and to help him learn to relax.

DISLOCATIONS

A dislocation is a disruption in the normal relationship of the bones that form a joint; so much force is applied to the joint that the bones separate from their articulation. A dislocation is not only a disruption of the joint capsule and its ligaments, it may also be associated with a wide variety of other injuries, including the tearing of the joint capsule, the stretching or rupture of collateral ligaments, and the stripping of the periosteum from the bone. Muscles, blood vessels, and nerves may also be torn. Children's soft tissue attachments are more lax than those of adults and their joint mobility is greater, making the joints the point of least resistance when parts of their bodies are subjected to trauma. Certain conditions, such as true hypermobility and Down syndrome, may also predispose them to dislocations.

Children dislocate their elbows more frequently than any other joint, most often when they fall on an outstretched hand with the elbow incompletely flexed.[1] Another common pediatric dislocation is an anterior dislocation of the head of the humerus, which can occur in football, skiing, and wrestling. Typically, the force applied to the joint not only displaces the head of the humerus under the coracoid process, but it also tears the anterior capsule of the shoulder joint and stretches the subscapularis and supraspinatus muscles.

The standard medical treatment for a dislocation begins with a careful evaluation of the injury. Because it takes so much force to cause a dislocation, there may also be fractures or other soft tissue injuries. Second, a reduction of the dislocation—putting the bones back in the normal position—is critical. Because dislocations and reductions can be painful, children may receive pain medication when the dislocation is reduced. Third, some degree of immobilization is almost always necessary while the ligaments heal. Depending on the joint and the extent of the injury, this could mean bed rest, traction, or simply wearing a splint or cast. For long-term instability, **prolotherapy** may be helpful, or surgery may be performed to shorten the ligaments.

The treatment for the two previously mentioned pediatric dislocations is as follows: For an elbow dislocation, swelling begins immediately and, if the joint is not reduced within approximately 15 minutes, there will be so much swelling, muscle spasm, and pain that an anesthetic will be needed during the reduction. (If a dislocated elbow joint is not reduced, there will be some type of soft tissue contracture within a few weeks, such as in the triceps, from the elbow being held in extension. If it is not reduced within several months or longer, the distal humerus, proximal radius, and proximal ulna may become progressively deformed.)[1] So the physician will first reduce the dislocation, then check for associated injuries (fracture of the medial epicondyle is common), and then prescribe immobilization, typically some type of splinting. This will be used for a few weeks until the ligaments are able to keep the joint in place. Elbow range-of-motion exercises should begin after 2 weeks, to minimize the risk of contracture and to eliminate stiffness. When damage to the joint capsule and surrounding ligament is too extreme and the ligaments will not support the joint, it is sometimes necessary to shorten them surgically.

An anterior shoulder dislocation will also be reduced as soon as possible, and the affected arm will be immobilized in a sling for approximately 3 weeks. Muscle strengthening exercises should begin as soon as the child's arm is out of the sling and range-of-motion exercises should begin as soon as the child is free of pain. Unfortunately, 60–85% of children have repeated dislocations within 2 years because their ligaments are not able to adequately support the joint.[2]

APPROACH AND GOALS

Massage will not strengthen the ligaments or the joint capsule and is contraindicated in the acute stage of healing. However, contrast treatments well above (proximal to) the injury can improve circulation and comfort in the acute stage. Hydrotherapy to the opposite limb can improve circulation in the immobilized limb by causing a reflex vasodilation.[3] Gentle Swedish massage can be done to enhance the circulation and relax the surrounding areas, although the dislocated joint should not be moved in any way.

Once the immobilization is removed, contrast treatments can be used directly over the dislocated joint to improve circulation. Also at this time, massage can be used for preventing muscular guarding in the area, treating trigger points, and releasing any fascial restriction or contractures caused by prolonged immobilization. It can also prevent scar tissue in the soft tissue around the joint and dramatically improve blood and lymph circulation.

MASSAGE AND HYDROTHERAPY FOR ELBOW DISLOCATIONS

The elbow is used as an example because it is the most common pediatric dislocation; however, these treatments may be used with any joint.

CONTRAST TREATMENT—ACUTE PHASE

Do not apply hydrotherapy on or near the injured elbow. A contrast treatment may be done on the same shoulder, which will improve the circulation proximal to the elbow. A contrast treatment with heat and ice may also be done on the noninjured elbow, using heat and ice to cause a reflex vasodilation.

Positioning: Have the child lay supine and completely support the injured elbow with pillows.

Step 1. Apply moist heat to the shoulder for 3 minutes.
Step 2. Apply an ice pack or perform ice massage on the shoulder for 1 minute.
Step 3. Repeat Steps 1 and 2.
Step 4. Repeat Steps 1 and 2, for a total of three changes.

CONTRAST TREATMENT—FOLLOWING ACUTE PHASE

Positioning: Have the child lay supine and completely support the injured elbow with pillows.

Step 1. Apply moist heat to the elbow for 3 minutes.
Step 2. Apply an ice pack or perform ice massage on the elbow for 1 minute.
Step 3. Repeat Steps 1 and 2.
Step 4. Repeat Steps 1 and 2, for a total of three changes.

MASSAGE SEQUENCE FOR DISLOCATIONS

Step 1. Basic relaxation sequence and passive touch over the dislocated joint.
Step 2. Apply oil or lotion.

Step 3. Effleurage above and below the dislocated joint. Begin stroking gently above and below the joint. Use your palms (or fingertips, if the area is small) and alternate hands. Stroke upward toward the heart. For a dislocated elbow, stroke up the forearm to the top of the humerus, then use your fingertips to stroke from fingers to wrist. Repeat for 5 minutes.
Step 4. Thumbstroke over the dislocated joint. Be extremely gentle. Make short strokes toward the heart. Massage the dislocated area and a few inches around it. Feel for scar tissue, muscle tension, and trigger points. If the child can tolerate deeper pressure without pain, deeper pressure may be applied after 2 to 3 minutes. Repeat for 2 to 5 minutes.
Step 5. Repeat Step 3.

 Consult with the child's physician before performing any range-of-motion exercises.

FRACTURES

Bone is generally thought of as a solid and static structure; in reality, it is a dynamic and responsive tissue. Especially in children, bones change in response to the individual's age, nutrition, general health, and level of activity (see Point of Interest Box 4–3). Emotional deprivation can even affect bone growth, as in the case of the children with growth retardation discussed in Chapter 1. During fetal life, the entire skeleton is formed of cartilage and consists of 330 separate bones. **Ossification** of the bones actually begins in utero, but is not complete until about age 25, when peak bone mass is reached. Even when the individual has reached full skeletal growth, bone is still a dynamic tissue that receives 5% of the body's total blood supply to meet its metabolic needs.[1-3]

The long bones of the body include the bones of the arms, hands, legs, and feet. During childhood, they grow from the shaft (diaphysis) out to the ends (epiphysis). At birth, the diaphyses are separate from the epiphyses. Growth occurs at the epiphyses, where new bone cells are made at a growth plate, an area of rapidly proliferating cells. Pediatric bone growth is amazingly rapid compared with that of an adult; for example, between birth and age 4, the spine, femurs, tibiae, and the bones of the arm and hand nearly double in length. Between the ages of 14 and 20, children reach full bone growth, the growth plates stop making new cells, the diaphyses fuse with the epiphyses, and the skeleton now consists of only 206 separate bones.

A fracture is any type of break in a bone. This term includes a range of damage to bones, from small

POINT OF INTEREST BOX 4–3
Bones Respond to Stress

Bones grow according to the demands placed upon them. For example, children with spastic cerebral palsy, whose muscles are constantly contracting, have strong bones due to the constant stimulation their bones receive from their muscles. So do athletic children. When children with hemophilia have bleeds into their joints, the hyperemia stimulates bone growth. This can lead to leg length differences as one bone grows more than the other, as well as to bony enlargements of the joints.[1] Joint inflammation in juvenile rheumatoid arthritis can cause bone growth for the same reason. Children with **hydrocephalus** may have enlarged cranial bones, because the bones grow to accommodate the greater volume of fluid around the brain.

Absence of active movement in the limbs due to muscle weakness (from such conditions as muscular dystrophy, floppy cerebral palsy, or polio or simply being in a wheelchair all day) can result in the opposite effect—weak bones caused by lack of stimulation. In one group of children with polio who had broken bones, 57 of 62 fractures were in severely paralyzed limbs and only five were in the children's nonparalyzed limbs. The most common cause of the fractures was having the paralyzed limb immobilized in a plaster cast to correct contractures, and losing bone strength while the limb was not used. A leg bone that is in a cast can become 30% decalcified within a few weeks.[2]

References

1. Anderson A, Hotzan T, Masley J: Physical Therapy in Bleeding Disorders. National Hemophilia Foundation booklet, 2000, p 9
2. Ogden J: *Skeletal Injury in the Child*. Philadelphia, PA: Lea and Febiger, 1982, p 183

cracks to complete breaks to thorough bone shattering. How badly a bone and its surrounding soft tissues are damaged depends on the force of the impact that caused the fracture. A force that just barely exceeds the bone's breaking point may crack the bone; with more force, it may break all the way through; and with extreme force, the bone may shatter.

Most children break at least one bone before reaching adulthood. Because they are not completely ossified, children's bones are more porous than adult bones. Fractures are more common in childhood compared with ligament injuries and dislocations, which are more common in adulthood. Fortunately, pediatric bones grow back together more rapidly than adult bones. The younger the child, the more rapid the healing. For example, a femur fracture may

heal in only 3 weeks in an infant, whereas 20 weeks is typical for an adult.

Point of Interest Box 4–4 identifies the bones most commonly fractured in children. Because the diaphysis and epiphysis are not yet fused, the growth plate may be the weakest point (or the point of least resistance) when a child suffers an impact. In fact, 15% of all pediatric fractures involve the growth plate. This can be a serious situation because, if the rapid cell proliferation at the growth plate is disturbed by injury, bone growth may be permanently halted. This can lead to a deformity of the bone, or a bone that is shorter than it would have been otherwise. This

POINT OF INTEREST BOX 4–4
Which Bones Are Children Most Likely to Break?

If you are giving massages to children, you will more likely treat some types of fractures more than others[1]; for example:

- Boys of all ages have more fractures than girls of the same age because they engage in more reckless and dangerous activities.
- During childhood, upper limb fractures are seven times more common than lower limb fractures. Clavicular fractures are common throughout childhood. Forearm and wrist fractures comprise 30–50% of all fractures. The rate of forearm fracture numbers increases progressively with age through the middle-school years, when it begins to decrease. The radius is the most frequently fractured bone. Complications of forearm fractures involve refracture; decreased forearm rotation; and synostosis, the growth of new bone between the radius and ulna.
- The majority of hand injuries result from crushing injuries in infancy or from sports injuries in adolescence.
- Pelvic fractures are rare. The immature pelvis is more malleable that that of an adult because a greater percentage of pelvis is still cartilage and pelvic joints are more flexible.
- Spinal, femur, ankle, and foot fractures are also uncommon, accounting for perhaps 15% of all childhood fractures.
- Tibial fractures account for 10–15% of all fractures. Most stress fractures in adolescents, which occur in the proximal third of the tibia, are associated with endurance running.

References

1. Morrissy R: *Lovell and Winter's Pediatric Orthopaedics*. Vol. 2. Baltimore, MD: Lippincott Williams & Wilkins, p 1355-1411, 2001

abnormality of the bone may have permanent consequences. For example, a fracture of the femur at the growth plate could cause it to be shorter and lead to leg length inequality, which can be a serious condition. A leg that is shorter on one side of the body than the other can lead to a tilted pelvis when standing; compensatory scoliosis; activation of trigger points in hip, torso, and neck muscles; and chronic back pain.[3-5]

As an adolescent approaches skeletal maturity, the bones become denser (more calcified) and the epiphyses fuse with the diaphyses. Hereafter, ligaments and musculotendinous structures will be more vulnerable to injury than bone and trauma will be transmitted through the soft tissue instead.

Fractures are treated in different ways, depending on their severity and location. As soon as possible after the injury occurs, the bone is splinted to prevent further damage and to prevent the cut ends from damaging blood vessels, nerves, and other tissue surrounding the bone. The muscles surrounding the fracture spasm as a result of the pain the child feels from the broken edges of the bone. Fractures are most often immobilized by applying casts; however, braces or rods, plates, and pins or screws may be necessary to hold the bone ends together. As new bone cells and calcium are deposited between the ends of the broken bones, they knit back together. Often, the bone heals so well that the healed fracture leaves the bone stronger than it was before the injury. In response to the injury, the child's bone will grow at an accelerated rate for 6 to 8 months.

When a cast is removed, the muscles around the break are usually weak. For each week of immobilization, it takes about 6 weeks of active use before the muscles regain full strength. There may be edema and poor circulation, as well. As children begin to use the body part again, they will actively move it through its normal range of motion and soft tissue and muscle strength will become normal. However, when a force sufficient to break a bone has been applied to an area, there may be lasting effects on the surrounding soft tissue (see Figure 4–2). These may include:

1. Stretching or tearing of surrounding muscles, tendons, or fascial sheaths.

2. Avulsion of the periosteum or stripping of the periosteum away from the bone.
3. Overstretching or complete tearing of the ligaments from the bone.
4. Tearing of cartilage.
5. Excess scar tissue, with possible permanent effects. For example, the condylar neck of the mandible is a relatively common place for a child to fracture, resulting from an injury such as a bicycle accident. If the fracture heals with extensive scar tissue and restriction, the mandible will not be able to grow down and forward as usual and one side of the mandible may not grow as much as the other side.[6]
6. Activation of trigger points in fascia, muscles, ligaments, and even in the periosteum. Trigger points in the muscles around the fracture site may be caused by stretching, tearing, or bruising, the instinctive contraction of muscles to splint a hurt area, or by reaction to the pain of the fracture. Short-term trigger points in the areas around a fracture will contribute to pain, swelling, and slow healing as a result of poor nutrition to the fracture site.[7]

The following are examples of trigger points subsequent to injury: Fracture of the proximal humerus can activate trigger points in the subscapularis; fracture of the upper ribs may activate trigger points in the pectoralis minor; an accident that causes a fracture of the ankle or leg may initiate or activate trigger points in the gastrocnemius and/or quadratus lumborum muscles; stress fractures of the tibia and fibula, usually associated with endurance running in adolescents, can activate trigger points in the extensor digitorum longus, extensor hallucis longus, and superficial and deep intrinsic foot muscles; and fractures of the small bones of the feet can activate trigger points in the intrinsic foot muscles.[3,4]

Immobilization of the fracture may also contribute to the development of trigger points. For example, immobilization of the arm in a sling or cast in an adducted position may initiate trigger points in the pectoralis major.[3] A walking cast, used for ankle or leg fractures, fixes the ankle and immobilizes and

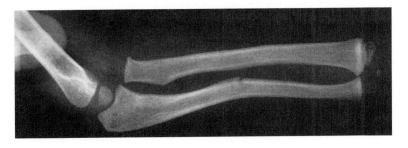

FIGURE 4–2 ■ The force that caused this child's ulnar fracture also caused an anterior dislocation of the radial head. Reprinted with permission from Morrissy R: *Lovell and Winter's Pediatric Orthopaedics.* Vol. 2. Baltimore, MD: Lippincott Williams & Wilkins, 2001, p 1357.

deconditions the gastrocnemius muscle, which promotes the development of trigger points. Immobilization after stress fractures of the tibia and fibula can activate trigger points in the extensor digitorum longus and extensor hallucis longus.[4]

APPROACH AND GOALS

After a broken bone has healed and the cast is removed, the muscles around the break are usually stiff and weak. For each week of being immobilized in a cast, it takes about 6 weeks for the muscles to regain their full strength. There may be edema in the tissue around the fracture and the muscles may be sore. Both massage and hydrotherapy can promote circulation to weakened muscles without fatiguing them and reduce muscle tightness and spasm caused by pain; this will help the child regain full movement. Massage helps the area relax, preventing chronic muscular guarding caused by trauma and pain. It also helps give the child a positive body sensation in an area that has had more than its share of negativity. It is important to massage above and below the fracture site, and to check the range of motion of the joints on either side as well. Trigger points and myofascial restriction may also need to be treated with other specific techniques.

MASSAGE AND HYDROTHERAPY FOR FRACTURES

Choose one hydrotherapy treatment to perform prior to massage:

CONTRAST TREATMENT—DURING IMMOBILIZATION

Hydrotherapy of the uninjured area on the opposite side of the body causes reflex vasodilation and may be done while the cast is still on. For example, if the left ankle is in a cast, perform a contrast treatment on the right ankle. Use the standard contrast treatment described in Chapter 3, with three changes of hot and cold.

CONTRAST TREATMENT—AFTER FRACTURE IS HEALED

After the cast has been removed, use a handheld shower attachment to give mechanical stimulation, as well as a circulatory effect.

Step 1. Spray the area with water for 2 minutes. The water should be as hot as the child can tolerate (about 105° to 110° F).
Step 2. Spray the area with water as cold as the child can tolerate for 30 seconds.

Step 3. Repeat twice more, for a total of three changes. This treatment can be done three times daily.

MOIST HEAT APPLICATION

Step 1. Dip a washcloth or small bath towel in hot water and then wring it out.
Step 2. Mold the towel over the area of the fracture and leave on for 3 minutes, then replace with another equally hot cloth for 3 minutes.
Step 3. Alternate washcloths for 9 to 12 minutes. Moist heat pads or Hydrocollator packs may also be used.
Step 4. Rub the area briefly with a washcloth wrung out in ice water or immerse the body part in a container of cold water for 10 seconds.

WATER EXERCISE

For clavicle, scapula, ribs, spine, pelvis, thigh, and upper arm fractures, use a full-body whirlpool and exercise the area underwater, at a temperature of about 94° F or warmer if tolerated. The water does not need to be as warm as for a hot bath because the child will be exercising and producing body heat.

MASSAGE DURING IMMOBILIZATION

Massage may be done above and below a cast, which decreases pain and swelling as it improves circulation. For a fracture of the tibia, for example, use effleurage and petrissage to massage above the knee to the top of the thigh and below the cast to the tips of the toes. This may be done as often as three times a day until the cast is removed. Massage of the opposite side causes a reflex vasodilation in the area of the fracture.

MASSAGE SEQUENCE FOR FRACTURES— AFTER HEALING

After the child's cast is removed, massage may be done one to three times every day. Do not cause the child any pain or discomfort!

Step 1. Basic relaxation sequence (see page 70).
Step 2. Passive touch over the fracture site.
Step 3. Apply oil or lotion.
Step 4. Gentle effleurage around the fracture site. Use your palms (or fingertips if the area is small) and alternate hands. Stroke upward toward the heart. If the fracture site is not sensitive, you may begin to stroke it gently. After 1 to 2 minutes, you may use more pressure, always working at the child's tolerance level. Effleurage for approximately 2 minutes.
Step 5. Thumbstroke around the fracture site. Stroke toward the heart. Cover the fracture site and a few

CASE STUDY 4–1

Background
Rosita is an 18-year-old girl who was injured in a fall off a cliff when she was 11 years old. Her fall fractured her T10 vertebrae and at least five ribs. Her back was surgically fused from T10 to L5. Rosita lived at home and used a wheelchair for mobility; she developed serious pressure ulcers and went to a clinic for children with disabilities to have the pressure ulcers treated. She had been in a lying-down wheelchair at the clinic for 7 months until returning to sitting in a wheelchair 3 days ago. Following her spinal cord injury, she has been in constant pain in her entire back and has pain in the area of the fractured ribs each time she inhales. After 3 days in a wheelchair, she is suffering from pain in her arms and increased pain in her lower back as she adjusts to a sitting position.

Impression
Pain secondary to vertebral fracture, rib fracture, injury of her spinal cord, and secondary compensations for restricted movement due to vertebral fusion. Recent pain due to muscular soreness. Chronic high stress level.

Treatment
Rosita transferred, with help, from her wheelchair to the treatment table. Shy and rather modest, she was treated with her tank top on and shirt and brassiere pulled up. A sheet was tucked into her underwear and her lower back was uncovered down to her gluteal cleft, leaving most of her back exposed. Superficial effleurage of the entire exposed back was used initially to evaluate her tissue. When her back was palpated, extreme tension was felt in her erector and intercostal muscles, as well as scar tissue around her fractured ribs; she had virtually no flexibility in her back. She reacted to the massage so happily that it was clear she was hungry for safe, nurturing touch, and that simple superficial effleurage was deeply comforting, both emotionally and physically. Her first 30-minute treatment consisted of this one stroke on her back. No effort was

made to use deeper pressure or a variety of strokes because she appeared so content. Rosita returned 2 days later and indicated that her back pain had been much reduced and that she was breathing with less pain. The next session again consisted of superficial effleurage of the back, with gradually deepening pressure. As this was well tolerated, thumbstroking was done around the scar tissue in the rib area, as well as stroking (raking) between the ribs to reduce the tension in her intercostal muscles. Abdominal effleurage was performed with her in the supine position, fully dressed and with only her abdomen exposed. The abdominal effleurage emphasized the abdominal muscles on the underside of her ribcage to release tension around the bottom ribs.

Rosita returned 2 days later for her third session full of enthusiasm and indicated that her back and rib pain were still further reduced. Her next three sessions were similar to the first two. At the end of her fifth session, her back and rib pain continued to be reduced, and she was able to breathe much deeper than before and with less pain. This concluded her treatment. Due to the severity of her injuries, the many years she had spent in a wheelchair, and her obvious hunger for nurturing touch, she would have benefited from more treatment. Once her muscle tension was further reduced and restricting scar tissue softened further, attention could have been directed to reducing muscle tension in other parts of her body and increasing her joint range of motion. However, her initial treatment was directed toward treating the soft-tissue effects of her spinal and rib fractures.

Discussion Questions
1. What tissues were injured or affected by Rosita's spinal cord injury?
2. What symptoms were present?
3. What other areas of Rosita's body were affected by her spinal cord injury?
4. How were Rosita's personal boundaries respected during her treatment?

inches around it. Use medium pressure. Thumbstroke for 2 minutes.
Step 6. Effleurage above and below the fracture site. Use your palms and massage farther away from the fracture site. For example, if the elbow was fractured, massage the entire upper arm, as well as the forearm and hand. Use medium pressure; massage for 2 or 3 minutes.
Step 7. Range-of-motion exercises for the joints above and below the fracture site.
Step 8. Basic relaxation sequence.

SCAR TISSUE

Scar tissue is an accumulation of collagen fibers that replaces damaged tissue at the site of an injury. Although scar tissue can present problems after a wound or burn has healed, the scar formation process, in which the body knits skin and fascia, is both sophisticated and complex. Wound-healing mechanisms include an increased number of fibroblast cells that form scar tissue and increased levels of the enzymes necessary for healing. These are in place about 7 to 10 days after an injury or surgical incision. Collagen fibers, which are denser than normal tissue, form 1 to 6 weeks after the injury; they orient around the injury and grow together, forming a thick, firm scar. Unfortunately, collagen growth across an injured area is random, without grain or definite orientation.

During a 1-year period, the enzyme collagenase digests extra collagen in the area of the scar, and scars begin to soften and fade somewhat. At that time, the scar is probably as soft as it will become by itself.

Problems with scar tissue include:

- Fibrous tissue can form adhesions from the skin to many layers of tissue below, preventing free movement of the area. Fascial layers must slide on each other for tissue to have the greatest possible degree of motion.
- Scars can feel uncomfortable, tight, and restricting. During growth spurts, the surrounding tissue expands and the scar does not; this may cause the child pain.
- Circulation may be poor around the scar.
- Trigger points in scar tissue can refer burning, prickling, or lightning-like jabs of pain to adjacent tissue.[1]
- Certain scars may contribute significantly to craniosacral dysfunction.[2]

APPROACH AND GOALS

Moist heat can relax the area around the scar and temporarily soften the scar tissue in preparation for massage.

Two types of massage are presented in this section. The first type is vitamin E application to the scar. The author has observed extensive scars that healed virtually without a trace when this regimen was followed. Vitamin E application may need to be repeated for up to 6 months. Another benefit of this application is that, when the child applies the oil and repeatedly touches the scar, the scar comes to feel more like a part of the child. This is important because, after surgery, the scar is typically sore or numb and has a reddish appearance that seems foreign to the child.

The second massage technique is to soften the scar tissue by breaking adhesions and loosening restricting fibers. The sooner the scar is treated with scar-tissue massage, the easier and more thorough the freedom of tissue movement and function. Massage also has an affirming quality, which helps the child incorporate the scar into his body image, rather than seeing it as ugly or foreign.

Scar tissue work may be painful for a child. The need to treat restriction in and around scars must be weighed against the need to prevent massage from being a negative experience for a child. Cross-fiber friction, a classic technique for scar tissue and adhesions, is generally done with, against, and diagonal to the direction of a scar. Deep friction helps break adhesions between fibers by forcibly broadening the tissue, producing a more parallel fiber arrangement. However, cross-fiber friction can be excruciatingly painful. If there is a pressing need to work with the scar and pain may be involved, the child, the parent, and the therapist should agree whether or not to proceed. The scar might possibly be painful after massage; if so, the child may be treated every second or third day. An ideal solution would be to have the massage therapist treat the child once a week and have the parent massage the child in between sessions. During a 30- or 60-minute session, you might try massaging the scar for 10 minutes, massaging other areas of the child for some time, then massaging the scar again for 10 minutes. The child's tolerance for massage around the scar should be the deciding factor.

MASSAGE AND HYDROTHERAPY FOR SCAR TISSUE

MOIST HEAT APPLICATION

Use heat before massaging scar tissue to soften the scar tissue.

Step 1. Apply a hot water bottle, moist heating pad, or Hydrocollator pack to the area for 10 minutes.
Step 2. Perform massage.

VITAMIN E OIL MASSAGE

The child or the parent can do this technique 2 weeks after surgery. This is not truly a massage technique, but an application of the vitamin E in the oil.

Step 1. Apply vitamin E oil to the scar.
Step 2. Rub oil gently into the scar for 1 minute, twice daily. Almost no pressure is used.
Step 3. Use gentle fingertip pressure and move the fingers in tiny circles over the scar.

MASSAGE SEQUENCE FOR SCAR TISSUE

This technique is particularly appropriate to teach to parents because the child may require only minutes a day of massage over a period of weeks. Massage may be done every day for 10 to 15 minutes. Although it may be tempting to begin massage sooner, it should begin no sooner than 6 weeks following the injury.

Step 1. Basic relaxation sequence.
Step 2. Apply oil or lotion.
Step 3. Begin by gently mobilizing the scar. With your fingertips, gently move the skin back and forth over

the underlying tissue. This gives you a "feel" for the amount of restriction or fibrous adhesions between the skin and the underlying tissue.

Step 4. Effleurage over the scar and a few inches around it by stroking with your palms (or fingertips, if the area is small). Stroke in the direction that the scar runs and at right angles. Do this for 2 minutes.

Step 5. Thumbstroke directly over the scar tissue, using as much pressure as the child can tolerate. Stroke in the direction that the scar tissue runs, diagonal to the scar, and at right angles to it, as well. Try to stretch the tissue between your thumbs. Repeat for 2 minutes.

Step 6. Effleurage over and around the scar tissue. Repeat for 2 minutes.

Step 7. Repeat thumbstroking directly over the scar tissue for 2 minutes.

Step 8. Gently mobilize the superficial tissue again, moving the skin back and forth over the deeper tissue. Teach the child to mobilize the scar tissue, as well. By feeling the scar and the tissue under it, the child can more readily accept the scar as part of himself.

Step 9. Stroke the area very lightly with your fingertips.

Step 10. Basic relaxation sequence.

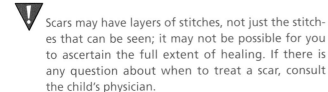

Scars may have layers of stitches, not just the stitches that can be seen; it may not be possible for you to ascertain the full extent of healing. If there is any question about when to treat a scar, consult the child's physician.

SPINAL CORD INJURIES

Almost all spinal cord injuries (SCIs) are caused by car accidents, falls, or violence (see Figure 4–3). Eighty-two percent of these injuries occur to males between the ages of 16 and 30.[1] In younger children, SCIs can also be caused by athletic injuries, abuse, or breech deliveries.[2] Spinal cord injury is less frequent in children than in adults because their spines are more flexible, allowing a greater deformation without fracture and a force to be dissipated over a larger number of segments. Should children be exposed to a great deal of force, their disproportionately large head size and other structural features make their cervical and upper spine at greatest risk for SCI. Trauma to the lower back rarely causes SCIs in children.[1,2] When trauma does occur, the spinal cord may be torn, bruised, or severed. When the cord is damaged, sensation and controlled movement may be partially or completely lost below the level of injury. Thirty-five percent of SCIs also involve some degree of brain injury and, possibly, other soft tissue injuries; 50% of children who have spinal fractures resulting from motor vehicle accidents have other associated injuries.[3]

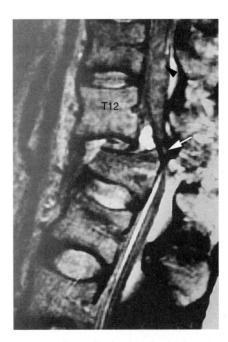

FIGURE 4–3 ■ Radiograph of Spinal Cord Injury. A crushing blow caused this injury. Note the compression of the cord caused by the posterior displacement of the first lumbar vertebrae. Reprinted with permission from Werner R: *A Massage Therapist's Guide to Pathology.* Ed. 2. Baltimore, MD: Lippincott Williams & Wilkins, 2002, p 213.

Common problems associated with SCIs include:

- Pain: pain is so severe among 40% of those with SCIs that it interferes with their daily routines.[3]
- Contractures and curvatures of the spine develop from spasticity or from the child's position in a wheelchair.
- Pressure ulcers can occur in body areas where sensation is lost (Chapter 6, page 191).
- Urinary infections are common in children who must use a catheter to urinate.
- Decalcification of the leg bones is possible because they are thin and weak from lack of exercise.
- Body temperature is difficult to control in hot weather.

APPROACH AND GOALS

Hydrotherapy can help prepare a child's tissue for massage; application of moist heat can relax muscles and increase local circulation. Muscle strength may be temporarily stimulated with hydrotherapy, allowing the child to do muscle strengthening exercises (see Muscle Weakness section, page 142).

Swedish massage has many benefits for the spinal cord injured child, including:

- a sense of body wholeness
- deeper breathing

- stimulation and increased circulation to paralyzed areas, helping to prevent atrophy
- prevention of edema
- less discomfort in the area of the spinal injury and/or a halo brace
- relief of muscle fatigue and strain caused by vigorous physical therapy
- relief of back pain caused by sitting in a wheelchair for long periods, as well as from pain caused by using upper body muscles to transfer from wheelchair to bed and back
- more supple muscle and connective tissue, helping to prevent contracture
- relief of muscle spasms in the legs
- maintenance of joint range of motion
- relief of constipation

A Touch Research Institute study compared the effects of massage and exercise with adults with SCIs at levels C5 to C7. Participants were given either a 40-minute Swedish massage, twice weekly for 5 weeks, or they performed an exercise routine, also twice weekly for 5 weeks. At the end of the study, the massage therapy group had greater muscle strength and range of motion than the exercise group and lower scores on anxiety and depression tests.[4] Although Swedish massage is highly beneficial for those with SCIs, other bodywork modalities may also be used at the same time, such as myofascial release and craniosacral therapy.[5] Massage therapists, including Patty Tipton-Sproul (therapist for the Seattle Seahawks football team) and Dr. Meir Schneider, have had good success with adults with SCIs when therapy began soon after the injury—even the next day—with physician approval (Tipton-Spradlin P, interview: Seattle, WA, May 2000).[6]

Larry Burns-Vidlak, a massage therapist who specializes in massage for the disabled, has massaged children with SCIs as young as age 2. He believes that the child's muscles, tendons, ligaments, and connective tissue need deep massage; however, he cautions that massage should only be done to the child's tolerance. If there is a painful area, use light pressure at first. Gradually, after a number of treatments, deeper massage will be tolerated (Burns-Vidlak L, personal communication, October 1992).

A daily massage of the entire body is ideal, using the Swedish massage techniques described in Chapter 3. Because parts of the body not directly affected by the SCI are likely to compensate for injured areas, they may be overworked and can become tense, stiff, sore, or uncomfortable. Parents should be taught to massage their children. Whenever the child is rolled over or moved, the parents should massage any areas that have been under pressure. However, they should not rub any areas with early signs of pressure ulcers, such as swelling, darkness, redness, or open skin (Chapter 6).

Despite having similar injuries, each child with an SCI is an individual with different concerns and different needs. When the child's medical history is being taken, be sure to find out what her greatest physical discomfort or concern is.

MASSAGE AND HYDROTHERAPY FOR SCIS

MOIST HEAT APPLICATION

Apply a moist hot pack or Hydrocollator pack for 10 minutes before massaging an area. Then, while that area is being massaged, apply it to the next part of the body that will be massaged. Use caution if an area is numb. Carefully monitor the area under the heat, so that the child's skin does not burn.

COLD WATER IMMERSION AND EXERCISE

See Muscle Weakness section in Chapter 5, page 142.

MASSAGE FOR SPECIFIC BODY AREAS OF THE CHILD WITH SCI

As stated earlier, a daily whole-body massage is ideal, using the Swedish massage techniques described in Chapter 3. Use the basic relaxation sequence to encourage deep breathing. Then ask the child to imagine that the area being massaged expands on inhalation and settles back to its normal size on exhalation. The child should breathe comfortably and without effort. This can help increase sensation in areas where the child has little feeling. Passive range-of-motion exercises are also important.

Neck Massage

If the injury was to the child's cervical vertebrae, his neck may feel strained, stiff, or uncomfortable, especially if the vertebrae were surgically fused. Massage the neck muscles on either side of the spine using the techniques described in Chapter 3 and the section on neck and shoulder tension in Chapter 5. If there is sensitivity or discomfort where a halo brace was in place, use gentle fingertip pressure until it is decreased.

Hand and Forearm Massage

For excessive tension of hands and forearms, use deep kneading, petrissage, and range-of-motion movements of all joints. Some children may have more pain from overusing their upper extremities propelling a wheelchair than from the SCI.

Leg Massage

To relieve muscle spasms in the legs, use the basic leg massage described in Chapter 3, but spend additional time massaging the front of the thigh and the buttock. Use deep

(Continued on page 114)

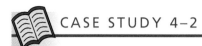

CASE STUDY 4-2

Background

Alejandro is a 13-year-old boy with a spinal cord injury (SCI) at the T6 level. He is one of 17 teenagers and young adults with SCIs being treated at a Mexican clinic for disabled children. Of those 17, 15 have back pain and discomfort from sitting in wheelchairs all day. Two patients, using lying-down wheelchairs while waiting for pressure ulcers to heal, have severe back discomfort and contractures in various joints from lying down for an extended time. All have poor circulation in their legs. Other than problems associated with the SCIs, nine patients have concerns related to associated injuries, such as fractures or gunshot wounds. All are dealing with the stress of being disabled at a time in their lives when they would normally be at the height of their physical vigor and strength, as well as being poor and disabled in a third-world country—they have an extremely high level of stress. Massage is being used to treat the effects of the SCIs and address pain from associated injuries; however, it is also addressing their touch deprivation and high stress levels.

When Alejandro was age 12, he was shot through the spine. The bullet entered through the right rhomboid area and exited through his left armpit. Soon after the injury, fluid was drained from his chest. He developed deep pressure ulcers (now healed) during his initial hospitalization. He uses a manual wheelchair and attends school. Severe pain in his shoulders and midback often keep him awake at night, probably caused by the combination of the spinal injury and using his arms to propel his chair through the sand and dirt roads of his town and to do transfers. His legs also feel stiff to him.

Impression

Pain secondary to SCI, other tissue injury and muscle strain, all possibly exacerbated by extreme stress.

Treatment

Alejandro transferred from his wheelchair to a treatment table. He began in the prone position, with only his shirt removed. Massage began with light effleurage stroking of the whole back to evaluate his tissue. Because his back was hypersensitive and his rhomboid area was hypersensitive and painful to the touch, only superficial effleurage was attempted for the first two sessions. At the third session, superficial effleurage of the whole back was done initially and, as Alejandro could tolerate it, deeper effleurage strokes of the whole back followed. Because his rhomboid area was so hypersensitive, deeper effleurage was begun around that area by stroking along the sides of the upper back. Range of motion of the shoulder

joints and pulling out of the scapulae to stretch the rhomboids was also done to encourage relaxation of the rhomboid region. Once this was done, superficial effleurage was cautiously followed by deeper effleurage.

As the author was able to palpate underneath the now-warmed superficial layers of tissue, deeper knots were encountered. There was a great deal of scar tissue and marked edema in the tissue around the bullet wound. It was also extremely sensitive. A gentle, but persistent approach, was tried; a variety of Swedish massage strokes, such as kneading and petrissage, were attempted at first around the rhomboid area and then over it. Each stroke began with superficial pressure, but was terminated immediately if not tolerated. Eventually Alejandro was able to tolerate one gentle effleurage stroke at a particular speed and in one particular direction (diagonal to the scar tissue); when this was established, no effort was made to go beyond it for this session. Subsequent sessions were similar, with gradually increasing pressure as tolerated. A variety of Swedish massage strokes were used on the back and later on the chest. Alejandro was seen daily for 8 days.

Response

After the third session, Alejandro reported he generally felt much better and had greatly reduced pain at night, which meant he slept better. The hypersensitivity in his rhomboid area was greatly reduced. He arrived early for his sessions and was eager to receive his massage therapy. He was seen for eight sessions and, each time, was enthusiastic about the improvement in his general well-being, reduction of pain, and greater ability to feel his upper body. Over time, Alejandro would have benefited from regular Swedish massage of his legs, in which he felt stiffness and had poor circulation due to his inability to move them. He certainly would have made greater gains in dealing with deeper levels of muscle tension and increased range of motion in his upper body. Eight sessions were only a beginning.

Discussion Questions

1. What tissues were injured or affected by Alejandro's spinal cord injury?
2. What symptoms were present?
3. What other areas of Alejandro's body might be affected by his spinal cord injury?
4. What was one way that Alejandro's personal boundaries were respected during his treatment?

kneading and effleurage as the tissue will be tight and dense. Swedish massage will have temporary effects on this problem; the use of craniosacral therapy or deeper techniques, such as myofascial release, may be more appropriate.

Back Massage

Spend extra time massaging the back if there is pain from sitting for long periods in a wheelchair. The techniques in Chapter 3 can be adapted to massage in a wheelchair, if more convenient. The neck, shoulders, and back can be massaged from behind the child. Roll the child's wheelchair up to a table and have him rest his head and arms on a pillow. The entire back is now accessible.

 A child with flaccid (limp) paralysis could be injured if a joint is moved or forced beyond its existing range of motion. The muscles could be stretched and joints dislocated without the child's awareness. If muscle spasticity occurs during passive range of motion, stop the movement temporarily but continue to apply slow, gentle pressure on the body part until the muscle relaxes; then proceed with the motion.[7]

SPRAINS

A sprain occurs when a joint is wrenched or twisted past its normal range of motion. As soft tissue is taken past the normal length, minute tears occur in the ligaments that stabilize the joint, with leakage of blood and fluid into the surrounding tissue. Trigger points may be immediately activated in the ligaments and joint capsules.[1] Sprains are classified by the number of torn ligament fibers. First-degree tears, involving only a few ligament fibers, are characterized by slight swelling, pain, and loss of function. Second-degree tears, involving many ligament fibers, are characterized by modest swelling, diffuse tenderness, and loss of function. For example, the child will have difficulty bearing weight on the injured ankle. In a third-degree tear, the ligament actually ruptures and is no longer attached to the bone, involving extensive bleeding, increased pain, and greater instability.[2]

Children are more prone to fractures than to joint sprains because their bones are not completely ossified. However, as an adolescent approaches skeletal maturity, his ligaments and musculotendinous structures become more vulnerable to injury. With ossification nearly complete and with the fusion of the epiphyses and apophyses, the bones can better withstand force, and trauma is instead transmitted through the soft-tissue structures.[3]

Ankle sprains are the most common pediatric sports injury, occurring in approximately 6% of all high school sports participants. Only 3% of these ankle sprains are of the medial ligaments; the remaining are sprains of the anterior talofibular ligament caused by inversion and supination of the foot (see Figure 4–4). Another common pediatric sports injury is the sprain of ulnar collateral ligament of the thumb. Forceful abduction (as can occur in football, skiing, hockey, wrestling, or baseball) tears the collateral ligament from its attachment at the proximal phalanx. Together with the tear of the specific ligament, there may be tearing of the entire joint capsule, stretching of nearby muscles, and even an associated chip fracture.[4]

Typical treatment for a sprain depends on severity. All degrees of sprain will cause pain, swelling, and loss of stability. There is always spasm of muscles near the sprained joint and, often, spasms farther away. With any sprain, the orthopedist will check to see if the child has simultaneously sustained a fracture. Specific attention will be given to the physeal growth plates, as an injury here can affect growth and final length of the tibia. As with any injury that involves a fair amount of force, other damage may be done to the soft tissue around the joint or to individual bones.[2]

First-degree sprains are treated with ice; additional support, such as braces or taping; compression; and elevation. Second-degree sprains are treated with additional support, ice, crutches, and isometric exercises. A third-degree sprain is treated with a rigid cast and possibly surgery to reattach the ligament in its proper place, followed by strengthening and stretching exercises when the cast is removed. It is vitally important that the child's joint regains stability because a chronically loose ligament may predispose the child to repeated sprains. Repetitive, unprotected ankle sprains in a young gymnast, for example, can lead to serious inversion injury with complete ligamentous disruption and a need for subsequent surgical reconstruction.[5] The child may also be more likely to develop osteoarthritis as an adult.

Prolotherapy, the injection of natural substances at the exact site of an injury to stimulate the person's immune system to repair damaged ligaments, has been shown to significantly increase ligament mass, thickness, and strength in children, as well as adults.[6]

APPROACH AND GOALS

Ice applications and contrast treatments can reduce swelling and pain, and ice massage can relieve muscle spasm. Massage can also relieve pain and swelling, which impair healing, and relieve muscle tightness and spasm, which hamper movement. Early massage of the area can prevent or reduce adhesions. Massaging will help the child relax the area, preventing chronic muscular guarding caused by trauma and pain.

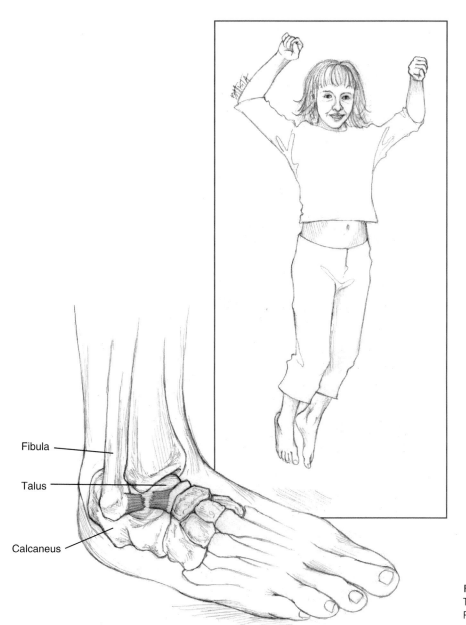

Fibula

Talus

Calcaneus

FIGURE 4–4 ■ Spraining of the Anterior Talofibular Ligament Following Forced Plantar Flexion and Inversion.

During the acute stages of a sprain (about the first 48 hours), massage should be done above and below the sprained joint to relieve swelling, increase circulation, and decrease muscle spasm and pain. After the first 48 hours, massage may be performed up to three times daily, as long as you are not causing discomfort or pain. Myotherapist Bonnie Prudden recommends trigger point therapy combined with exercise to treat a sprain immediately after injury; however, this should only be done by those with special training.[7]

MASSAGE AND HYDROTHERAPY FOR SPRAINS

ICE APPLICATION

Cold (in the form of ice packs) is generally used to treat a sprain in the first 24 hours. Ice massage may also be performed. Use an ice cup (see page 91) to massage the painful area and about 4 inches surrounding it. Continue ice massage for about 8 minutes.

CONTRAST TREATMENT

This treatment may be done on any joint; however, a contrast treatment for the ankle is discussed because ankle sprains are the most common pediatric sprains. Contrast treatments may be done three or more times daily.

Step 1. Fill two deep buckets or washtubs with water, one at 110° F and one at 50° F.

Step 2. Place the child's feet in the hot water for 3 minutes.

Step 3. Place the child's feet in the cold water for 30 seconds.

Step 4. Repeat steps 2 and 3.

Step 5. Repeat steps 2 and 3.

Step 6. Repeat steps 2 and 3.

Step 7. Remove the child's feet from the water and dry them.

MASSAGE SEQUENCE FOR SPRAINS

Step 1. Basic relaxation sequence (see page 70).

Step 2. Apply oil or lotion.

Step 3. Begin gentle stroking above and below the sprain. Use your palms (or fingertips, if the area is small) and alternate hands. Stroke up toward the heart. For a sprained ankle, stroke up the shins, over the knee, and up the thigh, then use your fingertips to stroke from toes to ankle. For a sprained wrist, stroke up the forearm and upper arm, then use your fingertips to stroke from fingers to wrist. Repeat for 5 minutes.

Step 4. Thumbstroke the sprain. Be extremely gentle. Make short strokes toward the heart. Cover the sprain and a few inches around it. Repeat for 1 to 2 minutes.

Step 5. Repeat step 3.

 Avoid moving the joint itself, which might put stress on the injured ligament and cause pain.

TRAUMATIC BRAIN INJURY

The most common way that children become disabled is by brain injury. A high percentage of children—one of 500—have a traumatic injury to the brain each year. Falls, motor vehicle accidents, assaults, child abuse, and sports and recreation injuries are the main causes of traumatic brain injury (TBI).[1] In 1999, the majority of children who died from TBI had collided with a motor vehicle when riding a bicycle.[2] Helmet use alone can prevent many of these injuries.[3]

Specific injuries to the brain include fracture of the cranial bones (fragments may injure the brain); damage or tearing of the nerve fibers of the brain; and bleeding from torn blood vessels (between the skull and the dura, beneath the dura, or inside the brain itself).

Depending on the nature of the damage and the care the child receives after the injury, a variety of impairments may result, including:

1. Motor impairments, such as spasticity, tremors, and ataxia (the inability to coordinate voluntary muscle activity during voluntary movement). Long-term, these impairments can lead to contractures, dislocations, and scoliosis.

2. Loss of oral motor skills.

3. Sensory impairments, such as **nystagmus** and eye muscle palsy.

4. Speech and language impairments.

5. Cognitive impairments, such as problems with attention, learning, judgment, and speed of information processing.

6. Changes in personality and behavior, such as irritability, a poor tolerance for frustration, aggression, poor emotional control, and apathy. The child's entire personality may appear to change. The child may also become depressed due to significant loss of abilities and ongoing struggles against impairments.

Traumatic brain injuries may have lifelong effects on an individual's functioning. One follow-up study of adults who had experienced severe TBI during their preschool years found that, although one-half had achieved average performance in school, only one-quarter were able to work full-time.[1]

APPROACH AND GOALS

Acute rehabilitation care following traumatic brain injury includes turning the child to prevent pressure ulcers, preventing contractures by performing passive range of motion, and carefully positioning and splinting limbs. In this acute phase, after checking with the child's physician, massage may be used to release tension, stimulate circulation, prevent muscular atrophy and contractures, and maintain joint range of motion.

Long-term rehabilitation includes dealing with musculoskeletal complications from immobilization or impairments, including pain, spasticity, and contractures. The large mechanical forces involved with this injury may damage not only the brain, but also soft tissue and bones of the head, spine, and other areas. As a result, children may develop headaches, neck pain; tension in the muscles of the scalp, jaw, and face; upper back or shoulder stiffness; shallow breathing; back pain; and other types of chronic myofascial pain.[4] Massage therapist Dianne Keanne, who treats adults with traumatic brain injury, has found they often have scar tissue and other soft tissue dysfunction around the bones of the spine (Keanne D, personal communication, September 2002). Osteopath John Upledger has found that head trauma can cause malalignment of the cranial bones as they are forced into each other. Upledger found a common pattern of malalignment—a lateral strain of the cranial base, nasal and zygomatic dysfunction, and an unleveling of the cranial base.[5]

Dr. Gail Denton is a psychotherapist, massage therapist, and brain injury survivor. In her book, *Brainlash: Maximize Your Recovery From Mild Brain Injury* (Attention Span Books, 1996), she relates how a number of bodywork modalities helped speed her recovery, including Swedish massage to reinforce the natural state of her muscles, craniosacral therapy to help repair her brain, and Aston-Patterning to undo the impact of the accident on her soft tissue.[4]

Because children with TBI are likely to have chronically high levels of stress, providing relaxing and nurturing touch and helping them to relax may be as helpful as dealing with any physical complaints they have. Massage may also be used as a pleasant relaxing treatment after rigorous or painful physical therapy. Musculoskeletal pain from associated injuries can be treated effectively with massage. Refer to the specific complaints discussed throughout this book. Any contractures may be treated with massage after discussion with the child's physical therapist (see Contractures, Chapter 6). Passive range-of-motion exercises are important to treat and prevent contractures, and to increase body awareness and relaxation.

MASSAGE SEQUENCE FOR CHILDREN WITH TBIS

MASSAGE

Use the full-body techniques described in Chapter 3 for general relaxation, as well as specific treatments in Chapter 4 and 5 for specific complaints. Be sure to perform all passive range-of-motion exercises.

A child with flaccid (limp) paralysis could be injured if a joint is moved or forced beyond its existing range of motion. The muscles could be stretched and joints dislocated without the child's awareness. If muscle spasticity occurs during passive range of motion, stop the movement temporarily but continue to apply slow, gentle pressure on the body part until the muscle relaxes. Then proceed with the motion (Keanne D, personal communication, September 2002).

REVIEW QUESTIONS

1. Explain why children are more prone than adults to amputations, burns, fractures, and traumatic head injuries.

2. Choose three acute injuries and explain their specific treatment with hydrotherapy and massage.

3. Choose three injuries that have long-term effects and explain their specific treatment with hydrotherapy and massage.

4. Discuss how musculoskeletal injuries such as dislocations, fractures, and sprains may leave lasting traces in the child's soft tissue. How might these lasting traces affect the child as an adult?

REFERENCES

1. Childhood Injury Fact Sheet. National SafeKids. Available at: www.Safekids.org. Accessed July 2001
2. Ogden J: *Skeletal Injury in the Child*. Philadelphia, PA: Lea and Febiger, 1982, p 4, 198
3. Cody BE, O'Toole ML, Mickalide AD, Paul HP: A National Study of Traumatic Brain Injury and Wheel-Related Sports. Washington, DC: National SafeKids Campaign, 2002, p 3, 5
4. Rivara FP: Epidemiology and prevention of pediatric traumatic head injury. *Pediatric Annals*, 23:12-17, 1994

Amputations

1. Percoraro D: Applications of massage for chronic health conditions. *Massage Therapy Journal*, Spring:52, 1986
2. Morrissy R: *Lovell and Winter's Pediatric Orthopaedics*. Vol. 2. Baltimore, MD: Lippincott Williams & Wilkins, 2001, p 1255

Birth Trauma

1. Dodson J: *Baby Beautiful: A Handbook of Baby Head Shaping*. Eugene, OR: Heirs Press, 1994, p 133, 137, 147, 250
2. Batshaw M: *Children With Disabilities*. Baltimore, MD: Paul Brookes Publishing, 1997, p 101
3. Ogden J: *Skeletal Injury in the Child*. Philadelphia, PA: Lea and Febiger, 1982, p 186
4. Cheek D: Maladjustment patterns apparently related to imprinting at birth. *American Journal of Clinical Hypnosis*, 18:390, 1975
5. Simons D, Travell JG: *Myofascial Pain and Dysfunction: The Triggerpoint Manual*. Vol. 1, Ed. 2. Baltimore, MD: Lippincott Williams & Wilkins, 1999, p 117
6. Morrissy R: *Lovell and Winter's Pediatric Orthopaedics*. Vol. 2. Baltimore, MD: Lippincott Williams & Wilkins, 2001, p 847
7. Hartsough CS, et al: Medical factors in hyperactive and normal children: prenatal developmental, and health history findings. *American Journal of Orthopsychiatry*, 55:190-210, 1985
8. Rockwell J, D.C., quoted in *Fibromyalgia and Chronic Pain Syndrome, A Survival Manual*. Berkeley, CA: New Harbinger Publications, 1996 p 151

9. Gillespie B: *Brain Therapy for Children and Adults: Natural Care for People With Craniosacral, Dental, and Facial Trauma*. King of Prussia, PA: Productions for Children's Healing, 2000, p 103

Burns

1. Colton H: *The Gift of Touch*. New York: Seaview/Putnam, 1983, p 109
2. Munster A: *Severe Burns: A Family Guide to Medical and Emotional Recovery*. Baltimore, MD: Johns Hopkins University Press, 1993, p xviii, xix, 11
3. Long T, Toscano K: *Handbook of Pediatric Physical Therapy*. Philadelphia, PA: Lippincott Williams & Wilkins, 2002, p 75
4. Olness K, Kohen D: *Hypnosis and Hypnotherapy With Children*. New York, NY: Guilford Press, 1996, p 273-279
5. Field T, et al: Burn injured benefit from massage therapy. *Journal of Burn Care and Rehabilitation*, 19:241-244, 1997
6. Field T: *Touch Therapy*. Edinburgh: Churchill Livingstone, 2000, p 58
7. Hernandez-Reif M, et al: Children's distress during burn treatment is reduced by massage therapy. *Journal of Burn Care and Rehabilitation*, 22:191-195, 2001

Dislocations

1. Ogden J: *Skeletal Injury in the Child*. Philadelphia, PA: Lea and Febiger, 1982, p 288, 290
2. Morrissy R: *Lovell and Winter's Pediatric Orthopaedics*. Vol. 2. Baltimore, MD: Lippincott Williams & Wilkins, 2001, p 1255
3. Thrash A: *Home Remedies: Hydrotherapy, Massage, Charcoal and Other Simple Treatments*. Seale, AL: Thrash Publications, 1981, p 45

Fractures

1. Morrissy R: *Lovell and Winter's Pediatric Orthopaedics*. Vol. 2. Baltimore, MD: Lippincott Williams & Wilkins, 2001
2. Ogden J: *Skeletal Injury in the Child*. Philadelphia, PA: Lea and Febiger, 1982
3. Simons D, Travell JG: *Myofascial Pain and Dysfunction: The Triggerpoint Manual*. Vol. 1, ed. 2. Baltimore, MD: Lippincott Williams & Wilkins, 1999, p 600, 828, 847
4. Simons D, Travell JG: *Myofascial Pain and Dysfunction: The Triggerpoint Manual*. Vol. 2, ed. 2. Baltimore, MD: Lippincott Williams & Wilkins, 1999, p 41, 410, 411, 481, 511, 533
5. Klein KK, et al: Asymmetries in the growth of the pelvis and legs of children: A clinical and statistical study 1964-1967. *Journal of the American Osteopathic Association*, 68:153-156, 1968
6. Proffit W, Fields H: *Contemporary Orthodontics*. St. Louis, MO: Mosby, 2000, p 117
7. Prudden B: *Fitness from Six to Twelve*. New York: Ballantine, 1987, p 416

Scar Tissue

1. Simons D, Travell JG: *Myofascial Pain and Dysfunction: The Triggerpoint Manual*. Vol. 1, ed. 2. Baltimore, MD: Lippincott Williams &Wilkins, 1999, p 43

2. Upledger J, Vredevoogd J: *Craniosacral Therapy*. Seattle, WA: Eastland Press, 1983, p 240

Spinal Cord Injury

1. Ogden J: *Skeletal Injury in the Child*. Philadelphia, PA: Lea and Febiger, 1982, p 186, 391
2. Morrissy R: *Lovell and Winter's Pediatric Orthopaedics*. Vol. 2. Baltimore, MD: Lippincott Williams & Wilkins, 2001, p 1367
3. Senelick R: *The Spinal Cord Injury Handbook for Patients and Their Families*. Birmingham, AL: HealthSouth Press, 1998, p 111
4. Diego M: Spinal cord patients benefit from massage therapy. *International Journal of Neuroscience*, 112:133-142, 2002
5. Brunie E: The road back—How bodywork and determination helped me recover from paralysis. *Massage Magazine*, January/February:73-83, 2001
6. Schneider D: Waking up from paralysis. School for Self-Healing Newsletter. Self-Healing Research Foundation, January 2000, p 847
7. Kozier B, Erb G, Bufalino, P: *Introduction to Nursing*. Redwood City, CA: Addison-Wesley Health Sciences, 1989, p 546

Sprains

1. Simons D, Travell JG: *Myofascial Pain and Dysfunction: The Triggerpoint Manual*. Vol. 1, ed. 2. Baltimore, MD: Lippincott Williams & Wilkins, 1999, p 43
2. Morrissy R: *Lovell and Winter's Pediatric Orthopaedics*. Vol. 2. Baltimore, MD: Lippincott Williams & Wilkins, 2001, p 1290, 1292
3. Waters P, Millis M: Hip and pelvic injuries in the young athlete. *Clinics in Sports Medicine*, 7, 1988, p 525
4. Birrer R, Brecher D: *Common Sports Injuries in Youngsters*. Oradell, NJ: Medical Economics, 1987, p 85
5. Ogden J: *Skeletal Injury in the Child*. Philadelphia, PA: Lea and Febiger, 1982, p 192
6. Hauser R: *Prolo Your Pain Away*. Chicago, IL: Beulahland Publications, 1992, p 39
7. Prudden B: *Fitness from Six to Twelve*. New York, NY: Ballantine, 1987, p 433

Traumatic Brain Injury

1. Batshaw M: *Children With Disabilities*. Baltimore, MD: Paul Brookes Publishing, 1997, p 596, 609
2. Cody BE, O'Toole ML, Mickalide AD, Paul HP: A National Study of Traumatic Brain Injury and Wheel-Related Sports. Washington, DC: National SafeKids Campaign, May 2002, p 3
3. Sinclair M: Going out to play? Don't forget the helmets! *Corvallis Gazette-Times*, April 2000, p 4
4. Denton G: *Brainlash: Maximize Your Recovery From Mild Brain Injury*. Niwot, CO: Attention Span Books, 1996, p 245-249, 255
5. Upledger J, Vredevoogd J: *Craniosacral Therapy*. Seattle, WA: Eastland Press, 1983, p 115, 199
6. Kozier B, Erb G, Bufalino P: *Introduction to Nursing*. Redwood City, CA: Addison-Wesley Health Sciences, 1989, p 546

MASSAGE AND HYDROTHERAPY FOR THE COMMON DISCOMFORTS OF CHILDHOOD

5

KEY POINTS

After reading this chapter, the student will be able to:

1. Understand the most common childhood discomforts and explain the causes.
2. Understand the effects of emotional stress on the most common childhood discomforts.
3. Explain the signs and symptoms of five different types of headache.
4. Explain the rationale for using massage and hydrotherapy to treat each common discomfort.
5. Explain the importance of teaching children how to approach these discomforts through wholistic, non-medication approaches.

In this chapter, the student will learn the background of many common childhood discomforts and how to use massage and hydrotherapy to relieve them. Although none of these conditions are dangerous to children's long-term health, they can still bother them very much. Unfortunately, physical pain is part of growing up. Injuries are a significant cause of pediatric pain. After injuries, headaches are the most common cause of nonpathologic pediatric pain, followed by stomachaches and then leg pain.[1] A surprisingly high percentage of children also have chronic musculoskeletal pain that directly affects their moods and behavior. Children cannot easily verbalize their body sensations; as a result, adults often do not know how much they hurt and may not seek treatment for their pain. Often it is discovered only when children have participated in a pain survey or other research where they are specifically asked if they have pain.[2] At some point during childhood, most children have bouts of pain resulting from earaches, constipation, or growing pains. Although other conditions do not cause pain, they can still be bothersome in other ways: considering that the average child has seven colds each year, the common cold may cause significant discomfort. Insomnia is yet another common complaint that does not involve pain but is bothersome to children. A dis-

cussion of depression has also been included in this chapter because it is extremely common in children and, although it does not cause physical suffering, it is terribly troubling.

The massage and hydrotherapy treatments in this chapter not only relieve common discomforts, but also provide the child with a positive model for wholistic, non-medication ways to care for themselves.

Many treatments in this chapter combine hydrotherapy, whole-body Swedish massage strokes, and pressure point massage. Refer to Chapter 3 for descriptions of basic techniques, if necessary. When you have learned the basic treatments discussed here, you may incorporate techniques from other styles of massage and bodywork, as well, because they promote relaxation. Many discomforts covered in this chapter may not be caused by emotional stress; however, stress will probably worsen the symptoms. Any techniques that help children release tension and learn to relax will promote healing.

THE COMMON COLD

Most healthy children have about seven colds a year. Cold symptoms include nasal discharge (runny nose); sore throat; dry cough; hoarseness; a general feeling of malaise; and, perhaps, a mild fever. Usually children feel quite ill for the first 3 or 4 days, gradually begin to feel better, and can expect to feel back to normal again in 1 to 2 weeks. About 20% of children will develop a bacterial infection in the last stages of the cold. An infection of the sinus or ear can occur if mucus cannot drain through swollen nasal passages, which then provides an excellent environment for bacteria to grow. A chest infection can develop if children have aspirated mucus into their lungs when swallowing mucus containing viral particles. The times most likely for a child to catch a cold are described in Point of Interest Box 5-1.

The following are simple preventive measures to prevent spreading a cold from one person to another:

- Cover the nose and mouth when coughing or sneezing to prevent spraying the cold virus onto others. Wash the hands immediately since they now have virus particles on them.
- Wash hands frequently throughout the day to prevent getting the virus on objects or on other people.
- Clean children's toys and household surfaces, such as faucet handles, light switches, doorknobs, and telephones, with a germicidal soap.
- Use disposable tissues and paper towels.
- Do not share towels, cups, dishes, utensils, or toothbrushes. These personal items should be washed in hot water to kill the cold virus.

APPROACH AND GOALS

A traditional hydrotherapy treatment at the very beginning of a cold is to raise the temperature of the whole body by a sauna, hot bath, or a hot foot soak. Raising the temperature of the body enhances the body's immune response and promotes the killing of the cold virus. However, you should not perform this treatment without special training and a physician's permission because it can raise the body temperature enough to create a mild fever. During the subacute phase of a cold, however, there are many massage and hydrotherapy treatments that can relieve symptoms of nasal and chest congestion and soothe and relax children who feel out of sorts. It is important to drink plenty of water to thin mucus and flush out the cold virus and to get extra rest to strengthen the immune system. Children should be seen by their physician if their fever is higher than 103° F; if they have a stiff neck, difficulty breathing, or are too sick to drink; or if they have had cold symptoms for longer than 7 to 10 days.

POINT OF INTEREST BOX 5–1
When Are Children Most Likely to Catch a Cold?

- Common colds begin in the nose because cold viruses grow best at 92° F and the temperature of the nose is cooler than the temperature of deeper body structures.[1] This may be why an old folk belief connects catching a chill to coming down with a cold.
- The cold virus thrives during the wet season because it can better survive outside the body when the humidity is high. Under the right conditions, it may survive for up to 3 hours.
- Children catch more colds in the winter because they spend more time indoors, where they can pass viruses around more easily. Children are notoriously unaware of such commonsense precautions as covering their mouths when they sneeze and washing their hands after sneezing.
- A high stress level nearly doubles the likelihood of becoming ill when exposed to a cold virus.[2]
- According to physician and author of *The Joy of Stress*, Peter Hanson, "Young children are usually brought to the physician with one infection after another for the first 5 or 6 years after starting day care or school. Partially, this is due to [contracting] contagious diseases from the other children, but mainly it is due to decreased resistance, from the stress of leaving the womblike comfort of the home."[3]

References

1. Thrash A: *Home Remedies*. Seale, AL: Thrash Publications, 1981, p 108
2. Roghman KJ: Daily stress, illness, and use of health services in young families. *Pediatric Research*, 7:520-526, 1973
3. Hanson P: *The Joy of Stress*. Kansas City, MO: Andrews, McNeel and Parker, 1986, p 22

MASSAGE AND HYDROTHERAPY FOR SINUS CONGESTION

Over-the-counter decongestants may give symptomatic relief but can make a child hyperactive and unable to sleep. In contrast, the following hydrotherapy techniques are highly effective for congestion of the sinus and nasal passages and have no adverse effects. One of the following techniques for sinus congestion can be chosen.

SINUS IRRIGATION WITH SALTWATER

Saltwater helps shrink swollen membranes and temporarily rinses the sinuses of mucus.

Step 1. Use ¼ teaspoon salt to 1 cup warm water.

Step 2. Instruct an older child to pour the warm saline into the palm, snuff up into one nostril, catch in the back of the throat, and spit out. (It is generally difficult to persuade a small child to try this, as they may not be able to do it without swallowing salt water).

Step 3. Repeat 5 times for each nostril. Do the entire irrigation 3 to 5 times a day.

Sinus irrigation may also be done with a sinus irrigator tip attachment to a pulsing electric toothbrush (Water Pik) or with a neti pot, which is available at health food stores.

CONTRAST TREATMENT

This treatment helps drain the sinuses and increase circulation to the area.

Step 1. Dip a washcloth in 110° F water and wring out. Place the cloth across the nose, leaving the nostrils exposed. Fold the ends of the cloth 90 degrees from the central point so that the ends lie alongside the nose. Leave on for 2 minutes.

Step 2. Replace the first washcloth with a washcloth or small bath towel that has been dipped in ice water and wrung out; leave on for 1 minute.

Step 3. Repeat hot and cold (Steps 1 and 2) two more times, for three changes.

STEAM INHALATION

Inhaling steam relieves nasal and sinus congestion, soothes the respiratory tract, and makes secretions looser and easier to spit up. The following two ways to inhale steam can be shown to parents:

• Pour six cups of boiling water into a heavy bowl that will not tip over. Have children sit at a table, drape a towel over their head to make a tent, and have them breathe in steam from the bowl, through the nose if possible. Continue for 5 to 10 minutes. A few drops of eucalyptus or peppermint oil may be added to the water to further open up the sinuses.

• Another way to help children inhale steam is to have them take a hot shower, inhaling the steam for as long as possible. If they feel weak, a plastic chair may be placed in the shower to sit on. Very small children go directly into the shower with their parents holding them.

COLD SOCKS

Step 1. Instruct the child's parents to wring out a pair of wool socks in very cold water and place the socks on the child's feet.

Step 2. Place a pair of dry, cotton socks on top.

Step 3. Leave the socks on all night. Initially, the feet will be cold, producing a vasoconstrictive effect on the blood vessels of the feet; however, the feet will gradually warm up as the socks trap the child's body heat. The blood vessels of the feet will then dilate and, eventually, will have a derivative effect similar to a hot footbath. This eases nasal congestion and helps the child get a good night's sleep.

MASSAGE SEQUENCE FOR SINUS CONGESTION

Positioning: Sit as you would for a head massage.

Step 1. Basic relaxation sequence (page 70).

Step 2. Apply a few drops of oil or lotion to the face.

Step 3. Forehead and eye circles (Figures 3–30 and 3–31). Repeat 10 times.

Step 4. Place your thumbs on either side of the nose at the level of the eyes; use firm pressure and stroke slowly down to the bottom of the nose. Repeat 10 times.

Step 5. Pressure points around the eyes (see Figures 5–1 and 5–2).

Step 6. Pressure points on the side of the nose (see Figure 5–3). Begin just below the bottom of the eye socket. Press on either side of the nose with your thumbs, as if you were trying to touch your thumbs together. Use gentle to moderate pressure, as much as the child can firmly tolerate. Do a second point in the middle of the nose and a third point at the bottom.

Step 7. Forehead and eye circles. Repeat 10 times.

Step 8. Basic relaxation sequence.

MASSAGE AND HYDROTHERAPY FOR CHEST CONGESTION

The application of heat to the chest increases local circulation; feels soothing; and loosens secretions, making them easier to cough up. Massage is also soothing for a sick child and helps relax the muscles of the ribcage. Releasing tension in the pectoral muscles, intercostals, diaphragm, and upper back muscles will help the child breathe more easily and deeply. Percussion of the chest loosens secretions as well.

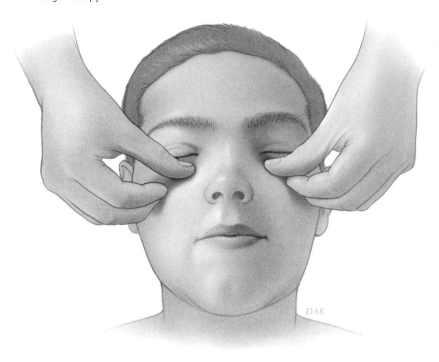

FIGURE 5–1 ■ Pressure Points Around the Eyes.

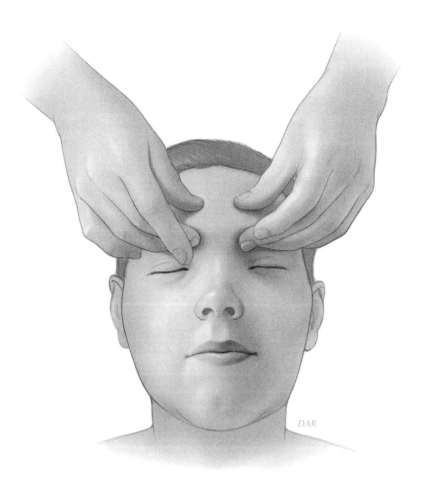

FIGURE 5–2 ■ Pressure Points Around the Eyes.

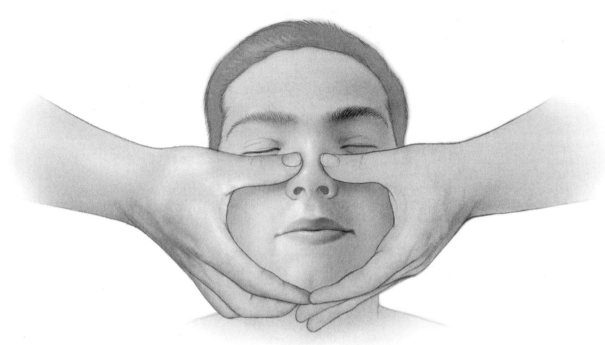

FIGURE 5–3 ■ Pressure Points on the Side of the Nose. These points are used to promote sinus drainage.

CONTRAST TREATMENT FOR THE CHEST

Equipment:

1. Linens: one plastic sheet; two cotton sheets; one blanket; and at least two pillowcases, washcloths, or terry cloth mitts.
2. A bowl (size: about 1 quart) containing ice cubes covered with water.
3. One moist heating pad for the child to lie on and one for the chest, or two Hydrocollator packs. A hot water bottle with a damp washcloth underneath is suitable for the chest of a small child.
4. Treatment table or covered massage surface on the floor.

Procedure (see Figure 3–55):

Step 1. Cover the treatment table with a blanket, cover the blanket with a plastic sheet, and cover the plastic sheet with one cotton sheet.
Step 2. Lay the moist heating pad on the sheet where the child's back will be and cover it with a pillowcase or towel. The moist heating pad should be positioned so that the child's entire upper back will be in contact with it. Lay the child on the pack. If it feels too hot to him, add another layer of cloth or towel. Monitor the heat carefully so he does not get burned.
Step 3. Put 1 or 2 pillowcases or towels on the child's chest, then the moist heating pad or Hydrocollator pack, then cover with the one more towel on top. Again, check with the child to make sure the heat is not excessive. Cover the child with a sheet.
Step 4. After 3 minutes, briskly rub the entire chest with a washcloth or terry cloth mitt that has been wrung

out in the ice water. First, tell the child what you are going to do, "Take a deep breath, and I'm going to rub your chest quickly with this cloth." Generally, the cold will feel good to the child because his chest will be very warm.
Step 5. After rubbing his chest with the cold cloth, quickly put the heating pad or Hydrocollator pack back on his chest, cover it with a towel, and cover the child with the sheet. After 3 minutes, briskly rub the chest with ice water and replace heat application.
Step 6. After 3 more minutes, remove the heat from the child's chest and rub it with an iced cloth. Dry his chest. Ask him to to sit up. Remove the heating pad from under his back and rub his back with the washcloth wrung out in ice water. Dry his back. Do not allow the child to become chilled. Replace any damp linen with dry linen.
Step 7. Ask the child to lay supine and begin the chest and upper back massage.

MASSAGE SEQUENCE FOR CHEST AND UPPER BACK

Step 1. Basic relaxation sequence.
Step 2. Chest and abdomen effleurage for 1 minute (Figure 3–34).
Step 3. Chest friction for 1 minute (Figure 3–35).
Step 4. Chest percussion (Figure 3–9). Cupping is used on the chest and upper back to help move mucus from the alveoli into the bronchial tubes, where coughing can expel the mucus from the body. As

you do cupping, ask the child to make a loud noise, and he will enjoy the resulting "funny sound." First, perform cupping on the chest for about 1 minute. Relax your hands and slightly cup them, then gently percuss the child's chest by alternately flexing and extending the wrists. This should not be painful—be firm but gentle. Avoid breast tissue on a girl.

Step 5.   Encourage the child to cough.

Step 6.   Repeat chest friction for 1 minute.

Step 7.   Repeat cupping for 1 minute.

Step 8.   Encourage the child to cough one more time.

Step 9.   Ask the child to turn on to his abdomen (prone position) and then perform back effleurage for 1 minute (Figure 3–2).

Step 10.   Perform cupping of the upper back for 1 minute. If there is mucus deep in the child's chest, while cupping have the child place his head over the end of the treatment table and prop his torso with pillows. A 30-degree angle is effective for allowing mucus to drain.

Step 11.   Encourage the child to cough.

Step 12.   Repeat back effleurage for 1 minute.

Step 13.   Have the child lie down to rest in a position where gravity will help the mucus to drain, such as the position in Step 10. Another effective position is to have the child lay down on one side, with pillows under where the ribcage touches the table. The chest is higher than the mouth in this position, and the mucus can drain from the lower part of the chest and be more readily coughed up.

CONSTIPATION

When a normally regular child has not had a bowel movement for 2 to 3 days or has difficulty having a bowel movement, she is considered constipated. If she has not had a bowel movement in 4 days, she should be seen by a physician to rule out any serious problems.

A diet high in fiber is the best way to prevent constipation. High fiber content is found in whole grains; food made with bran, such as cereal or muffins; beans; popcorn; fresh fruit and vegetables; and dried fruit, such as prunes and figs. Prune, apricot, and papaya juice are mild laxatives. Drinking plenty of water is important; doubling a child's water intake for a few days will often resolve constipation. Diuretics, bulk-forming laxatives, methylphenidate hydrochloride (Ritalin), and certain seizure medications and medications that affect peristalsis may cause the child to need more fluids and can contribute to constipation.[1]

APPROACH AND GOALS

The child's parent may try a simple hydrotherapy treatment for constipation: have the child drink one to two large glasses of lukewarm water first thing in the morning, at least one-half hour before breakfast. This often stimulates the intestines to move. If you have

taught the parents to perform abdominal effleurage, it can be done immediately.

Massage can relieve constipation by relaxing the abdominal musculature and stimulating peristalsis. If a child is chronically constipated, massage can be an important part of a regular program to resolve the problem. For some children, chronic tension in the gluteal muscles prevents them from relaxing the anal sphincter and having a bowel movement. Sandra Wheeler, an infant massage instructor, taught massage to the mother of a 6-month-old infant who was chronically constipated. The infant's pediatrician had told the mother that the child's constipation appeared to be caused by an anal sphincter that was too small and had prescribed suppositories for the infant. During massage instructions, however, Ms. Wheeler noticed that the infant's gluteal muscles were extremely tight. Infant massage strokes for the abdomen and simple Swedish massage of the buttocks completely resolved the infant's constipation (Wheeler S, personal communication, April 1992). Although infant massage is not discussed in this book, this story illustrates that children, even very young children, may have chronic gluteal tension that needs to be treated before constipation can be resolved.

MASSAGE AND HYDROTHERAPY FOR CONSTIPATION

HOT WATER BOTTLE OR HOT PACK APPLICATION

Place bottle or pack on the stomach for 10 minutes. This will not affect constipation, but will relieve discomfort and relax the abdomen in preparation for massage.

MASSAGE SEQUENCE FOR CONSTIPATION

Step 1.   Basic relaxation sequence (see page 70).

Step 2.   Apply oil or lotion.

Step 3.   Perform abdominal effleurage (Figure 3–36). Repeat 20 times.

Step 4.   Thumbstroke the stomach (see Figure 5–4). Sit at the child's right side. Begin just inside the right hipbone and thumbstroke straight up to the ribcage, across the top of the abdomen, and down the left side. Stop just above the left hipbone. Go slowly and thoroughly; the entire stroke should take 2 minutes to do one time. Use medium pressure. This stroke is extremely effective for constipation. Occasionally, infants and small children may have a bowel movement during abdominal massage. Older children may need to get up and go to the bathroom immediately.

Step 5.   Perform abdominal effleurage. Repeat 20 times.

Step 6.   Basic relaxation sequence (see page 70).

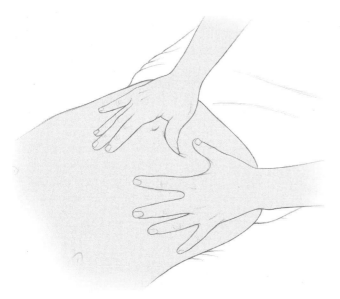

FIGURE 5–4 ■ Thumbstroking the Stomach. A deeper stroke that follows the path of the large intestine.

DEPRESSION

> I was giving a 20-year-old girl her first massage. When she was 14, she was severely depressed after her parents divorced. She ran away from home, lived on the streets, became addicted to heroin, and then went through a detox program. Now, 6 years later, although she was still free of her heroin addiction, she continued to struggle with depression. I was seeing her to treat severe muscle spasm and pain in her back. As soon as I began to massage her back, she turned around, looked up at me, and said, 'This is better than *any* drug!' Before this, she had equated something that made her feel good with something that was morally and physically bad for her. Sadly, after she went through the detox from heroin, she thought she would never experience pleasure again.
>
> —*Annie Siemens, massage therapist*
> *(personal communication, June 1999)*

It is estimated that 2% of American children and 8% (3 million) of adolescents are depressed.[1] Depression is a mood disorder characterized by feelings of hopelessness, sadness, loneliness, despair, low self-esteem, and social isolation. Depression is most often seen after a child has experienced a serious loss, such as a dear friend moving away, a death in the family, or a change of neighborhoods or schools. Known as reactive or situational depression, this is a normal reaction to loss.

When a child suffers more extreme depression that continues for an extended period, it changes from a normal, distressing reaction to something more serious. When the child not only feels sad, but also has sleep and appetite disturbances; feelings of worthlessness, guilt, and hopelessness; fatigue; and an inability to concentrate lasting 2 weeks or longer, the child is considered clinically depressed.

Signs of depression in infants and toddlers include depressed or irritable moods, excessive whining, sleeping and eating disturbances, weight loss, a loss of interest in activities, and decreased social interaction. In older children, some or all of the following signs may be seen: overactivity or underactivity, a sad appearance, irritability, anxiety, apathy, and difficulty dealing with frustration. Children will often have physical complaints, such as increased muscle tension, stomachaches, headaches, insomnia, diarrhea, or fatigue.[2] Blood tests may show increased levels of cortisol, a stress hormone. The signs of depression in teenagers are similar to those of children, but may also include substance abuse if teens begin using drugs or alcohol to soothe or escape from painful feelings. Teens who smoke may use nicotine to deal with feelings of depression and are more likely to become depressed than their nonsmoking peers. This may explain why antidepressant drugs can help adults quit smoking.[3]

Depression is linked to genetics and to the environment. You are at a higher risk for depression if you have a sibling or relative with depression.[2] The greater a child's total life stress, the greater the likelihood that she will be depressed. Major trauma in the first 4 years predisposes an adolescent to psychological problems, including depression, when stressful situations occur in the teen years.[4] Any child with a higher than average score on a life stress scale may be at risk for depression (Chapter 1).

Standard medical treatment for depression includes antidepressant medications and psychotherapy. Medication as a first-line course of treatment is used for children and adolescents with symptoms so severe that they would prevent effective psychotherapy, children with chronic depression, and children with chronic or recurring episodes. Following the remission of symptoms, treatment with medication and/or psychotherapy is normally continued for at least several months.[1] Between one-half million and one million prescriptions are written for antidepressants every year for American children and adolescents, and the number is growing.[5]

A mind-body approach that has had positive effects on depression in children is relaxation training. It can reduce anxiety and acting-out behavior and may be more effective than "talk" therapy. Many hypnotherapeutic techniques that treat **conversion disorders** in children combine hypnotherapy to help the child cope with her immediate anguish with long-term treatment. Children may learn self-hypnosis for relaxation and continue psychotherapy to treat long-term depression and other emotional problems.[6] In one study, children who were depressed and hospitalized in a psychiatric hospital were trained in relaxation techniques (yoga and progressive relaxation) and received massage therapy. The children in the study reported decreased anxiety, and they were observed by nurses to be less anxious and in more positive moods. Because more than one relaxation technique was used, it is not possible to tell which technique helped the most, although all three techniques have been shown to alleviate stress in children.[7]

APPROACH AND GOALS

Massage therapy alone is not a primary treatment for depression but can be an excellent adjunct treatment. Three Touch Research Institute studies assessed the effect of massage therapy on children who were depressed. In the first study, children ages 7 to 18, who were hospitalized for depression and other emotional disorders, were given 30 minutes of Swedish massage a day for 5 days. They were less anxious and depressed, slept better, and had lower levels of stress hormones.[8] In the second study, children ages 5 to 10, who had been through Hurricane Andrew in Florida in 1990 and had posttraumatic stress disorder, were given 30 minutes of Swedish-type back massage twice a week for 4 weeks; subsequently, they were less depressed.[9] In the third study, adolescent mothers, who had recently given birth and were depressed, were given a 30-minute Swedish massage 2 days a week for 5 consecutive weeks. They were less anxious, less depressed, and had lower stress hormones after their sessions.[10]

The author has treated a number of teenagers and young adults with depression, and found that massage not only offers relief from the pent-up physical tension that is such a major component of depression, but also helps by giving them another person to talk to and be part of their support system. A 15-year-old girl with severe depression was referred by a counselor to massage therapist Jane Megard. The counselor wanted to help the girl find ways to nurture herself. Over a 2-year period, a combination of medication, psychotherapy, and massage proved highly effective in relieving her depression (Megard J, personal communication, June 1999). Acupressure is also reported to relieve depression in children.[11]

The daughter of physical therapist Martha Pauly was a happy and highly functioning child until age 13, when she began to seem sad and withdrawn, and suffered from stomachaches and fatigue. Her family physician originally diagnosed her stomachaches as caused by anxiety and stress. When her stomachaches did not improve, she was seen by a social worker and a psychiatrist; both diagnosed her as seriously depressed. For months, she was prescribed powerful psychiatric medications and hospitalized, and her condition deteriorated dramatically. She became **catatonic**, paranoid, and

suicidal. Her family then decided to make a drastic change in the way the girl's depression was being treated. Gradually, she was weaned from psychiatric medications. Her new treatment was based on craniosacral therapy, herbs and supplements, and counseling. After a period of months, she gradually recovered from her depression, reentered school, and now continues to function at a high level. Her family believes that her original depression was triggered by hormonal imbalances, combined with a perfectionist personality.[12] Osteopath John Upledger has treated many depressed adults with craniosacral therapy and has never seen a case of severe depression without a severe anterior-posterior compression of the cranial base.[13]

MASSAGE THERAPY FOR CHILDREN WITH DEPRESSION

Massage therapy, while helpful, is not a cure for depression. Children should receive some type of regular psychotherapy as well as massage. The techniques presented in Chapter 3 may be used, as well as many other forms of massage and bodywork. Begin each massage with a progressive relaxation sequence to help the child learn to relax and release tension. Perform whole-body massage for several sessions before doing concentrated massage on any particular area, so that children get a clear sense of their total physical self. Any hands-on therapy that offers relaxation, nurturing touch, and personal contact with a caring adult will be beneficial. Regular massage will be required for at least a few months for a seriously depressed child. The therapist should be aware that the child may have a need to talk as much as a need to be massaged.

EARACHE

Ear infections are the most common cause of pediatric ear pain. Almost 35% of children have one or more ear infections in the first year of life, which can predispose them to recurring ear problems that may continue long into childhood.[1] Risk factors for pediatric ear infections are identified in Point of Interest Box 5–2. Earaches may also be caused by exposure to severe cold or injuries such as minor head trauma. At age 7, for example, the author's son fell from a diving board into a swimming pool in such a way that his entire body weight landed on one ear. He subsequently had pain in that ear in cold weather and when swimming underwater.

APPROACH AND GOALS

Massage and hydrotherapy treatments for earaches are not a substitute for medical treatment. When a child

POINT OF INTEREST BOX 5–2
Risk Factors for Ear Infections

Infants and children have more ear infections than adults because their eustachian tubes are wider, shorter, and more horizontal. As a result, children's middle ears are not able to drain as well as those of adults, and the eustachian tube opening may more easily be obstructed by mucus or debris. This allows bacterial infections to take hold more easily, as bacteria from the throat breed in the moist environment of a blocked eustachian tube. Common contributors to ear infections include:

- Upper respiratory problems, such as colds, asthma, or nasal congestion, precede nearly 50% of all ear infections.[1] Infants and toddlers in day care are twice as likely to contract an illness that lasts more than 10 days, causes a fever of 102° F for more than 3 days, or requires medical attention than children in home care.[1]
- High levels of certain toxic industrial chemicals.[2]
- Food allergies.
- Vitamin or mineral deficiencies.
- Being bottle-fed as a baby. Breast-fed babies have fewer ear infections than bottle-fed babies because their eustachian tube muscles are better developed and their eustachian tubes do not as easily fall shut.
- Living in a home where one or more adults smoke cigarettes.
- Being fed while lying flat on the back with a bottle propped in the mouth, or being put to bed with a bottle at night. Swallowing while lying down allows fluids to more readily enter and pool in the eustachian tube.
- Having fetal alcohol syndrome.
- Having Down syndrome.

References

1. Schmidt M: *Childhood Ear Infections: What Every Parent Should Know About Prevention, Home Care, and Alternative Treatment.* Berkeley, CA: North Atlantic Books, 1996, p 11, 179
2. Steingraber S: *Having Faith: An Ecologist's Journey to Motherhood.* Cambridge, MA: Perseus Publishing, 2001, p 271

1996), recommends that the front and sides of the neck be massaged to enhance tonsil and adenoid function, improve the environment of the eustachian tube area, and enhance lymphatic drainage.[1]

There is a special massage technique to drain the eustachian tube which is effective for congestion, called endonasal technique, that is often taught to the parents of a child with ear congestion. It is not covered in this book because it may not be in the scope of practice for massage therapists in many states. To learn more about this technique, contact a naturopathic physician.

MASSAGE AND HYDROTHERAPY FOR EARACHE

Use one of the following four treatments prior to massage:

MOIST HEAT APPLICATION TO THE EAR

Place heat on the ear for 30 minutes, using a small heating pad, washcloths wrung out in hot water (as hot as the child can tolerate), or a partially filled hot water bottle. Using a standard hot footbath at the same time will help alleviate congestion and pain.

HOT WATER GARGLE

Gargle with water that is as hot as can be tolerated for 10 minutes. This is a more appropriate treatment for an adult because it is too difficult for most young children to do without choking on the water; however, a teenager may be able to gargle without difficulty. The heat will relieve nasal and sinus congestion.

STEAM INHALATION

Refer to directions in the Common Cold section, page 121.

CONTRAST TREATMENT

Step 1. Wring out a washcloth or small towel in hot water. With the child lying on his side, apply the hot towel over the painful ear for 3 minutes. To keep the towel hot, cover it with a plastic bag and another towel.
Step 2. Wring out another washcloth or small towel in ice water. Apply it to the child's ear and leave on for 30 seconds.
Step 3. Repeat hot and cold (Steps 1 and 2) twice, for three changes.

has ear pain, only a physician can determine if an ear infection is present, and, if so, how it should be treated. Massage and hydrotherapy treatments can relieve pain, comfort a child and, possibly, promote faster healing.[2,3] Massage, if done gently and sensitively, will soothe and relax the area and improve the circulation of blood and lymphatic fluid. Dr. Michael Schmidt, author of *Childhood Ear Infections* (North Atlantic Books,

STERNOCLEIDOMASTOID MASSAGE

Positioning: Have the child lay supine, with a pillow under his head.

Step 1. Basic relaxation sequence.

Step 2. Gently apply oil or lotion.

Step 3. Perform superficial effleurage of the sternocleidomastoid muscle. Begin by placing your fingertips on the sternocleidomastoid, about 1 inch above the clavicle. Stroke down the muscle to the clavicle. The pressure should be directed as if to lengthen the muscle, and pressure should not be directed up against the neck. Repeat 10 times. Then move up about 1 inch and again stroke down the muscle toward the collarbone. Repeat 10 times. Again move up about 1 inch, and stroke toward the collarbone 10 times. Work your way gradually up the muscle toward the ear. Massage for about 1 minute, then repeat on the other side.

Step 4. Apply pressure to points on the sternocleidomastoid muscle (Figure 5–5). Do one side at a time. Begin at the base of the muscle and press four separate points between the base of the muscle at the clavicle and the top. Gently pinch the muscle between your thumb and middle finger and pull it away from the neck. Hold each point for about 10 seconds. Do not push down into the child's neck or on the child's throat. Press each point just until the beginning of pain. Ask the child for feedback. You might say, "Tell me when this just begins to hurt, and I will stop right there." You establish trust with the child when you work at his tolerance

level and listen carefully to his feedback. Hold all the points on the left sternocleidomastoid and then repeat on the right side.

 Parents of a child with an earache should check with the physician if they suspect the child has an ear infection. A child with ear pain should always be seen by a physician if he has a temperature higher than 103° F, if he refuses to drink liquids, or if he has a stiff neck or headache.

EYE FATIGUE AND STRAIN

Children are not born with adult visual capabilities. The visual system at birth is so immature that everything appears blurred (acuity is 20/600; 30 times worse than 20/20) and almost all adult visual skills are absent. These include the ability to distinguish color, to move the eyes without moving the head, to use both eyes together, to locate objects in space, to detect contrasts, to follow moving objects, and to perceive depth. All these skills will develop as the connections between the eye and brain mature. 20/20 vision is not reached until children are ages 3 to 5; their visual system typically does not fully mature until age 12.[1,2] Visual development is an ongoing process that is deeply affected by children's physical and emotional states and by the environment in

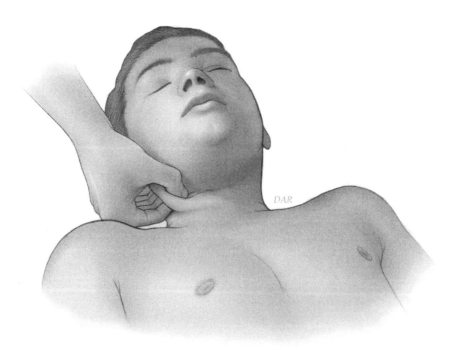

FIGURE 5–5 ■ Pressure Points on the Sternocleidomastoid Muscle.

which they live. Natural vision improvement teacher Janet Goodrich describes eyesight as "a living, changing expression intimately reflecting the child's inner life."[3] Any problem that obscures vision or interferes with the normal coordination of the eyes can affect a child's visual development.

Eye fatigue and eyestrain may occur to any child, with or without a normal visual system. Their complaints may include eyes that are tired, sore, dry, or itchy; blurred vision; headaches; double vision; body fatigue; or tension in the eyes, temples, forehead, neck, shoulders, or back. They may complain of headache or eye pain after an extended period of near-vision tasks, such as working at a computer or reading a book. Or they may simply seem overly tired for no obvious reason. Chronic tension in the muscles of the head and upper body may be a sign of chronic overwork or inappropriate use of the visual system.

CAUSES OF EYE FATIGUE

What causes eye fatigue and strain?

1. Trying to use the eyes when there is an uncorrected vision problem. Up to 5% of infants are born with some kind of visual abnormality or will develop one in the first few years of life. In young children, the most common visual deficiencies are **myopia, hyperopia, astigmatism,** and **strabismus.** Older children may or may not outgrow these problems. One national health survey of 7,000 American youths, ages 12 to 17, found that one of 12 had significant visual problems and 43% were unable to read at a 20/20 level.[4] Many of the causes of the common visual deficiencies are unknown. Other than mechanical eye problems, nutrition, illness, trauma at critical stages of visual development, and even misalignment of the cranial bones may affect the child's vision.[5-7]

2. Emotional stress. "One day, when I was 7 years old, I was playing alone in my bedroom. I decided to go downstairs for a snack. I remember coming down the stairs and opening the door to the kitchen. As I stepped in, I realized that my mother, father, and sister were in the kitchen. I watched as my father threw my sister into a corner of the room. She fell on the floor and he began to kick her. My sister and father were both screaming, and my mother and I were paralyzed. I wonder now if I was going into shock. I heard knocking and looked over at the sliding glass door in the living room. My friend Ann was behind the glass door and was trying to look through. She could see me. I remember being terrified that she would see what was happening in the kitchen. I still could not move and then I realized that my vision was changing. Everything went blurry and objects became less clearly defined. I have never regained the visual acuity I lost that day. I got my first pair of glasses soon afterward and have needed glasses for the last 40 years." (Author's client, personal communication, October 2002)

Emotional stress may be manifested by chronic tension in the internal muscles of the eye (those that change the shape of the lens and the size of the pupil) or in the external muscles that move the eyeballs, close the eyelids, furrow the brow, and squint. For example, emotional stress causes the pupillary muscles to dilate to allow better peripheral and night vision. Many optometrists, individuals with vision problems, teachers of natural vision improvement, and psychiatrists have observed that the eye may become the target organ for the expression of a variety of emotional conflicts and stress.[8,9] A period of high stress caused by such events as a death or divorce in the family, a move to a new home, or a negative learning situation in school may interfere with a critical phase of normal visual development.[2,5,10-13]

3. Excessive close work, such as reading, doing computer work, or performing other near-vision tasks, can cause tremendous stress on an immature visual system. A study at the University of California at Berkeley of 253 children found that multiple-hour computer use leads to focusing problems and nearsightedness or farsightedness. Before children were spending so much time on the computer, a similar pattern was seen in those who were reading chapter books before fourth grade.[14] An overload of schoolwork in the primary grades may stress the vision system to the point of causing a breakdown in the child's visual skills. To perform near-vision work, the child's visual system must be mature enough to perform a variety of visual tasks, such as focusing, tracking a line of print across the printed page, using the two eyes together, converging, and recognizing different shapes.

To prevent visual strain when performing near-vision tasks, children should pause at the end of each page to look out a window, take a deep breath, and blink. This will rest and moisten the eyes. A big yawn will stimulate the eyes to water. The eyes should also be rested at least every 20 minutes when writing, watching TV, or using a computer. If things look blurry when children look up, they should get up and move around before attempting to read again.

MUSCULOSKELETAL ADAPTATIONS TO VISUAL PROBLEMS, EMOTIONAL STRESS, AND EXCESSIVE CLOSE WORK

The musculature of the head and neck can be affected and, in certain ways, shaped by the child's vision. For example, movement teacher Moshe Feldenkrais observed that, with a dominant eye, the muscles that turn the head are very different. "The left sternocleidomastoid muscle in a left-eyed person will be softer. The right sternocleidomastoid, which contracts to turn the head to the left, will be stronger, stiffer, and less nimble."[15]

Holding the head in unusual positions to accommodate visual problems may cause chronic tension in the upper back, cervical, or facial regions. Uncorrected myopia, for example, can activate trigger points in the suboccipital muscles as a result of sustained forward flexion of the head and neck.[16] If a myopic child slouches forward and strains to see, he or she may have deep tension in the jaw, neck, shoulders, and erector spinae muscles.[17] Vertical strabismus, when one eye is higher than the other, will cause the child to tilt the head in an attempt to keep the eyes level. This can cause a type of torticollis in which the head is persistently laterally flexed and rotated on the neck and the sternocleidomastoid and other cervical muscles are overcontracted on one side.[18] The child with decreased visual acuity, for any reason, is likely to activate trigger points in the occipitalis muscle by persistently contracting the forehead and scalp muscles.[16] Anyone who is light-sensitive or has astigmatism is likely to squint, which can activate trigger points in the orbicularis oculi.[16] Astigmatism is often accompanied by tension in the muscles of the neck, particularly the muscle around the top cervical vertebrae.[19]

Wearing glasses for correction of visual problems may also cause tension in the upper body. Cocking the head to avoid the reflection of overhead lights can chronically strain the sternocleidomastoid.[16] If the lenses have too short a focal length, causing the child to tilt the head in sustained flexion in order to read or do other close work or if the frames of the eyeglasses are improperly adjusted (causing the child to tilt his head too far forward to read), trigger points can be activated in the suboccipital, semispinalis, capitis, semispinalis cervicis, and multifidi muscles.[16] All children who wear glasses should be checked for tension in the muscles of the head, neck, and face.

APPROACH AND GOALS

Massage and hydrotherapy can increase circulation and ease muscle tension in and around the eyes. Heat applications over the eyes are soothing, increase circulation, and relieve pain and inflammation. Cold applications initially cause vasoconstriction, which is then followed by vasodilation. Cold is effective in relieving pain and promoting healing in the eyes.[20] Alternating hot-and-cold applications causes a dramatic increase in the blood flow to the eyes. The goal of massage is to relieve muscle tension and improve circulation in the eyes and the surrounding area. Because eyestrain may cause tension, not only in the eyes but also in other parts of the child's body, a massage for eyestrain includes techniques for the face, especially around the eyes, and techniques for the neck and upper trapezius. Children may be taught to massage around their eyes to relieve tension.

Many teachers of natural vision improvement have successfully reduced or eliminated strabismus, myopia, hyperopia, and astigmatism in children using exercises that relax and stimulate the eyes and with massage that treats tension of the eyes and the entire upper body. Helping the child understand the contribution stress makes to vision problems has been an important part of therapy.[3] Osteopath John Upledger has successfully treated cases of strabismus and problems with visual acuity with craniosacral therapy; he believes that malalignment of the cranial bones, such as lateral strain lesions of the cranial base, and atlanto-occipital dysfunction, may be directly related to visual problems.[7]

Palming is another way to relax the eyes. The child cups her hands over the eyes, crossing the fingers over the middle of the forehead. Pressure is not put on the eyes or on the eyebrows; the eyes are simply covered to block out the light. The child should then take deep comfortable breaths and let the eyes relax. And, last but not least, the child can learn to massage his or her own face, especially around the eyes.

MASSAGE AND HYDROTHERAPY FOR EYE FATIGUE AND STRAIN

CONTRAST TREATMENT

Step 1. Have the child lie down. Fold a washcloth into a narrow strip, and dip it into a bowl of water (temperature, 110° F). Wring the cloth out and place it over the child's eyes. Because the skin over the eyes is very thin, ask the child if the washcloth is too hot and, if so, let it cool a moment before reapplying. Leave it on the eyes for 3 minutes. If the washcloth appears to be cooling off too much, replace it with another cloth after 2 minutes.

Step 2. Fold another washcloth into a narrow strip and dip it into a bowl of very cold water (put ice cubes in the water to make it as cold as possible). Wring the cloth out and cover the eyes, making sure the nostrils are exposed. Leave it on for 1 minute.

Step 3. Repeat hot and cold (Steps 1 and 2) twice, for three changes.

MASSAGE SEQUENCE FOR EYE FATIGUE AND STRAIN

Positioning: The child should be supine on the treatment table or the floor, with the therapist seated at the child's head.

Step 1. Basic relaxation sequence (see page 70).

Step 2. Apply oil or lotion to face.

Step 3. Perform forehead and eye circles (Figures 3–30 and 3–31). Repeat 10 times.

Step 4. Make small circles on the temples; go slowly and use as much pressure as you can without causing pain. Repeat for 1 minute or more.

Step 5. Thumbstroke between the eyebrows. Thumbstroke toward yourself instead of away. Place your thumbs next to each other between the eyebrows. Stroke up with one thumb, then the other. Return your first thumb to the starting position and stroke upward; return your second thumb to the starting position and stroke upward. Continue for 30 seconds or more.

Step 6. Perform forehead and eye circles. Repeat 10 times.

Step 7. Pressure points around the eyes. Do both sides at once (Figures 5–1 and 5–2). Begin at the inside corner of each eye socket, just below the beginning of the eyebrow. With your index fingers, gently curl underneath the ridge of bone and press upward. (Do not press on the eye.) Press to the point of soreness, not pain; back off a bit and maintain that pressure for 10 seconds. Do a second and a third point, evenly spaced in the middle part of each socket, and finish with a fourth point at the outside corner. Hold each point for 10 seconds. Using your thumbs, press on a fifth and sixth point in the middle of the socket below the eye, and finish with a seventh point at the inside corner.

Step 8. Face effleurage (Figures 3–32 and 3–33).

Step 9. Petrissage of the scalp (Figure 3–29).

Step 10. Pressure points on the base of the occiput (Figure 5–6). Let the child's head rest in your hands, as in scalp petrissage. Curl your fingertips under the bony ridge at the base of the skull (close to the hairline). Begin with a pressure point just a little to either side of the midline. Do both sides at once. Press upward with your middle fingers. Press just to the point of soreness (not pain), then back off slightly and hold for 15 seconds. Do two more points, moving out toward the ear. Ask the child to help you locate points that are tight or sore. Hold each point for 15 seconds.

Step 11. Pressure points on the sternocleidomastoid muscle (Figure 5–5).

Step 12. Pressure points on the upper trapezius (Figure 5–7). Begin this stroke where the neck intersects the shoulder, and do both sides at once. With your thumbs, press directly down (toward the feet) just to the point of soreness (not pain), then back off slightly and hold for 10 seconds. Do three more points along the top of the shoulder (as if you were following the shoulder seam on a shirt), moving away from the neck. Ask the child to help you locate points that feel tight or sore. Hold for 10 seconds each.

Step 13. Face effleurage; repeat six times.

Step 14. Cup your hands gently over the child's eyes, with fingertips pointing toward each other. Be careful not to press on the eyeball. Remind the child to relax the eyes. Hold for 30 seconds, then slowly take your hands away.

Step 15. Basic relaxation sequence.

GAS PAIN

A couple years back, I took care of a 9-year-old boy who was a quadriplegic and had been on a respirator for 5 years. He would swallow a lot of air trying to talk around his respirator and have terrible stomachaches. Massaging his stomach helped relieve the pain and gas. I would also massage his legs, arms, and chest. He really enjoyed the massage. It gave him a lot of sensory stimulation, as well as relaxation.

—*Julie Fronzuto, RN (intensive care nurse, personal communication, December 1991)*

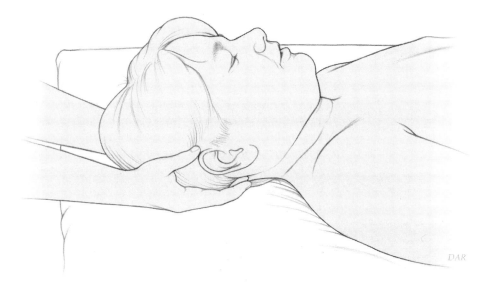

FIGURE 5–6 ■ Pressure Points of the Base of the Occiput. These points are useful in tension headache massage.

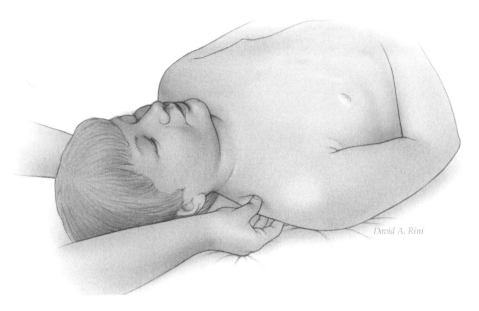

David A. Rini

FIGURE 5–7 ■ Pressure Points on the Upper Trapezius.

Gas pain is caused by the excessive collection of gas in the stomach or intestines. Many a parent has been faced with a small child with such severe abdominal pain that he or she has called their family physician, worried that the child might have appendicitis or another severe problem, only to have the child pass gas while waiting to hear the physician's voice! For children prone to severe gas pain, a few simple suggestions to parents may help:

- Food should be eaten slowly and not gulped down.
- Children should move around after eating rather than sitting still—this moves gas.
- Foods that are known to cause gas in a particular child should be avoided.
- Hot drinks, especially peppermint tea, may help children pass gas.

APPROACH AND GOALS

Hydrotherapy can help prepare the child's abdomen for massage by relaxing the abdominal musculature. Abdominal massage is effective for gas pain because it relaxes the abdominal musculature even further, and stimulates movement of gas through the intestine.

MASSAGE AND HYDROTHERAPY FOR GAS PAIN

MOIST HEAT APPLICATION

Step 1. Wrap a hot towel wrung out in hot water and covered with wool or polar fleece, a moist heating pad, or a hydrocollator pack around the waist area, and leave it on for 10 to 15 minutes.

MASSAGE SEQUENCE FOR THE ABDOMEN

Step 1. Use the same strokes used to treat constipation (see page 124).
Step 2. Concentrate the massage on less sensitive areas (if the child's abdomen is sensitive to pressure) until his abdominal muscles begin to relax and the gas begins to move. Pressure should be to the child's tolerance level.
Step 3. A few drops of essential oil of peppermint may be added to the massage oil or lotion.

GROWING PAINS IN THE LEGS

Growing pains are defined as deep and recurring aches, typically felt by children in their legs. Although the pains have no known cause, growing pains are clearly not related to any disease process. Approximately 15–30% of children experience them between the ages of 4 and 12. Usually growing pains are experienced late in the day or at night, often with such severity that the children are awakened from sleep. Days, weeks, or months may go by without the pains occurring.[1]

Although no cause has been proven, most physicians attribute them to muscle spasms that result from fatigue and ischemia of leg muscles that have been active during the day or to inflammation of the leg muscles as a result of overexercise. Either theory explains why a child could be active until bedtime, go to sleep without leg pains, and wake up with them in the night. Some physicians believe that emotional stress may also contribute to growing pains.[2] Medication and warm soaks are the standard treatment.

APPROACH AND GOALS

Treatment of the leg muscles has shown success in treating growing pains. Pediatricians Talcott Bates and Edward Grunwaldt relate the case of a 3-year-old boy who had such severe calf pain that he napped poorly during the day and awoke screaming at least five times each night. Treatment of trigger points in the vastus lateralis and gluteus minimus muscles of both legs was performed four times at 2-day intervals, using ethyl chloride spray and stretching. The child no longer complained of pain and slept well at nap and nighttime.[3] Another muscle treatment that has been successful is stretching of the quadriceps, gastrocnemius, soleus, and hamstring muscles (Figure 5–8). A study was made of 34 children between the ages of 5 and 14 who were divided into either a control group that received no stretching exercises or a muscle-stretching group. Parents of children in the second group were taught to stretch their childrens' leg muscles for 10 minutes twice a day. Children in the muscle-stretching group had a significant decrease in growing pains compared with the children in the control group.[2]

Massage therapy and hydrotherapy can relieve growing pains by decreasing muscle tension and increasing circulation in the legs. These soothing treatments are especially appropriate to teach to parents because they need to be done when the child is in pain, which is usually at night.

MASSAGE AND HYDROTHERAPY FOR GROWING PAINS

WARM BATHS

Simply taking a warm bath at about 102° F for 20 minutes will soothe growing pains for many children; however, this will not stimulate the circulation in the legs as much as a contrast treatment.

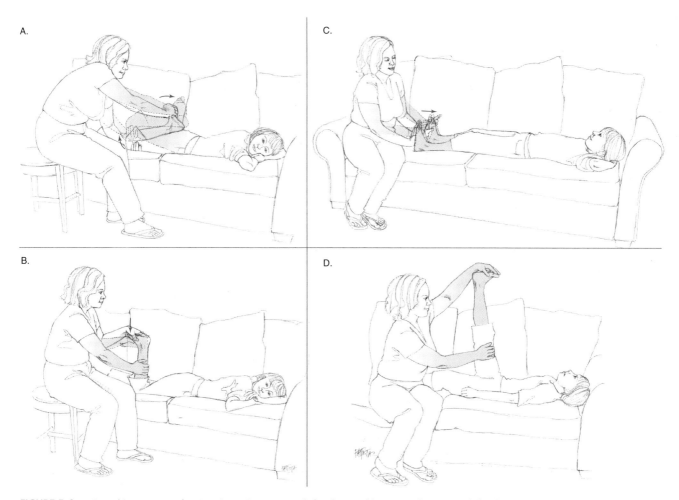

FIGURE 5–8 ■ Stretching Program for Growing Pains. **A,** Stretch for the quadriceps muscle; **B,** Stretch for the gastrocnemius and soleus muscles; **C,** Stretch for the gastrocnemius and soleus muscles; **D,** Stretch for the hamstrings.

CONTRAST TREATMENT

Step 1. Fill two deep buckets or washtubs with water; one tub with water at 110° F and one tub with water at about 60° F. It may be necessary to add ice cubes to the tap water to reach this temperature.

Step 2. Place the child's feet in the hot water for 2 minutes.

Step 3. Place the child's feet in the cold water for 1 minute.

Step 4. Repeat hot and cold (Steps 2 and 3) twice, for three changes.

Step 5. Dry the child's feet.

MASSAGE SEQUENCE AND STRETCHING OF THE LEGS (FIGURE 5–8)

Step 1. Basic relaxation sequence.

Step 2. Apply oil or lotion.

Step 3. Effleurage the back of the leg, 1 minute (Figure 3–21).

Step 4. Rake the back of the leg, 2 minutes (Figure 3–22).

Step 5. Thumbstroke the back of the leg, 1 minute (Figure 3–23).

Step 6. Effleurage the back of the leg, 1 minute.

Step 7. Stretch the quadriceps. Hold for 15 to 20 seconds and repeat 10 times.

Step 8. Stretch the gastrocnemius and soleus, with child prone. Hold for 15 to 20 seconds and repeat 10 times.

Step 9. Stretch gastrocnemius and soleus, with child supine. Hold for 15 to 20 seconds and repeat 10 times.

Step 10. Stretch the hamstrings. Hold for 15 to 20 seconds and repeat 10 times.

Step 11. Basic relaxation sequence.

HEADACHE

As many as two-thirds of children complain of headaches severe enough to seek medical attention at some time during childhood.[1] More than 40% of all children have had a headache by the age 7 and, by age 15, 20% will have experienced frequent headaches.[2] In this section, we discuss five common types of headaches. You should never try to diagnose the cause of a child's headache because a headache can have many causes, some more serious than others. The child's family physician should be consulted when a child has repeated headaches or even one severe headache.

DEHYDRATION HEADACHE

Water makes up 60% of the human body and is critical for body function. It is needed to digest and absorb the nutrients in food; circulate blood; excrete wastes; transport nutrients to cells; carry waste materials and salts to the kidneys; build tissue; maintain body temperature; cushion joints; and keep body tissues, such as the eyes and air passages, moist. Body fluids, such as blood, lymphatic fluid, and cerebrospinal fluid, are 80% water. Nutritionists consider water one of the 6 major nutrients; the others are carbohydrates, fat, protein, vitamins, and minerals.[1]

Dehydration, the loss of water in body tissue, is a common and often unrecognized cause of headaches in children and can also be a contributing factor in other types of headaches. Dehydration can also cause daytime fatigue and irritability in children and may contribute to constipation as well. A mere 2% drop in body water can lower mental alertness and trigger fuzzy short-term memory, trouble with basic math, and difficulty focusing on a computer screen or printed page. More severe dehydration can occur when children have high fevers, diarrhea, frequent vomiting, or if they overexercise in hot weather. Major clinical signs of dehydration, including decreased peripheral perfusion, occur at 3–4% body dehydration in young children and indicate admission to the hospital for treatment with intravenous fluid.[2]

When children are dehydrated, their bodies make less saliva and their mouths get dry, which should be a signal to drink fluids. Unfortunately, many children do not feel thirsty until they have become very dehydrated. Children need to acquire the habit of drinking water, and plenty of it, early in life. The average amount of water a child needs in a single day is:

- five 8-ounce glasses of water for the average 3-year-old (30 pounds)
- six glasses of water for the average 6-year-old (60 pounds)
- six and one-half glasses of water for the average 8-year-old (75 pounds)
- eight glasses of water for the average 12-year-old (90 pounds)

Approach and Goals

When seeing a child who has a headache for any reason, encourage him or her to drink water or rehydration drinks as if he or she had a dehydration headache. At the least, a child who has any type of headache will feel better when well-hydrated and, possibly, the headache will be greatly diminished.

When the author's son was age 10 and weighed 90 pounds, he suffered from excruciating dehydration headaches that were associated with taking hot baths or exercising in hot weather. If he drank two full glasses of water, waited 20 minutes, and drank one more glass of water, his headaches would disappear.

Massage and Hydrotherapy for Dehydration Headaches

DRINKING WATER

As soon as possible, have the child drink one to two glasses of water, depending on body size. Repeat 20 minutes later.

MASSAGE SEQUENCE FOR MUSCLE CONTRACTION HEADACHES

(See page 137)

EYESTRAIN HEADACHES

A full discussion of eye fatigue and strain was given earlier in this chapter. To treat an eyestrain headache, follow the massage and hydrotherapy treatment sequence for eyestrain, page 131.

MIGRAINE HEADACHES

A migraine is a severely painful headache, usually limited to one side of the head and accompanied by vertigo, nausea, hypersensitivity to light, a perception of flashing lights, or other visual disorders. Migraine headaches begin with extreme vasoconstriction of the blood vessels of the brain on the affected side of the head. During this warning phase, children may have feelings of dread, blurred vision, or other sensations indicating they are about to have a migraine. After 2 to 4 hours, the vasoconstriction phase ends and the next phase of a migraine begins. This is an extreme vasodilation of the blood vessels of the brain, and it causes the actual pain of the migraine. The brain is encased in the bones of the skull, and the increased blood in its vessels causes increased pressure on the structures of the brain. This pressure not only causes the pain but also causes the neurologic symptoms; both typically last for several hours. Compared with adults, pediatric migraines are of shorter duration and less likely to have a visual aura, but more likely to be accompanied by nausea and vomiting.[1]

Most adults with migraines had their first migraine as a child. Between 4% and 11% of children have migraines headaches,[1,2] and 70–80% of children with migraines have other family members who experience migraines, as well.[3]

Many things can trigger migraines in susceptible children. Triggers do not necessarily start a migraine every time they occur, and it may take a combination of triggers to start an attack. For example, if a child is tense and dehydrated and eats a food that is a trigger for him, it may be this combination that precipitates a headache. High levels of emotional stress, including immediate stress, anxiety, depression and, especially, repressed anger, are potent triggers. Individuals prone to migraines appear to have a generalized hypersensitivity to emotional stress, which they react to with their vascular system.[3,4]

Other migraine triggers in susceptible children include dehydration, altitude changes, fatigue, fluctuations in hormone levels related to menstruation, certain foods (probably due to food allergies), anxiety, low blood glucose levels, and minor head trauma.[3] Upledger believes that malalignment of the cranial bones contributes to migraine as well.[5] Trigger points in the temporalis, occipitalis, and posterior cervicals muscles are also known migraine inducers.[6,7] Talcott Bates treated a 9-year-old boy who had "severe prostrating headaches accompanied by nausea, vertigo, and vomiting." His headaches were eliminated with trigger point therapy of his right sternocleidomastoid muscle.[8]

Childhood migraine headaches have been successfully decreased through a variety of nonmedication methods, including progressive relaxation, cognitive coping, self-hypnosis, progressive relaxation, and autogenic relaxation. Some techniques have been more effective than standard migraine medication, indicating that the mind-body connection can be used to good advantage.[2,9] At the Diamond Headache Clinic in Chicago, Illinois, patients learn different types of biofeedback to control migraines, including increasing the temperature of the hands by visualization (i.e., relaxing at the beach with their hands in hot sand) and using electromyograph biofeedback to reduce tension in different muscle groups. Biofeedback also helps them identify common physical signs of stress, such as tooth grinding or shoulder tightening. Clinic director Seymour Diamond states, "Children with headaches are excellent candidates for biofeedback training. They are more receptive to learning new techniques and have not learned the pain behavior so often seen in adult headache patients."[3]

Approach and Goals

Although some therapists have reported success in relieving migraine headaches with deep tissue massage or craniosacral therapy (Nelson C, personal communication, July 2002),[10] when a migraine headache begins, massage treatment will not always relieve it; the longer the migraine continues, the less likely that massage will help. However, the classic hydrotherapy treatment for a migraine headache, a hot footbath, can be effective in the early stages of a headache. By immersing the feet in hot water, the blood vessels dilate and blood is drawn from congested areas. The hands may be immersed in hot water at the same time. An ice pack on the back of the neck will assist with vasoconstriction of blood vessels to the brain. Point of Interest Box 5–3 describes one woman's success with hydrotherapy for migraines.

Although massage may not relieve a migraine, children still find massage soothing, especially massage of the upper body. For 4 years, the author treated a boy who had his first migraine at age 10. Some effective treatments for this boy were:

POINT OF INTEREST BOX 5–3
Hot Water Can Dilate Blood Vessels to Relieve Migraine Headaches

This quotation illustrates the way that the derivative effect of hot water can work:

> For years, I have suffered from recurring migraine headaches. I believe I tried every medication and vitamin on the market to ease the migraine pain and all except B complex vitamins gave either no pain relief or caused such unwanted side effects as insomnia and stomach distress. The B complex vitamins eased the pain so that I could at least crawl out of bed, but I had to take the vitamins every few hours round-the-clock for 3 or 4 days just to tolerate the lingering pain. Raising an active 2-year-old girl, I decided I needed more relief.
>
> Somewhere in the jungle of headache books I had read, I learned that, during a migraine, the head's blood vessels are dilated and swollen and that biofeedback could teach me to move that excess blood down to my hands, constricting the head's blood vessels back to normal and relieving the headache. Well, that was fine, but where do I go to learn biofeedback? During my search for a biofeedback training center, I was struck by another migraine. I was determined to keep functioning—feeding my daughter, doing the laundry, and washing the dirty dishes. I ran hot, hot water to rinse off my dishes and, while rinsing, I felt my headache ebb. I could feel the blood draining out of my head like the tide washing away from the shore. It dawned on me that I was practicing my own biofeedback, by immersing my bare hands in the hot water. The blood vessels in my hands were dilating to allow blood to rush to the area and carry away the heat. That took the pressure out of my head. The dishes were clean and my headache was gone.
>
> *JLT (California), quoted in Bricklin M: Rodale's* Encyclopedia of Natural Home Remedies. *Emmaus, PA: Rodale Press, p 256*

1. A very hot bath, in which only the boy's lower body was immersed.
2. A hot footbath, combined with the massage strokes for tension headache. In this case, the boy would lie on the treatment table and receive a hot footbath while getting a massage.
3. Massage alone, using the strokes for tension headache.

Typically, these treatments did not eliminate the migraine, but greatly decreased the amount of pain the boy was experiencing, and he found them both soothing and nurturing.

Regular massage therapy, as part of a stress-reduction program, may also help susceptible children prevent tension buildup that can trigger migraines. A study at the Touch Research Institute included adults with migraines. They received ten 30-minute Swedish massages for 5 weeks. This regular massage therapy significantly reduced the number and severity of the study participants' migraines. Hopefully, this research will be repeated with children.[11]

Massage and Hydrotherapy for Migraine Headaches

HOT FOOT SOAK AND ICE PACK

Step 1. Make sure the child is well hydrated.
Step 2. Give him a 20-minute footbath (temperature, 110° F), combined with a cold compress to the forehead and an ice pack to the back of the neck (Figure 3–52). The child may be seated in a chair; at a counter with his feet in a sink, if he is small enough; or lying down on a treatment table with his knees up and his feet in a basin. The water in the footbath must be kept at 110° F for the entire treatment; as the water cools, more hot water must be added. The hot water should be added carefully so that it is not poured directly on the child's feet, and the cold compress should be changed every 3 minutes.
Step 3. Pour cold water over his feet, dry them off, and have him lie down and rest for at least 20 minutes.

MASSAGE SEQUENCE FOR MIGRAINE HEADACHE

Same as for Muscle Contraction Headache, see page 137.

MUSCLE CONTRACTION HEADACHES

In younger children, the cause of head pain is frequently stress. Stress and tension can cause headaches even in 5-year-olds; in older children, most headaches are due to stress. Muscle spasms in the neck and scalp

cause these pains, aggravated possibly by a widening of blood vessels inside the brain. Tension headaches can occur in any part of the head, produce a dull or swollen feeling inside the head, and usually come on slowly. Headaches are often the first symptom of stressful problems at school, at home, or with friends.[1]
—*R. Pantell*

A muscle contraction headache is caused by muscle contraction, spasm, and irritation of trigger points in the face, head, neck, or upper back. Tension in the neck and shoulder muscles can have many causes, as discussed previously in this chapter, and emotional stress may combine with this tension to produce a headache.

Approach and Goals

Hydrotherapy treatments can increase circulation to the neck and head muscles. Massage treatment, by relieving muscle tension, is frequently successful at relieving the pain of a muscle contraction headache. It can also provide nurturing, comforting personal contact.

Massage and Hydrotherapy for Muscle Contraction Headaches

These treatments are especially appropriate to teach to parents because they will often be with the child when he has a headache.

COLD APPLICATION TO THE NECK OR SCALP

Choose one:

1. Run cold water in the sink. Stand the child in front of the sink, on a stool if necessary, and put his head in the sink. Let the water run over his scalp for 3 minutes. Towel the hair dry. It will be difficult to persuade most children to tolerate the cold water; a more tolerable treatment is an ice application.
2. Place an ice pack on the back of the child's neck for 10 minutes.

MASSAGE SEQUENCE FOR TENSION HEADACHE

Positioning:

This sequence can be done sitting at a treatment table or on the floor, while you sit cross-legged at the child's head.

Step 1. Basic relaxation sequence (see page 70).
Step 2. Apply oil or lotion.
Step 3. Effleurage shoulder and neck 10 times (Figures 3–26 and 3–27).
Step 4. Perform diagonal neck stroke, 10 times (Figure 3–28).
Step 5. Effleurage shoulder and neck, 10 times.

Step 6. Petrissage scalp, 1 minute (Figure 3–29).
Step 7. Knead the upper trapezius (Figure 3–17). Knead each side for 30 seconds or more. Myofascial trigger points in the fibers of the upper trapezius are sources of temporal headache, tension neckache, and referred pain to the side of the neck, mastoid process, temple, occiput, and back of the eye orbit. Of all the muscles in the body, the trapezius is most likely to harbor trigger points.[2]
Step 8. Perform diagonal neck stroke, 10 times.
Step 9. Pressure points on the base of the occiput (Figure 5–6).
Step 10. Effleurage shoulder and neck, 10 times.
Step 11. Basic relaxation sequence.

SINUS HEADACHE

Sinus headaches are caused by sinus congestion, and they may be either acute or chronic. They can also be caused by inflammation resulting from allergies or infections, which often develop in the later stages of a cold.

Approach and Goals

Massage and hydrotherapy can reduce sinus congestion and increase circulation to the face and sinuses, relieving the pain of congestion.

Massage and Hydrotherapy for Sinus Headache

HYDROTHERAPY FOR SINUS CONGESTION

See treatments for sinus congestion described in the common cold section of this chapter. A hot foot soak may be given to the child on the treatment table while he is receiving massage.

MASSAGE SEQUENCE FOR SINUS HEADACHE

Positioning:

Position yourself as for a head massage.
Step 1. Basic relaxation sequence.
Step 2. Apply oil or lotion.
Step 3. Perform diagonal neck stroke (Figure 3–28). Repeat 20 times.
Step 4. Pressure points on the upper trapezius (Figure 5–7).
Step 5. Petrissage scalp (Figure 3–29).
Step 6. Perform forehead and eye circles (Figures 3–30 and 3–31).
Step 7. Put your thumbs along either side of the nose, level with the eyes; stroke slowly and firmly down to the bottom of the nose. Repeat 10 times.
Step 8. Pressure points around the eyes (Figures 5–1 and 5–2).

Step 9. Pressure points on the side of the nose. Begin just below the bottom of the eye socket. Press with your thumbs on either side of the nose just below the eye socket, as if you were trying to touch them together. Use gentle to moderate pressure, as firm as the child can tolerate. Press at a second point in the middle of the nose and a third point at the bottom.

Step 10. Perform forehead and eye circles. Repeat 10 times.

Step 11. Basic relaxation sequence.

 If the child has a sinus infection (not just sinus inflammation) or a fever, massage is contraindicated.

INSOMNIA

Insomnia is a common problem for children and can be a sign of stress, anxiety, or depression. In children who are highly active and have trouble falling asleep in general, however, insomnia is not necessarily a sign of stress but may simply reflect a nervous system that is "wired" differently. When these children are overtired, they have great difficulty falling asleep; allowing them to stay up too long will make it difficult for them to unwind and fall asleep. To go to sleep easily, all children need regular bedtimes and environments that are calm and quiet.

APPROACH AND GOALS

Hydrotherapy and massage are soothing, nurturing, relaxing, and helpful for children with sleep problems. Bedtime rituals help a child learn to gradually slow down and, when taught to parents, massage and hydrotherapy can be incorporated into them. Regular therapy can also be part of a stress-reduction program for a child with insomnia who is tense, anxious, or depressed.

MASSAGE AND HYDROTHERAPY FOR INSOMNIA

WARM BATHS

Have the child take a warm bath (temperature, 100° F) for 20 minutes.

MASSAGE SEQUENCE FOR INSOMNIA

Positioning:
Begin with the child lying in the prone position.

Step 1. Basic relaxation sequence (page 70).

Step 2. Apply oil or lotion.

Step 3. Perform back effleurage (Figure 3–2). Repeat 20 times.

Step 4. Ask the child to turn over into the supine position and reapply oil or lotion.

Step 5. Perform shoulder and neck effleurage (Figures 3–26 and 3–27). Repeat 10 times.

Step 6. Perform diagonal neck stroke (Figure 3–28). Repeat 10 times.

Step 7. Face effleurage (Figures 3–32 and 3–33). Repeat 10 times.

Step 8. Scalp petrissage (Figure 3–29). Repeat for 1 minute.

Step 9. Pressure points around the eyes (Figures 5–1 and 5–2).

Step 10. Shoulder and neck effleurage. Repeat 10 times.

Step 11. Basic relaxation sequence.

LEG CRAMPS

Muscle cramps are painful, but short-lived, muscle spasms. Leg cramps in the hamstrings, calves, or feet muscles can be painful. Leg cramps that occur at night (nocturnal leg cramps) are clearly associated with trigger points in the gastrocnemius muscle. One study found that 50–75% of adults and 16% of healthy children experience these cramps. Many people who suffer from painful leg cramps may be deficient in calcium and/or magnesium. Dehydration and electrolyte imbalance may also contribute to cramps in the calf.[1]

APPROACH AND GOALS

When the cramp occurs, stretching the cramping muscle and then massaging it as soon as the cramp has subsided is an effective emergency treatment. To prevent cramping, do massage regularly to increase the circulation to leg muscles and decrease muscle tension. Teach the child or his parents to do the stretches located in the "Growing Pains" section daily. Depending on the child's age, the parents may need to supervise this stretching. If massage and stretching are not effective, his parents may wish to evaluate a need for supplementation.

MASSAGE AND HYDROTHERAPY FOR LEG CRAMPS

WARM SOAKS

There is no time for hydrotherapy when the child has a cramp; however, soaking the area in a hot bath and then stretching it can help prevent future cramping.

MASSAGE FOR LEG CRAMPS

Step 1. Have the child lie face down on a bed or the floor. There is no time to use the basic relaxation sequence or to apply oil or lotion.

Step 2. In the event of a hamstring, calf, or foot muscle cramp, stretch the cramping muscle by engaging the antagonistic muscle. For example, in the case of a gastrocnemius cramp, ask the child to contract the tibialis anterior.

Step 3. When the cramp subsides, effleurage and knead the muscle briefly, using moderate pressure.

Step 4. When the cramp is gone, do a few more warming strokes, gradually lightening your pressure.

LOWER BACK PAIN

Children can have sacroiliac dysfunction and lower back pain; however, when younger children complain of pain in the lower back, it is usually a result of injuries, such as falls on the coccyx.[1] Low back pain is not a common complaint in children before adolescence.[2] There is probably a combination of factors that causes adolescents to experience more lower back pain than younger children, including:

1. Previous musculoskeletal injuries, resulting in muscular compensations or in damage to the spine. Damage may often show up only after a child goes through the adolescent growth spurt. Disc protrusions and degeneration are frequent in adolescents. Researchers, using magnetic resonance imaging (MRI) to evaluate pain and disc degeneration in 15 year olds, found that 16% of those with no low back pain had disc protrusions and 26% of those with low back pain had disk protrusions. In a follow-up study 4 years later, repeat MRIs of the same two groups of young people, now age 19, indicated increased rates of disk protrusion and degeneration.[3,4]

2. Muscle strain. Injuries to the low back, including lifting injuries and falls, may strain the supporting muscles alongside the spine, which may cause them to spasm. Adolescent athletes who are playing at a high level, may have extreme tension in the muscles of the lower back. The author has treated many adolescents who developed significant back pain after beginning athletics early in childhood and competed constantly for many years.

3. Emotional stress. The lower back can become the target organ for the expression of emotional conflicts. The contribution of stress to low back pain is underappreciated.[5] Children, as well as adults, may store emotional tension in the muscles of their low back. Psychiatrist David Williams successfully treated a 13-year-old boy with emotionally based, severe lower back pain by teaching him self-hypnosis. The boy learned to repeat phrases such as "Cooped-up feelings can cause tension" and "By relaxing, I can reduce the tension and eliminate the pain."[6] Any time a child presents with back pain that is not from an acute injury, stress may be a factor. Information about the contribution of stress to lower back pain can be shared with the parent and child, without intruding on their privacy, by telling them that stress can contribute to lower back pain for some children.

4. Structural or postural problems. For example, if one leg is shorter than the other, it can contribute to trigger points and muscle spasm in the muscles of the lower back.

APPROACH AND GOALS

Hydrotherapy can relieve muscle spasm and increase circulation to the muscles of the lower back. This greatly enhances the beneficial effects of massage for lower back pain. Ice massage, for example, can be effective in the acute stage of a low back strain. It will often do more to relieve spasm than any medication. Contrast treatments improve the circulation to the lower back. Heat alone should never be used in the acute phase of a lower back injury.

A salt glow will improve the circulation to the back muscles and remove the most superficial layer of tension in the lower back; children find it novel and interesting, as well. It can be done in the acute stage of injury because heat is not used on the area. Massage can release tension and improve circulation in the lower back.

MASSAGE AND HYDROTHERAPY FOR LOWER BACK PAIN

Choose one to perform prior to massage:

ICE MASSAGE

Use an ice cup (see page 91) to massage the painful area and the surrounding 4 inches. Continue ice massage for about 8 minutes.

CONTRAST TREATMENT

Step 1. Apply a moist heating pad or Hydrocollator pack to the lower back for 3 minutes.

Step 2. Apply an ice pack to the lower back or do ice massage for 1 minute.

Step 3. Repeat hot and cold twice, for a total of three changes.

SALT GLOW OF THE LOWER BACK (FIGURES 3–53 AND 3–54)

Positioning:

The child's back should be uncovered, with the underwear moved down to expose the iliac crest; the gluteal cleft is covered. To prevent salt crystals from getting in the underwear, tuck in a towel. Follow directions for a local salt glow (page 93).

MASSAGE SEQUENCE FOR LOWER BACK PAIN

Step 1. Basic relaxation sequence (page 70).

Step 2. Apply oil or lotion.

Step 3. Back effleurage (Figure 3–2). Use firm pressure, especially in the lower back area. Repeat the full stroke 20 times.

Step 4. Thumbstroke the lower back (Figure 3–19) slowly and thoroughly, working as deeply as possible without causing discomfort to the child. Thumbstroke for approximately 2 minutes.

Step 5. Knead the buttock muscles, through the underwear, using medium pressure, from the sacrum out to the side of the hip. Knead each buttock for about 1 minute (Figure 3–20).

Step 6. Pressure points along the posterior iliac crest (Figure 5–9). Press against the back of the iliac crest, beginning just lateral to the spine. Use your thumb and press downward (toward the feet).

This will contact the large back and gluteal muscles that attach on the posterior iliac crest. Do four points along the hipbone, each one further away from the spine. Use the maximum pressure that the child finds comfortable. Do first one to the posterior iliac crest, and then cross to the opposite side and do the other.

Step 7. Pressure points on the sacrum (Figure 5–10). If working on the floor, kneel next to the child opposite his or her lower back. Beginning at the coccyx, press with the flat of your thumbs along the side of the vertebrae. Begin with slight pressure and gradually increase to the point of soreness, but not pain. Back off a bit, then hold for 10 seconds. Go from the tailbone up the sacrum to the level of the waist, moving upward about a thumb's width each time.

Step 8. Knead the buttock, same as above.

Step 9. Back effleurage, 10 times.

Step 10. Basic relaxation sequence.

 Any child with severe or chronic lower back pain should be examined by a physician to rule out any conditions that might contraindicate massage.

MENSTRUAL CRAMPS

Menstrual cramps are mild to severe cramping pains in the pelvic and abdominal areas. They can last from a few minutes to a few days, just prior to or at the onset of menstruation. For some girls, pain causes several days of disability each month because the pain is severe enough to interfere with activities. Menstrual

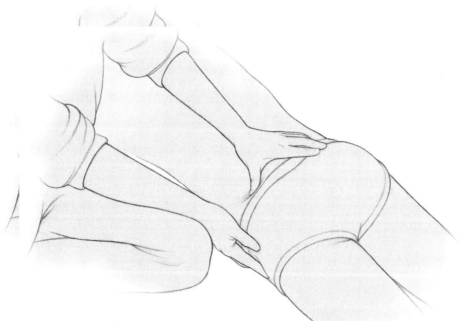

FIGURE 5–9 ■ Pressure Points Along the Posterior Iliac Crest. These points are useful in low back pain massage.

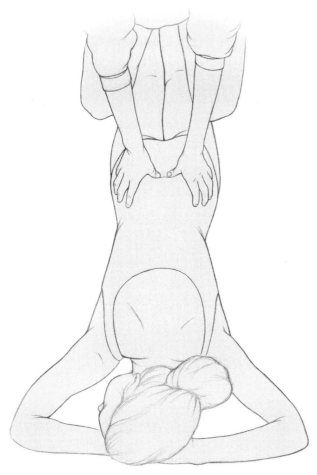

FIGURE 5–10 ■ Pressure Points on the Sacrum. These points are useful in massage for low back pain and menstrual cramps.

pain or dysmenorrhea is caused by a combination of uterine muscle spasm, ischemia, referred pain to groin and low back dermatomes, and mechanical tugging on uterine ligaments. Heredity, stress, diet, constipation, and many other factors contribute to this condition.

APPROACH AND GOALS

Hydrotherapy, in the form of a sitz bath, can relieve the pain of menstrual cramps because it increases circulation and relaxes the muscles in the pelvic area. A sitz bath is a partial bath, involving only the pelvic region. Traditionally, a sitz bath was given in a specially constructed tub that allowed only the pelvic region to be submerged in water, but a regular bathtub may be used if the girl puts her feet out of the tub during the treatment. Sitz baths may be given with either hot or cold water, or as a contrast treatment of heat followed by cold. A hot sitz bath followed by an application of cold water, such as a cold friction to the area, will stimulate the circulation, although not as much as a hot bath followed by a cold bath. (However, it may be difficult, if not impossible, to persuade an adolescent girl to plunge her pelvic area into cold water after a hot bath!) Contrast treatments to the pelvic area can also increase circulation and relieve pain.

Massage can be an excellent emergency treatment to relieve menstrual cramps in adolescent girls; the massage sequence for menstrual cramps given below may give relief for a few minutes to a few hours. Regular massage may also be effective in reducing menstrual symptoms. In a Touch Research Institute study, adult women receiving a 30-minute Swedish massage, twice a week for 5 weeks, had less menstrual pain, less water retention, and a marked improvement in mood.[1]

MASSAGE AND HYDROTHERAPY TREATMENTS FOR MENSTRUAL CRAMPS

HOT SITZ BATH WITH COLD FRICTION

Hot sitz bath: Have the girl take a 15-minute hot bath with her feet out of the water. The water should be about 105° F, depending on individual tolerance. When she gets out of the bath, quickly rub her lower abdomen with a washcloth or terrycloth mitt that has been wrung out in ice water. This treatment may be done by the girl or her mother at home before coming to your facility for a massage treatment or at your facility if there is access to a bathtub.

CONTRAST TREATMENT TO THE PELVIC AREA

Step 1. Apply a moist heating pad or Hydrocollator pack to the lower abdomen for 3 minutes.
Step 2. Apply an ice pack to the lower abdomen for 1 minute or quickly rub the lower abdomen with a washcloth or terrycloth mitt that has been wrung out in ice water.
Step 3. Repeat hot and cold (steps 1 and 2) twice, for three changes.

MASSAGE SEQUENCE FOR MENSTRUAL CRAMPS

Positioning: Stand at the child's right side, opposite the waist.

Step 1. Basic relaxation sequence.
Step 2. Apply oil or lotion.
Step 3. Abdominal effleurage (Figure 3–36). Use gentle pressure. Repeat 20 times.
Step 4. Pressure points on the pubic bone (Figure 5–11). Begin at the center of the pubic bone. Using the middle finger of your right hand, press directly on top of the bone. Go just to the point of soreness (not pain), back off a bit, and hold for 10 seconds.

Then move outward approximately one-half inch, until you find a sensitive spot, and hold for 10 seconds. Be gentle; these points can be extremely sensitive during the menses. Move outward another one-half inch and hold, then one more time, for a total of four points. Cross over to the left side, beside the left hipbone, and repeat, using the middle finger of your left hand.

Step 5. Abdominal effleurage. Repeat 20 times.
Step 6. Pressure points on the sacrum (Figure 5–10).
Step 7. Basic relaxation sequence.

MUSCLE WEAKNESS

Muscle weakness can be a temporary condition caused by fatigue, minor illnesses, low blood glucose levels, dehydration, or emotional stress. It can also be a chronic condition when the child lacks the muscle strength and endurance to carry out the normal activities of daily living. Chronic muscle weakness is a feature of different disabilities, including muscular dystrophy, spinal cord injury, polio, stroke, and certain types of cerebral palsy. In this section, we discuss the chronic type of muscle weakness caused by these disabilities. One problem arising from muscle weakness is the chronic tension that can develop in children's muscles when they are constantly straining to move or substitute stronger muscles for weaker ones.

APPROACH AND GOALS

Both massage and hydrotherapy can be beneficial for children with muscle weakness. For example, exposure to cold can stimulate the action of extensor muscles. A weak or paralyzed hand or foot can be immersed in cold water and exercised while the strength of the muscles is stimulated. A contraction will be noticed at the moment of immersion, even if it is weak or inhibited by spasticity. The first contraction will be the strongest, and the successive contractions, which occur each time the part is immersed in cold water, will be weaker. However, the extensors will be stimulated and the flexors inhibited for about 20 minutes following the treatment.[1] This is the time to have children do strengthening exercises. Massage after the hydrotherapy and exercise session can ensure that children's muscles have not been strained by contractions that are too vigorous. Strengthening exercises recommended by the physical therapist can also be incorporated into a massage treatment, as long as the session is enjoyable and not extremely taxing. Alternating massage and visualizations with muscle strengthening helps the child relax and recharge, and the variety will maintain interest. Try to make the session as much fun as possible and give positive reinforcement for even small improvements.

Dr. Meir Schneider has developed special massage techniques to develop muscle tone (see Muscular Dystrophy section). He recommends having children visualize doing a movement as a way to augment the strengthening. It is important that they not be asked to do a movement that would clearly be impossible, but have them try one that they can barely do. Have them picture the movement as smoother, easier, or lighter.[2] Exercising in water can help children develop muscle strength without fighting gravity and can be combined with Watsu massage techniques.[3]

Whole-body massage is recommended for children with any type of chronic muscle weakness to reduce chronic tension that may have developed as they try to compensate for deficiencies in their ability to move.

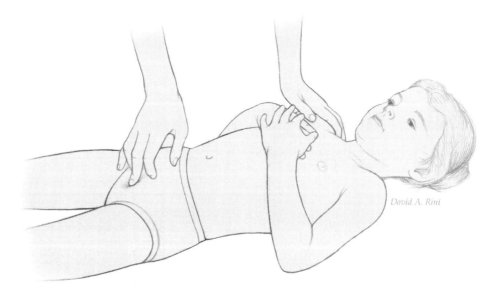

FIGURE 5–11 ■ Pressure Points on the Pubic Bone. These points are useful in massage for menstrual cramps.

COLD WATER IMMERSION AND EXERCISE

Step 1. Begin with a large bowl or bucket of water (temperature, 35° to 40° F). Ice cubes will be needed to achieve this temperature. Make sure that the child is comfortably warm before beginning the cold water immersion.

Step 2. Immerse the part in the water for 3 seconds.

Step 3. Remove the body part out of the water and have the child do isometric contractions or contractions against resistance for 30 seconds. If she becomes fatigued, stop the exercises until after the next cold water immersion.

Step 4. Repeat Steps 2 and 3 two to five times.

MASSAGE

Use Swedish massage of the part, using the techniques in Chapter 3 and conclude with lots of tapotement, which can be more stimulating to muscle tone. If the child is not fatigued, more strengthening exercises may be performed at this time. The stimulating effect of the cold water will last 10 to 20 minutes.

NECK AND SHOULDER TENSION

Tension in the neck and shoulder muscles is common in children as well as in adults and is probably the most common complaint for which adults seek massage therapy. Because chronic neck and shoulder tension is such a widespread problem, this section goes into greater detail about its causes than of many discomforts in this chapter. Although massage is an effective short-term treatment for chronic neck and shoulder tension, true resolution may involve referring the child to an appropriate specialist, such as a counselor, dentist, or optometrist. Parents will be grateful to learn what can address the cause of their children's discomfort. Common causes of neck and shoulder tension include:

- A poor position in utero. This can activate trigger points in the neck and shoulder muscles and cause such problems as torticollis, which is a result of the child's head being twisted to one side for an extended period (see Torticollis in this chapter, page 147).
- Birth trauma. This can cause strain to the muscles and bones of the neck and upper spine (see Chapter 4).
- Falls and motor vehicle accidents. These are the two most common injuries to children, and can establish patterns of neck and shoulder tension.

Falling on the head or striking it by diving into shallow water, for example, can activate trigger points in the posterior cervical muscles.[1]

- Malocclusion of the teeth and jaw (improper fitting together of the upper and lower teeth). In the United States, 50% of children ages 8 to 11 have well-aligned incisors; the rest have varying degrees of malalignment and crowding, and 14% have severe malocclusion. This percentage increases during adolescence until adulthood, when only 34% have well-aligned incisors.[2] Malocclusion may have many causes. Injuries to the jawbone or teeth can cause malocclusion and one-half of all children have a traumatic injury to their baby or permanent teeth by the time they graduate from high school. Massage therapist and craniosacral dentist Clint Nelson believes that a great percentage of malocclusions are a consequence of poor alignment of the cranial bones (Nelson C, personal communication, July 2002). Poorly aligned teeth cause children to use extra muscular effort to chew their food and may change the way children swallow, leading to teeth clenching and grinding as a response to stressful conditions.[2] Dental malocclusion can overload masticatory (chewing) muscles, such as the pterygoids, temporalis, and masseters, and perpetuate their trigger points.[1] When the masseters are chronically overcontracted, they fatigue; this contributes to a forward head posture, which leads to tension in the upper trapezius, sternocleidomastoid, levator scapulae, scalene, and upper pectoral muscles. For neck and shoulder tension caused by problems with the bite, massage will be an effective short-term solution, but the long-term solution may be treatment of the malocclusion by a dentist (Nelson C, personal communication, July 2002).
- Eyestrain caused by too much reading, working at a computer, or other near-vision tasks, or straining to see because of vision problems causes compensations in many of the neck and shoulder muscles. Some of the affected muscles may be the sternocleidomastoid, occipitalis, suboccipital, or erector spinae muscles (see the section on Eyestrain, page 128).
- Poor ergonomics while working at a computer or while playing video games. The average child spends at least several hours a day sitting in front of a computer screen. Extended forward posture of the head may cause tension in the upper trapezius, scalene, sternocleidomastoid, posterior cervical, and pectoral muscles. A position with the head turned to one side and projected forward can activate trigger points in the splenius cervicis muscle; typing with the head and neck

turned toward the side of the keyboard can activate trigger points in the levator scapulae.[1]

- Compensations for postural imbalance elsewhere in the body. Chronic neck and shoulder tension can result from trying to maintain good posture when there is a structural problem. For example, when one leg is shorter than the other, the pelvis tilts down on the side of the short leg and the shoulders are tilted as well. Then, to maintain the eyes at an even level, the child must tilt his or her head, and this can activate trigger points in the sternocleidomastoid, scalene, levator scapulae, and upper trapezius muscles.[1]

- Emotional stress. Deep tension in the muscles of the entire upper body can be caused by emotional stress, especially anxiety. When the child is under stress, trigger points may be aggravated from other causes discussed above.

APPROACH AND GOALS

Massage and hydrotherapy are excellent short-term treatments for chronic neck and shoulder tension because they relax the muscles of the head and neck and increase local circulation. They are also excellent for acute neck and shoulder tension resulting from physical strain, such as unaccustomed exercise.

MASSAGE AND HYDROTHERAPY FOR NECK AND SHOULDER TENSION

MOIST HEAT APPLICATION

With the child lying prone, place a hot water bottle, moist heating pad, or Hydrocollator pack on the upper back and neck for 5 to 10 minutes.

CONTRAST TREATMENT

Step 1. Have the child prone and place a hot water bottle, moist heating pad, or Hydrocollator pack on the child's upper back and neck for 5 to 10 minutes.

Step 2. Have the child turn over. Place an ice pack under the back of the neck for 1 minute. Make sure the rest of the child's body is warm; the ice pack should not cause chilling.

MASSAGE SEQUENCE FOR NECK AND SHOULDER TENSION

Step 1. Basic relaxation sequence.
Step 2. Apply oil or lotion.
Step 3. Shoulder and neck effleurage (Figures 3–26 and 3–27). Repeat 20 times.

Step 4. Diagonal neck stroke (Figure 3–28). Repeat 20 times.
Step 5. Shoulder and neck effleurage, repeat three times.
Step 6. Scalp petrissage (Figure 3–29).
Step 7. Shoulder and neck effleurage, repeat three times.
Step 8. Knead the upper trapezius (Figure 3–17). Perform for 1 minute.
Step 9. Pressure points on the upper trapezius (Figure 5–7).
Step 10. Pressure points on the occiput (Figure 5–6).
Step 11. Shoulder and neck effleurage, repeat three times.
Step 12. Basic relaxation sequence.

SORE THROAT

A sore throat is one of the most common complaints of childhood. Frequent and recurrent sore throats are especially common between ages 5 and 10. (There is no evidence that removing the tonsils helps decrease sore throats.[1]) A sore throat can be caused by anything that irritates the sensitive mucous membranes at the back of the throat and mouth, including viruses, bacteria, allergies, mouth breathing, excessively dry air, and overuse of the voice. Fully 90% of childhood sore throats are caused by viruses, which, of course, cannot be treated with antibiotics and must run their course.

APPROACH AND GOALS

Massage is contraindicated in the acute stage of any bacterial or viral sore throat. However, parents may wish to perform the following treatments when their child is recovering from strep throat. Massage and hydrotherapy treatments may not only relieve the discomfort and pain of sore throat in the subacute stages of a viral or bacterial infection by increasing blood circulation and improving lymphatic drainage, but also may speed healing. Children often feel immediate and dramatic relief of sore throat pain. Massage and hydrotherapy are also useful for simple sore throats that are not caused by an infection, and for tension and stress in the muscles of the anterior neck.

MASSAGE AND HYDROTHERAPY FOR SORE THROATS

Choose one hydrotherapy treatment for the child prior to massage:

HYDROTHERAPY

1. Gargle using warm saline (½ teaspoon of salt to 1 cup of warm water) for 5 to 10 minutes, four times a day. This is an effective treatment for children; however,

smaller children may not be able to gargle without choking on the water.

2. Drink plenty of water to keep the throat moist.
3. Contrast Treatment

Step 1. Have the child lie supine. Fold a washcloth into a narrow strip, and dip it into a bowl of water at 110° F. Wring out cloth and place on the child's throat. A small, moist heating pad may also be used. Leave the hot application on the throat for 3 minutes. If the washcloth appears to be cooling off, replace it with another cloth after 2 minutes.

Step 2. Fold another washcloth into a narrow strip and dip it into a bowl of very cold water (add ice cubes to the water to make it as cold as possible). Wring out and cover the throat. Leave the cold application on for 1 minute.

Step 3. Repeat hot and cold (steps 1 and 2) twice, for three changes.

MASSAGE SEQUENCE FOR SORE THROAT

Positioning: Have the child lay supine, with a pillow under his head

Step 1. Basic relaxation sequence.
Step 2. Passive touch on the shoulders or throat.
Step 3. Superficial effleurage of the sternocleidomastoid.
Step 4. Pressure points on the sternocleidomastoid muscle (Figure 5–5).
Step 5. Basic relaxation sequence.

If the sore throat is severe; persists for more than 2 days; or is accompanied or followed by fever, headache, rash, nausea, or vomiting, the child's physician should be consulted promptly. These may be symptoms of strep throat, a serious bacterial illness for which antibiotics are customarily prescribed. Left untreated, strep throat can lead to serious complications, including rheumatic fever. It is also highly contagious.

SORENESS AFTER EXERCISE

Muscle soreness is generally felt 24 to 36 hours after strenuous exercise. Working muscles very vigorously results in microscopic tears to muscle fiber, local swelling, and pain messages being sent from the nerves in the muscles to the brain.

APPROACH AND GOALS

When a child experiences muscle soreness after strenuous exercise, gentle movement, Epsom salt baths, and massage will increase the circulation to the muscle,

relieve swelling and pain, and help the muscle repair. Use caution when massaging a sore area, so that massage does not become unpleasant or stressful for the child.

MASSAGE AND HYDROTHERAPY FOR SORENESS AFTER EXERCISE

Choose one hydrotherapy treatment to do prior to massage:

HYDROTHERAPY

1. Ice massage. Use an ice cup (see page 91) to massage the painful area and the surrounding 4 inches. Do not press hard. Continue ice massage for about 8 minutes.
2. Epsom salts bath. For an adult, use 1 cup Epsom salts in a tub of warm water. Adjust the amount of Epsom salts to the size of the child; for example, use 1 cup salts for a 150-pound adult, ½ cup for a 75-pound child, and ⅓ cup for a 50-pound child. The temperature should be 100° to 105°F—whatever is comfortably warm to the child. Have the child stay in the tub for at least 20 minutes.

MASSAGE FOR SORENESS AFTER EXERCISE

Perform effleurage and thumbstroking of the sore area for 10 minutes. If the area is tender, begin with light pressure and gradually increase pressure to the child's tolerance.

TENSION STOMACHACHE

When we refer to recurrent abdominal pain, we are talking about repeated bouts of abdominal pain for which no explanation is obvious. Somewhere between 10–20% of all children will complain of these recurrent problems. The most common cause of abdominal pain in adults and children alike is stress. It is only natural for us to react to the environment in which we live. A bad day, the loss of a pet, or an argument with a friend would create stress in all of us. It is a common misconception that children's feelings are not as complex and sensitive as adults. Children become just as angry, anxious, and depressed as we do.[1]

Recurring abdominal pain is one of the most common somatic complaints of children, although a specific organic cause is found in only 5–10% of those children.[2]

In some children, recurring stomachaches can be linked to family factors. For example, two studies of 3 year olds found a link between stomachaches in the child, maternal depression, maternal health problems, and parental marital problems. Temper tantrums and a high level of fearfulness were also associated with recurrent stomachaches.[3,4]

One study admitted children from ages 6 to 16 to a pediatric gastroenterology clinic for evaluation of abdominal pain. The children had all experienced at least three episodes within 3 months of abdominal pain severe enough to interfere with their activities. Researchers found that these children tended to be more anxious and to internalize their emotions more than the average child. In addition, a high percentage of the children had experienced the death of a family member or friend shortly before their pain began. Children in this study were better able to cope with their pain when they were able to understand its connection with emotional stress.[2]

APPROACH AND GOALS

Massage therapy can provide immediate relief for some tension stomachaches, and regular massage may release chronic tension and associated emotional stress and teach the child to relax. Massage therapy may be especially important in treating stress-related abdominal pain because one-third to one-half of children experiencing such pain continue to have pain as adults.[2] Giving them tools to cope with the tendency to store stress in the abdomen may help them for life.

MASSAGE AND HYDROTHERAPY FOR TENSION STOMACHACHE

MOIST HEAT APPLICATION

Place a hot water bottle, moist heating pad, or Hydrocollator pack on the stomach for 10 minutes.

MASSAGE SEQUENCE FOR TENSION STOMACHACHES

Step 1. Basic relaxation sequence (see page 70).
Step 2. Apply oil or lotion.
Step 3. Abdominal effleurage (Figure 3–36).
Step 4. Abdominal smoother. Begin with one palm on the upper abdomen, just below the ribs. Do not push on the xyphoid process. Glide to the bottom of the abdomen using gentle, even palm pressure over the entire area. Repeat with your other hand. Continue alternating hands in a slow, steady rhythm. Do 20 times.
Step 5. Abdominal effleurage, 20 times.
Step 6. Abdominal smoother, 20 times.
Step 7. Abdominal effleurage, 20 times.
Step 8. Basic relaxation sequence.

 There are many causes of abdominal pain. If a child is suffering from recurring abdominal pain, the family physician should be consulted to rule out any pathology.

TIRED FEET

This section presents a simple treatment for muscular fatigue of the feet, but not for conditions caused by poor alignment, bad shoes, or any type of pathologic condition. It is most appropriate for children who have been walking or running long distances or competing in games that involve a lot of running, such as basketball or soccer.

APPROACH AND GOALS

Competitive runners frequently use hydrotherapy to ease muscular fatigue and rejuvenate muscles. Unfortunately, no studies have been done on the effect of hydrotherapy on the muscles of the feet; however, the leg muscles, many of which insert on the feet, have been studied. One study found that cold baths greatly increased the strength of leg muscles. Subjects were given leg baths (temperature, 54° F) for 30 minutes. Each subject was tested for leg strength 11 times during the 30 minutes, as well as every 20 minutes for 3 hours after the treatment as they were relaxing. Their leg muscles had increased in strength during the cold bath and afterward for as long as 6 hours. The researchers felt that the increased strength was a result of increased blood flow to the deep muscles caused by restriction of peripheral blood flow during the treatment.[1]

Massage can bring great relief for feet that ache or are fatigued from vigorous exercise. If a young athlete is taking a rest and then going back on the field, massage can have a rejuvenating effect by improving the circulation and relieving muscle tension. A study at the University of North Carolina found that a 10-minute leg massage after vigorous leg weight lifting was more successful at reducing muscular fatigue than just sitting quietly.[2] Massage of the feet feels soothing, improves circulation, and stretches tight muscles, especially those of the arch. Because tension and fatigue in the leg muscles are often related to the condition of the feet, leg massage will also help relieve fatigue in the feet muscles. Massage of the fronts or backs of the legs could easily be done along with the sequence for the feet. Refer to massage for the front and back of the legs discussed in Chapter 3.

MASSAGE AND HYDROTHERAPY FOR TIRED FEET

CONTRAST TREATMENT

Step 1. Fill two deep buckets or washtubs with water, one hot and one cold (put in a few ice cubes).
Step 2. Put the child's feet in the hot water for 3 minutes.
Step 3. Put both feet in the cold water for 1 minute.
Step 4. Repeat steps 2 and 3.
Step 5. Repeat steps 2 and 3.
Step 6. Dry the child's feet.

MASSAGE SEQUENCE FOR TIRED FEET

Positioning:

Position yourself as for massaging the front of the leg. Begin with the right foot.
Step 1. Basic relaxation sequence (see page 70).
Step 2. Apply oil or lotion.
Step 3. Foot friction (Figure 3–47). Repeat for 30 seconds or longer.
Step 4. Thumbstroke the top of the foot (Figure 3–48). Thumbstroke for at least 1 minute.
Step 5. Foot friction, 30 seconds.
Step 6. Stretch the sole of the foot. Hold underneath the heel with your right hand and grasp the toes with your left hand. Bend them back firmly but gently. Hold for 10 seconds.
Step 7. Knuckling the sole. Make a loose fist with your right hand. Hold the top of the foot with your left hand. Rub rapidly up and down the sole from heel to great toe, using firm pressure. Continue for 15 seconds.
Step 8. Rotate the ankle (Figure 3–13F). Hold the heel with the left hand. Using the heel of the right hand against the ball of the foot, gently rotate the foot, making a large circle. Encourage the child to relax and try to not help make circles. Do 10 slow circles, reverse direction and do 10 more.
Step 9. Knuckling the sole, 15 seconds.
Step 10. Foot friction, 30 seconds.
Step 11. Stretch and stroke each toe (Figure 3–49).
Step 12. Foot friction, 30 seconds or longer.
Step 13. Basic relaxation sequence.
Step 14. Move to the left foot and repeat, using the opposite hands.

TORTICOLLIS

Torticollis means *twisted neck*. In this condition, there is an exaggerated lateral flexion of the child's head to one side, and a rotation of the head to the opposite side (Figure 5–12). The most common cause of torticollis is fibrous shortening of the sternocleidomastoid

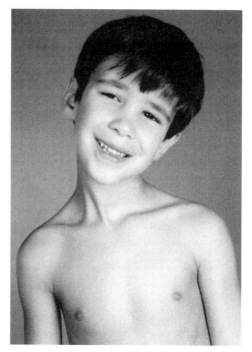

FIGURE 5–12 ■ A Young Boy with Torticollis. Reprinted with permission from Morrissy R: *Lovell and Winter's Pediatric Orthopaedics.* Vol. 2. Baltimore, MD: Lippincott Williams & Wilkins, 2001, p 810.

muscle, which may be caused by a number of different factors, including a twisting of the head to one side in utero during the late stages of pregnancy, birth trauma, visual difficulties that cause the child to tilt the head, inflammatory conditions of the tissues of the neck such as pharyngitis or cellulitis, and very rarely, malformations of the occipital or cervical bones.[1]

It is important that torticollis be treated early in life for two reasons: one, it is annoying to the child and can slow down the learning of new skills such as crawling and walking; and two, children can have discomfort and referred pain from triggerpoints in this muscle, which will persist into adulthood if they are not treated. Triggerpoints in other neck muscles may develop, such as in the scalenes, trapezius, levator scapulae, and posterior neck muscles.[2] Adults with uncorrected torticollis have very restricted mobility of the cervical spine.

When a child is born with torticollis, therapy for the shortened sternocleidomastoid muscle is often prescribed for parents to do at home. It consists of gentle but persistent head flexion and rotation to stretch the muscle. Three or four times daily, the parent or therapist does ten to twenty repititions, each time holding momentarily at the maximal range. Physical therapy may involve having the child do exercises which stretch the muscle. such as rolling towards the ipsilateral side and doing midline activities in different positions. Parents are taught to carry the infant outward to encourage her to position her head and neck in the midline, and to turn her crib so that looking at interesting objects will stretch the involved sternocleidomastoid.[3] If this gentle stretching is not successful, children with torticollis may have surgery to release the muscle, with postoperative physical therapy and splinting. This is usually done between the ages of 1 and 4 years.[4,5]

APPROACH AND GOALS

Torticollis, which is related to muscle spasm and triggerpoints, can be addressed with massage, and may be an excelllent adjunct to the therapy the child is receiving for torticollis, even with an infant. Thorough massage of the entire neck and shoulders is advised, because a change in the length of the sternocleidomastoid muscle may have affected many other muscles as well.

MASSAGE SEQUENCE FOR TORTICOLLIS

Step 1. Use the treatment for neck and shoulder tension discussed in this chapter.
Step 2. Superficial effleurage of the sternocleidomastoid muscle. (Step 3, Sternocleidomastoid Massage, page 128).
Step 3. Pressure points on the sternocleidomastoid muscle.
Step 4. Shoulder and neck effleurage, repeat 10 times.
Step 5. Basic relaxation sequence.
Step 6. Stretching of the sternocleidomastoid as prescribed by the child's physician. Because this therapy may be difficult to do at one time with a small child, you may teach the child's parents to do some or all of this massage and stretching sequence on a daily basis and have the child brought in for weekly massage.

Because torticollis may have other causes besides the shortening of the sternocleidomastoid muscle, consult with the child's physician for approval to treat the child's torticollis.

REVIEW QUESTIONS

1. Choose three discomforts and explain their causes. Explain how specific treatment with massage and hydrotherapy can work together to treat each discomfort.

2. Explain the causes and manifestations of five different headache types. How are they treated differently with massage and hydrotherapy?

3. Discuss the common causes of neck and shoulder tension. Can massage be a symptomatic treatment for neck and shoulder tension, or can it help deal with the cause? Explain.

4. Name three discomforts discussed in this chapter in which stress may be a major contributor, and explain why. Name three in which stress has nothing to do with the condition, and explain why.

5. Discuss the lifelong lessons that children learn by using massage and hydrotherapy to treat the emotional and physical aspects of the discomforts discussed in Chapter 5, that is by using simple, holistic techniques before trying medications.

REFERENCES

Introduction

1. Sanell L: *Fundamentals of Pediatric Orthopedics.* Philadelphia, PA: Lippincott, Raven, 1998, p 68
2. Mikkelson M, et al: Psychiatric symptoms in preadolescents with musculoskeletal pain and fibromyalgia. *Pediatrics*, 100:116, 1997

Constipation

1. Sinclair M, Weller A: Don't let the well run dry: The importance of water to the child's health. *Exceptional Parent Magazine*, May:4, 2001

Depression

1. Depression in Children and Adolescents. National Institute of Mental Health. Available at: http://www.nimh.nih.gov/publicat/depchildresfact.cfm. Accessed January 2003.
2. Fassler D: *Help Me, I'm Sad—Recognizing, Treating, and Preventing Childhood and Adolescent Depression.* New York: Viking, 1994, p 23, 44-49
3. Goodman E, Capitman J: Depressive symptoms and cigarette smoking among teens. *Pediatrics*, 106:748-755, 2000
4. Dumont L: *Surviving Adolescence*, p 6
5. Guthrie E: *The Trouble With Perfect: How Parents Can Avoid the Overachievement Trap and Still Raise Successful Children.* New York: Broadway Books, 2002, p 93
6. Olness K, Kohen D: *Hypnosis and Hypnotherapy With Children.* New York, NY: Guilford, 1996, p. 256
7. Platania A, et al: Relaxation therapy reduces anxiety in child/adolescent psychiatry patients. *Acta Paedopsychiatrica*, 55:115-120, 1992
8. Field T, et al: Massage therapy reduces anxiety in child adolescent psychiatric patients. *Journal of the American Academy of Adolescent Psychiatry*, 131:125-131, 1992
9. Field T, et al: Alleviating posttraumatic stress in children following Hurricane Andrew. *Journal of Applied Developmental Psychology*, 17:37-50, 1996

10. Field T, et al: Massage and relaxation therapies' effects on depressed adolescent mothers. *Adolescence*, 31:903-911, 1996
11. Zibart R: Acupressure study may pinpoint kids' needs. *Sage Magazine*, September:11, 2000
12. Pauly M: A child's second chance. *Natural Health*, May-June, 1998, p 70
13. Upledger J, Vredevoogd J: *Craniospinal Therapy.* Seattle, WA: Eastland Press, 19083, p 120

Earache

1. Schmidt M: *Childhood Ear Infections: What Every Parent Should Know About Prevention, Home Care, and Alternative Treatment.* Berkeley, CA: North Atlantic Books, 1996, p 11, 151
2. Thrash A: *Home Remedies—Massage, Hydrotherapy, Charcoal and Other Simple Treatments.* Seale, AL: Thrash Publications, 1981, p 110
3. Austin P, Thrash A: *More Natural Remedies.* Sunfield, MI: Family Health Publications, 1985, p 83

Eye Fatigue and Strain

1. Eliot L: *What's Going On in There? How the Brain and the Mind Develop in the First Five Years of Life.* New York, NY: Bantam Books, 2001, p 212
2. Berne S: *Creating Your Personal Vision—A Mind-Body Guide for Better Eyesight.* Santa Fe, NM: Color Stone Press, 1994, p 42, 58, 137
3. Goodrich J: *Help Your Child to Perfect Eyesight Without Glasses.* Berkeley, CA: Celestial Arts, 1999, p 33, 158, 176
4. Neinstein L: *Adolescent Health Care: A Practical Guide.* Ed. 3. Baltimore, MD: Lippincott Williams & Wilkins, 1996, p 129
5. Kavener R: *Your Child's Vision: A Parent's Guide to Seeing, Growing, and Developing.* New York, NY: Simon and Schuster, 1985, p 102, 188, 202
6. Dobson J: *Baby Beautiful—The Handbook of Baby Head Shaping.* Carson City, NV: Heirs Press, 1994, p 137
7. Upledger J, Vredevoogd J: *Craniosacral Therapy.* Seattle, WA: Eastland Press, 1983, p 210, 269
8. Williams D, Singh M: Hypnosis as a facilitating therapeutic adjunct in child psychiatry. *Journal of the American Academy of Child Psychiatry.* 15:332, 1976
9. Rada R, et al: Visual Conversion Reaction in Children. I. Diagnosis. *Psychosomatics*, 10:23-28, 1969. II. (Follow-up) *Psychosomatics*, 14:271-276, 1973
10. Lieberman J: *Take Off Your Glasses and See.* New York, NY: Three Rivers Press, 1995, p 61
11. Lieberman J: *Light, Medicine of the Future.* Santa Fe, NM: Bear and Co, 1991, p 81-83, 145
12. Grossman M: *Greater Vision.* Los Angeles, CA: Keats Publishing, 2001
13. Hanson P: *The Joy of Stress.* Kansas City, MO: Andrews, McNeel and Parker, 1986, p 65
14. Moses A: Heavy Computer Use May Strain Eyes. *Reuters Health Newsletter*, March 18, 2002
15. Feldenkrais M: *The Master Moves.* Cupertino, CA: Meta Publications, 1984, p 93

16. Simons D, Travell J: *Myofascial Pain and Dysfunction: The Triggerpoint Manual.* Vol. 1, ed. 2. Baltimore, MD: Lippincott Williams & Wilkins, 1999, p 316, 421, 456, 476
17. Gallup C, Schneider M: That person in the wheelchair needs your touch. *Massage Magazine*, 64:36, 1996
18. Burg F, et al: *Gellis and Kagan's Current Pediatric Therapy.* Philadelphia, PA: W.B. Saunders, 1999, p 945.
19. Schneider M, Grossman M: National Association of Vision Improvement Instructors Conference, Forest Grove, OR, October 2001
20. Rodin F: Heat and cold in the therapy of the eyes. *Archives of Ophthalmology*, 32:296-300, 1944

Growing Pains

1. Sanell L: *Fundamentals of Pediatric Orthopedics.* Philadelphia, PA: Lippincott, Raven, 1998, p 117
2. Baxter M, Dulberg C: Growing pains in childhood—A proposal for treatment. *Journal of Pediatric Orthopedics*, Philadelphia, PA: 8:402, 1988
3. Bates T, Grunwaldt E: Myofascial pain in childhood. *Journal of Pediatrics*, 53:198-209, 1958

Introduction to Headache

1. Pantell R: *Taking Care of Your Child: A Parent's Guide to Medical Care.* Reading, MA: Perseus, 2002, p 304
2. Stafstrom C, et al: The usefulness of children's drawings in the diagnosis of headache. *Pediatrics*, 109:460, 2002

Dehydration Headache

1. Sinclair M, Weller A: Don't let the well run dry: The importance of water to the child's health. *Exceptional Parent Magazine*, May 2001, p 66
2. Vellas B, Albarede J, Garry P: *Hydration in Aging.* New York, NY: Springer Publishing, 1998, p 50

Migraine Headache

1. Stafstrom C, et al: The usefulness of children's drawings in the diagnosis of headache. *Pediatrics*, 109:460-461, 2002
2. Richter I, et al: Cognitive and relaxation treatment of pediatric migraine. *Pain*, 25:195-203, 1986
3. Diamond S: *Conquering your Migraine—the Essential Guide for Understanding and Treating Migraines for All Sufferers and Their Families.* New York, NY: Fireside, 2001, p 55-56, 138
4. Lynch J: *The Language of the Heart: The Body's Response to Human Dialogue.* New York, NY: Basic Books, 1986, p 214-220
5. Upledger J, Vredevoogd J: *Craniospinal Therapy.* Seattle, WA: Eastland Press, 1983, p 110.
6. Cheek D: Maladjustment patterns apparently related to imprinting at birth. *American Journal of Clinical Hypnosis*, 18:390, 1975
7. Simons D, Travell JG: *Myofascial Pain and Dysfunction: The Triggerpoint Manual.* Vol. 1, ed. 2. Baltimore, MD: Lippincott Williams & Wilkins, 1999, p 117
8. Bates T, Grundwalt E: Myofascial pain in childhood. *Journal of Pediatrics*, 22, 1952

9. Olness K, Kohen D: *Hypnosis and Hypnotherapy in Children*. New York, NY: Guilford Press, 1996, p 243-245
10. Milne H: *The Heart of Listening*. Berkley, CA: North Atlantic Books, 1995, p 393
11. Hernandez-Rief M, et al: Migraine headaches are reduced by massage therapy. *International Journal of Neuroscience*, 96:1-11, 1998

Muscle Contraction Headache

1. Pantell R: *Taking Care of Your Child: A Parent's Guide to Medical Care*. Reading, MA: Perseus, 2002, p 304
2. Simons D, Travell JG: *Myofascial Pain and Dysfunction: The Triggerpoint Manual*. Vol. 1, ed. 2. Baltimore, MD: Lippincott Williams & Wilkins, 1999, p 184

Leg Cramps

1. Simons D, Travell JG: *Myofascial Pain and Dysfunction: The Triggerpoint Manual*. Vol. 1, ed. 2. Baltimore, MD: Lippincott Williams & Wilkins, 1999, p 407

Lower Back Pain

1. Mierau DR, Cassidy JD: Sacroiliac joint dysfunction and low back pain in school aged children. *Journal of Manipulative and Physiological Therapeutics*, 7:81-84, 1984
2. Pantell R: *Taking Care of Your Child: A Parents Guide to Medical Care*. Reading, MA: Perseus, 2002, p 96
3. Tortii MO, et al: Low-back pain and disc degeneration in children: A case-control MR imaging study. Department of Diagnostic Radiology, University of Turku, Finland. *Radiology*, 180:503-507, 1991
4. Kintalo ER: Development of degenerative changes in the lumbar intervertebral disc: Results of a prospective MR imaging study in adolescents with and without low-back pain. Department of Diagnostic Radiology, University of Turku, Finland. *Radiology*, 196:529-533, 1995
5. Sarno J: *Healing Back Pain—The Mind-Body Connection*. New York, NY: Warner Books, 1991
6. Williams D, Singh M: Hypnosis as a therapeutic adjunct. In: Noshpitz JD, ed. *Basic Handbook of Child Psychiatry*. Vol. 3. New York, NY: Basic Books, 1979

Menstrual Cramps

1. Hernandez-Reif M, et al: Premenstrual syndrome symptoms are relieved by massage therapy. *Journal of Psychosomatic Obstetrics and Gynecology*, 21:9-15, 2000

Muscle Weakness

1. Thrash A: *Home Remedies—Massage, Hydrotherapy, Charcoal and Other Simple Treatments*. Seale, AL: Thrash Publications, 1981, p 32

2. Schneider M, Gallup C: That person in the wheelchair needs your touch. *Massage Magazine*, November/December:28, 1996
3. Campion M: *Hydrotherapy in Pediatrics*. Rockville, MD: Aspen Systems, 1985, p 200

Neck and Shoulder Tension

1. Simons D, Travell JG: *Myofascial Pain and Dysfunction: The Triggerpoint Manual*. Vol. 1, ed. 2. Baltimore, MD: Lippincott Williams & Wilkins, 1999, p 179, 186, 315, 383, 436, 453, 494
2. Fields H: *Contemporary Orthodontics*. St. Louis, MO: Mosby, 2000, p 10

Sore Throat

1. Pantell R: *Taking Care of Your Child: A Parent's Guide to Medical Care*. Reading, MA: Perseus, 2002, p 204

Tension Stomachache

1. Pantell R: *Taking Care of Your Child: A Parent's Guide to Medical Care*. Reading, MA: Perseus, 2002, p 356
2. Wasserman P, et al: Psychogenic basis for abdominal pain in children and adolescents. *Journal of the American Academy of Child and Adolescent Psychiatry*, 27:179, 183, 1988
3. Stevenson J, et al: Research note: Recurrent headaches and stomachaches in preschool children. *Journal of Child Psychology and Psychiatry*, 29, 1988, p 897-900
4. Zuckerman S, et al: Stomachaches and headaches in a community sample of preschool children. *Pediatrics*, 79:677-682, 1987

Tired Feet

1. *Physical Therapy Review*, 39:598-599, 1959
2. The recuperative effects of sports massage as compared to passive rest. *Massage Therapy Journal*, 29:57-66, 1990

Torticollis

1. Sanell L: *Fundamentals of Pediatric Orthopedics*. Philadelphia, PA: Lippincott, Raven, 1998, p 22
2. Simons D, Travell JG: *Myofascial Pain and Dysfunction: The Triggerpoint Manual*. Vol. 1, ed. 2. Baltimore, MD: Lippincott Williams & Wilkins, 1999, p 311
3. Long T, Toscano K: *Handbook of Pediatric Physical Therapy*. Baltimore, MD: Lippincott Williams & Wilkins, 2002, p 49
4. Burg F, et al: *Gellis and Kagan's Current Pediatric Therapy*. Philadelphia, PA: W.B. Saunders, 1999, p 945
5. Morrissy R: *Lovell and Winter's Pediatric Orthopaedics*. Vol. 2. Baltimore, MD: Lippincott Williams & Wilkins 2001, p 805

MASSAGE AND HYDROTHERAPY FOR CHILDREN WITH DISABILITIES

6

I cringed at the thought that another qualified professional would be touching me. Since my infancy, an army of doctors, therapists, and nurses had poked, probed, and punctured me in the name of therapy. Professional hands, in large part, had produced pressure, pain, and protest. To be touched meant I was sick, different, vulnerable. I remember cold, impersonal hands in hospitals and doctors' offices. They always lacked the warm reassurance of my mother's touch. Their touching was more torment than treatment. After hearing my chronic complaints of leg cramps and neck pain, a friend recommended massage. My fears immediately surfaced when the massage therapist arrived at my door. I steeled myself for her touch. As she delicately rested her hands on my back, tears filled my eyes. Her touches were tender, calm, and sensitive. Each stroke was punctuated with acceptance and understanding. My body had never felt such a sense of reverence and spiritual harmony. It was as if this were an anatomic apology for my decades of physical struggle. My body was no longer alone and abandoned. It had found a refuge of nurturing and renewal. And in those hands, I discovered the healing art of touch.[1]

—*Steve Mikita, Assistant Attorney General,*
State of Utah, who has muscular dystrophy

KEY POINTS

After reading this chapter, the student will be able to:

1. Explain the general value of massage for children with disabilities.
2. Distinguish between a birth defect and an acquired disability.
3. Describe common problems facing disabled children.
4. Discuss the origin and background of each disability discussed in this chapter.
5. Describe how the specific effects of massage may be tailored to meet the needs of children with each disability.
6. Explain when hydrotherapy may be appropriate.
7. Discuss the effects of massage on different body systems for various disabilities.

Between 9% and 15% of all children in the United States have some type of disability.[2] Before we continue, the definition of disability may be helpful. Disability is defined as *a physical or mental impairment that substantially limits one or more of an individual's major life activities.* By this definition, orthopedic, speech, visual, and hearing impairments; mental retardation; cerebral palsy; muscular dystrophy; learning disabilities; injury-caused impairments, such as spinal cord injuries; and chronic illnesses, such as HIV/AIDS, are

all disabilities. A disability can be present at birth or acquired later (see Point of Interest Box 6–1). A number of disabilities are brought together in this chapter, not necessarily because they are similar conditions, but because they impose similar limitations and challenges on the individual child. To function with the least restriction, many disabled children require assistance with special needs. For example, a child with attention deficit disorder may need extra help with academics; a child who walks with difficulty as a result of chronic

POINT OF INTEREST BOX 6–1
Disabilities Present at Birth (Birth Defects) Versus Acquired Disabilities

Birth defects are body imperfections, malformations, and dysfunctions or an absence of something normally present at birth. Approximately 5% of all children are born with birth defects, and one-half of those are congenital malformations such as cleft palate.[1] Subtle alterations in the brain's structure and mild developmental delays may be detectable during infancy or they may only become evident when the child begins school. During pregnancy, birth defects can be caused by environmental factors, such as radiation; malnutrition; certain prescription medications; certain infections, such as German measles (rubella); maternal substance abuse; chronic illness, such as diabetes; or the mother's exposure to toxic chemicals, such as certain solvents, pesticides, and heavy metals such as lead or mercury.[2,3] Birth defects may also be caused by genetic factors. In more than one-half of the cases of a child with a birth defect, the cause is unknown.

Acquired disabilities are not present at birth, but are caused later by injury or exposure to an infectious agent, such as amputations, burns, brain damage from a head injury, juvenile rheumatoid arthritis, and polio. Certain disabilities may have both a genetic and an environmental basis. Attention deficit disorder is inherited in many cases; however, it can also be caused by exposure to high levels of lead or head trauma. Depression tends to run in families, but the amount of stress experienced during childhood will influence whether or not the child becomes chronically depressed.

References

1. Batshaw M: *Children with Disabilities.* Baltimore, MD: Paul Brooks Pub., 1997, p 11
2. Batshaw M: *Children with Disabilities.* Baltimore, MD: Paul Brooks Pub., 1997
3. Steingraber S: *Having Faith: An Ecologist's Journey to Motherhood.* Cambridge, MA: Perseus Publishing, 2001

pain may need elevators and pain medication; and a child who has Down syndrome may need help with vision and hearing problems. Massage cannot replace these essential forms of assistance. Although massage helps meet physical therapy needs—while children are benefiting from increased range of motion or a higher level of stimulation—it can, at the same time, help them be nurtured and comforted. Massage can make a significant and unique difference in improving a child's quality of life.

COMMON PROBLEMS FOR CHILDREN WITH DISABILITIES

Many problems discussed are common to all children who are disabled; however, the disabilities covered in this chapter are so different from each other that not all problems will apply to all children. A brief discussion of the applicability of massage for each problem is included.

UNDERSTIMULATION

Understimulation is common with many disabilities. For example, if children's hearing impairments are identified early in life and treated appropriately, through hearing aids, speech-language therapy, sign language training, and special education services, they may develop normally. If they don't receive the treatment they need, children may be slower to develop because they not only lack the stimulation of sound, but also that of social interaction. Massage can benefit children who are deaf by providing another mode of sensory stimulation and by helping them develop greater body awareness, giving them more of a connection with a body they cannot hear. A pilot program funded by the New York State Education Department found that 17 children who were both blind and deaf had a 69% increase in language skills after 3 months of receiving massage (Guyer E, personal communication, January 1990).

Lack of visual stimulation may also affect a child's development. For example, children with severely impaired vision may be slow to develop physically because they have no visual enticement to reach, crawl, or walk. They need additional stimulation, especially that of touch and sound, to reach the same level of development as fully sighted children.[1] Several studies of children who are blind have shown that tactile stimulation encourages them to explore visually (in the case of partial blindness) and tactilely (Guyer E, personal communication, January 1990).

Children who experience limited mobility, such as those with muscle weakness, chronic pain, cerebral palsy or paralysis, may also be deprived of stimulation to their skin, nerves, joints, muscles, and proprioceptors, resulting in decreased body awareness. Lack of movement usually results in poor circulation, especially to the legs. Without exercise, certain muscles atrophy and certain other muscles may be overused. When joints do not regularly move through normal range of motion, **contractures** may develop. Over time, bones that are not bearing weight may become decalcified. In addition, constipation may result from hypotonic abdominal muscles. Children may become stiffer and more limited in their

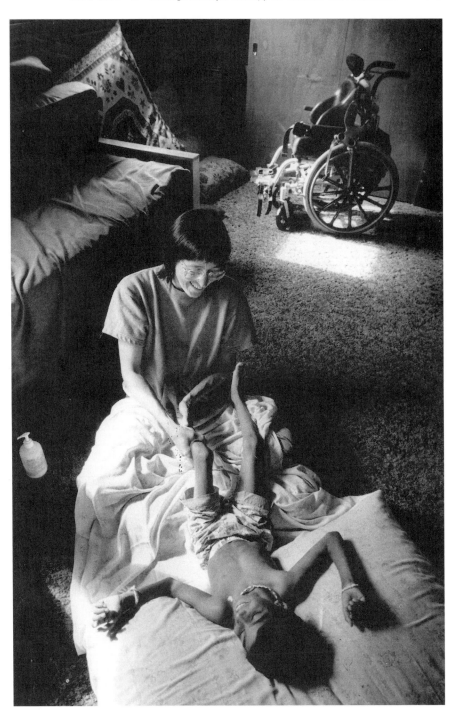

FIGURE 6–1 ■ Massaging a Child With Cerebral Palsy. Reprinted with permission from Wind J: Massage Therapist Soothes Disabled. *Corvallis Gazette-Times*, Corvallis, OR, July 9, 1991.

ability to move freely. Massage can give the tissue of children with limited movement the extra stimulation they need. During massage, children can benefit from being in positions that they may have forgotten were possible, and stretch or stimulate tissue that has not been challenged for a long time. Muscles, joints, blood vessels, nerves, and other tissue will receive extra information and greater activity.

Finally, because many individuals do not understand disability and fear touching them, many children will be deprived of tactile stimulation. Children with limited movement have fewer opportunities to be exposed to different types of touch sensations, and so they need more tactile stimulation than the average child.

SOCIAL ISOLATION

Some people do not realize that hearing-impaired children have difficulty hearing and they treat these children as if they were mentally slow. Children who are hearing impaired may be slow learning to relate to others, have difficulty in social situations and school, and feel lonely or forgotten. Hearing impairment can be a lonely and difficult disability, causing long-term stress.[2] Babies who are visually impaired and left alone tend to tune out and ignore the people and sounds around them. If children have difficulty playing and interacting with others, their social development may be also be delayed. Often, after a period in the hospital, a visually impaired child will seem unhappy about being held and will resist cuddling. If the child is permitted to remain in this isolation, development can be affected and the child will remain at that level.[3] Children with chronic physical disabilities may have similar problems, such as social isolation and difficulty with peers.[4]

According to the authors of *Can't the Child See?: A Guide for Parents and Professionals About Young Children Who Are Visually Impaired*, parents can show love to their visually impaired offspring with lots of holding, cuddling, patting, stroking, rocking, and just plain enjoying. "The child's name should be used a lot so that he or she learns it. The parents should hold the child upright and talk against a cheek so he or she can feel the puffs of breath. . . . Parents should not worry about spoiling the baby with too much loving. Whenever the baby is awake, the parents should carry it from room to room as they go about the daily household routine and talk to and touch the child with little pats, hugs, and kisses, so he or she knows they are there." After blind children are hospitalized, it is vitally important for the parents to cuddle them.[3]

Massage is a positive and pleasurable way of giving social contact and caring personal attention to the child with a disability. Massage therapist and educator Meir Schneider was born with cataracts and was severely visually impaired from birth. As a child, his grandmother frequently massaged him, and he remembers that massage gave him a sense of being truly supported and a strong sense of self-esteem (Schneider M, personal communication, May 1989).

SOCIAL DISCRIMINATION

People's attitude toward someone in a wheelchair can be very annoying and upsetting. Shopping on a Saturday can become a nightmare. People stand and stare at me or they give me funny looks. People never talk to you, they talk to whoever is pushing you. People think that just because you can't walk you can't talk either. I don't know why they think like this but they do and it is very annoying. I would like to be treated normally, like everyone else, and one of my ambitions is to be able to go from one end of the street to the other without one person turning around to look at me.[5]

—*Heather Jones, age 13*

Many disabled children constantly face discomfort and the uncertainly of dealing with persons who fear their disability. The mere presence of a disabled person forces many individuals to realize that they too might be vulnerable to disability, unsightliness, or even death. They find this frightening and threatening. Also, many nondisabled people are uncertain what type of behavior is appropriate. There are strong societal norms to be especially kind and careful with a disabled person; however, there are equally strong norms that disabled persons should be treated like everyone else to avoid condescension. Even when unintentional, children who are disabled are often treated differently, in a way that makes them uncomfortable. The quotation above shows how children in wheelchairs are deeply affected by the awkwardness, discomfort, and tension many nondisabled people show. Experiments conducted at Stanford University found that if a disabled person acknowledges his disability when he first meets a nondisabled person, the nondisabled person feels more comfortable and less awkward. If a child in a wheelchair simply uses the word "wheelchair" early in a conversation, he or she is likely to reduce the nondisabled person's tension and discomfort and make them more likely to treat the child in a normal way.[6] Unfortunately, in this situation it is up to the child who is disabled to cope with this awkwardness.

LOSS OF A POSITIVE BODY IMAGE

Another hazard of many illnesses and disabilities is the loss of a healthy and normal body image. Extensive bandages, painful and invasive medical procedures, restraints, or casts may decrease the tactile, kinesthetic, and visual perceptions that children use to define body boundaries. Without nursing interventions designed to provide them with adequate perceptual feedback, they may lose a sense of their bodies being whole and strong.[7] Evy McDonald, RN, came to hate her body after a childhood bout with polio that left her with one spindly, ill-shaped leg, and she came to have a "relentless obsession" with her weight. As an adult, McDonald decided to correct her "habitual and ingrained negativity" toward her body, but it required many months of concentrated daily effort to single out acceptable aspects of her body, repeating them to herself many times before she came to accept her body as it was.[8]

Regular massage therapy can help meet the need for caring and appropriate touch. It also supplies much-needed sensory stimulation, which informs the brain about the position of the body in space, its muscle tension, its movements, and its relationship to other people and objects in the environment. This additional information helps develop a healthy body image. People with disabilities often say they feel better about their bodies after massage therapy. Helen Rowe, an infant massage instructor who has worked with a variety of disabled children, found massage can help form a more positive body image. She worked with a girl who had spina bifida and tended to negate the entire lower part of her body; massage encouraged her to have a sense of body wholeness.[9] For another example, see the drawing of the boy whose body image improved after receiving acupressure (Chapter 1).

PHYSICAL OR SEXUAL ABUSE

Children with disabilities are two to three times more likely to be physically or sexually abused than nondisabled children because: (1) disabled children with communication problems may be unable to understand or verbalize episodes of abuse; (2) extra stress is placed on the parents and caregivers of disabled children, who need significantly more care than the average child and may act out with tantrums, aggressiveness, and noncompliance that exhaust the children and caregivers; and (3) children at special schools and residential care facilities are significantly more likely to be victims of sexual abuse than mainstreamed children because these settings, where children lack the protection of their natural home environment, often attract pedophiles. Perpetrators may include teachers, dormitory counselors, clergy, classroom aides, babysitters, custodians, and others.[10-13]

DEPRESSION

Chronic stress in children challenged by some or all of the problems discussed above can lead to depression. Additional stressors may include discomfort or pain, special diets, unpleasant medical procedures, and medications, all of which may make the child feel different at a time when, for most children, belonging is a driving force in their lives. For more information on depression, see Chapter 5, page 125.

CHRONIC DEHYDRATION

Children with some disabilities may be at an even greater risk of dehydration than nondisabled children. They may not be able to ask for water or get it themselves; they may not want to drink because of difficulty with swallowing or urinating; they may not cognitively identify thirst messages; or they may need more fluid due to constipation or medications. Diuretics, bulk-forming laxatives, methylphenidate hydrochloride (Ritalin), and some medications that affect peristalsis or treat seizures can lead to dehydration.

Chronically dehydrated children may be chronically tired and irritable. Many health problems worsen with dehydration. Signs of dehydration that you might observe when massaging a chronically dehydrated child include irritability, lethargy, and crying without shedding any tears. Two simple actions you can take in this case are to alert parents to the importance of their child being sufficiently hydrated and to offer children water before, during, and after the massage sessions. If parents suspect their children are not getting enough fluid, they should consult their pediatrician.[14]

CONTRACTURES

About 50% of physically disabled children develop **contractures,** especially children who are paralyzed, have severe joint pain, have been in bed for a long time, or have severe spasticity.[15] When an arm or leg is bent for a long time, some soft tissue around a joint becomes shorter and the limb cannot fully straighten. This persistent flexion of the joint is a "contracture." If a limb has been straight for too long and will not bend, this persistent extension of the joint is also referred to as a contracture. Any limb or joint that does not regularly move through its full range of motion can develop a contracture. Chronically tight muscle fibers eventually atrophy, to be replaced by thick, tough connective tissue.

GENERAL PRINCIPLES OF MASSAGE FOR CHILDREN WITH DISABILITIES

General principles for massaging children with disabilities include:

1. Learn the causes, symptoms, and contraindications of massage for each condition presented in this chapter. Remember that you are treating young people, not pathologies. Children are not defined by their disabilities and the specific challenges they represent; this is only part of who they are. Seeing each child as an individual is part of being fully present and caring; the mind-body connection in every child is more readily accessed when you do.

2. Although massage therapy may not affect the primary condition, the therapist can often help with secondary effects. For example, cerebral palsy is a problem deep in the brain. Although massage may impact the brain—particularly massage in the first 2 years of life when brain growth is occurring at a phenomenal pace—the massage techniques in this book do not address

brain dysfunction. This does not mean that massage is not of value. A child with cerebral palsy, for example, may develop **contractures,** scoliosis, limitations in movement, and a lack of stimulation from being in a wheelchair. Addressing these problems makes a significant improvement in the child's quality of life. Working with the child during the formative years, when body image, habits of relating to others, and ways of dealing with stress are being learned, ensures that the effects of massage are not just temporary. Some lessons that massage teaches children will be beneficial throughout their lives. The following is an example of massage treating a secondary symptom and not the primary condition: Eric Dalrymple was born 3 $1/2$ months premature. He weighed only 1 pound, 12 ounces and was only 12 $1/2$ inches long. In the hospital, he had pulmonary and gastric problems. His long-term disabilities, included **hydrocephalus, quadriplegic spastic cerebral palsy,** and visual impairment. Eric was age 15 when he began receiving massage therapy. His mother, Denise, feels that massage therapy had a profound effect on her son's life. "Because of his medical problems, most of Eric's early years were spent in the hospital with a ventilator in his mouth. Because the ventilator tube entered his mouth from the left, his head was always turned that way. With the ventilator removed and able to breathe on his own, Eric still held his head turned all the way to the left. This position increased his breathing difficulties. Through massage therapy, Eric learned to relax his neck. At first, it meant that I could position his head straight or to the right. With time and continued massage therapy, he began to turn his head on his own. Eric's breathing became easier. His frequent trips to the emergency department for breathing difficulties became a thing of the past. With improved breathing, Eric learned to speak. He now makes his wants and needs known. Talking allows him to interact with family, teachers, and fellow students at school. His personality has blossomed. If his head had remained locked to the left, I do not know that this would have ever happened."[1]

3. Contact the child's primary care physician or physical therapist before beginning massage with a child who is disabled. Both are excellent resources for understanding the child's specific needs, as well as any contraindications to massage. Work with the child's physical therapist, if possible, and consider both as part of the child's health care team. For example, the effec-

tiveness of any kind of massage will be diminished if the child is heavily medicated, but medication should never be stopped unless approved by the child's physician.

4. If a condition is not discussed in this book, be sure to consult with the patient's physician prior to massage. Due to space limitations, certain common pediatric disabilities that respond positively to massage were not included.

5. Never force massage on a child, especially a child who has already experienced many medical procedures over which he or she has no control. Begin with a little massage, use relaxation techniques whenever possible, and give lots of positive reinforcement. Some children may need to simply play in the therapy room at first or even watch a parent receive massage before they are comfortable. See the section on tactile defensiveness for additional suggestions. More than anything else, you should be prepared to meet children at their developmental level and let their responses guide the therapy. It may take some time but, gradually, children learn to respond to and to appreciate massage. Frequent short sessions may be better than fewer long ones.

6. The basic Swedish massage techniques covered in Chapter 3 work well with children with disabilities, and other successful therapies will be noted in each section. With any hands-on therapy, however, use caution and avoid causing pain by excessive pressure or movements that are too vigorous. Be especially gentle over sensitive areas, such as bony areas or where there has been surgery, pain, or trauma. If children have prescribed exercises, such as range of motion, they may be incorporated into the massage time. Range of motion is often substantially increased after massage.

7. Most children will benefit when their parents are taught how to massage them (see Appendix A). The Swedish massage techniques presented in Chapter 3 may be used, with the aid of handouts; however, individual practitioners may wish to teach other bodywork modalities, as well. Others who participate in a child's care, including siblings and caregivers, can also learn massage techniques. Parents also benefit tremendously from massage therapy, not only to relieve their own considerable stress, but also to help them understand how massage benefits their children.

8. Psychological factors may be paramount in understanding a child's condition and response to your treatment. Stress of any type (including physical pain, separation from parents or fami-

ly, neglect, or abuse) may damage a child's physical or emotional health. High levels of stress exacerbate or even initiate many conditions. A child's response to stress-reduction therapies, such as **medical hypnosis,** relaxation training, and biofeedback, indicates that the mind-body connection is more influential than often recognized. Examples of these therapies are included in Chapter 6. Massage may offer significantly more help in the mind-body realm than physical therapies that involve electrical devices or mechanical repetition. Through touch, a massage therapist helps children, not only by treating symptoms, but also by treating the whole person.

9. Treat each child as an individual. Even different children suffering from the same condition may have significantly different concerns. For example, three children with spinal cord injuries may need therapy for sensory stimulation; however, one may also have a major issue with constipation, one needs help in preventing pressure ulcers, and one experiences significant pain or restriction. It is important to listen carefully to the parents and child.

10. It is generally better to treat children with two short massages each week rather than one long massage. It is important not to tire the child's nervous system.

11. Any therapist working with children who are very ill should be aware that it can be emotionally demanding. It is important to network with other health professionals and to monitor and treat your own stress.

12. Nonmedicinal treatments that are helpful to children have been included under the "Complementary Treatments." Because all children are individuals, these treatments may not be effective for all children with a specific condition.

PHYSICAL AND SEXUAL ABUSE

My siblings and I were beaten for various transgressions: refusing to eat the lima beans in our soup, failing to clean our rooms, scrub our hands, or maintain silence at church. My mother's preferred instrument, a wooden paddle, inflicted a broad flash of pain that soon subsided. My father used his belt, a thinner, more flexible instrument capable of inflicting welts and bruises that lasted for weeks. Neither parent ever touched me in any other way. I have no memories of being kissed, hugged, rocked in my mother's arms, or even patted on the head. Still, throughout my childhood, I thought it was normal, that all kids were raised this way.

It wasn't until I studied domestic violence in a college sociology class that I realized what I'd endured fit the definition of child abuse. Suddenly a lot of things began to make sense, from my bouts of depression and low self-esteem, to my discomfort with touch, to my relationships with men. Throughout adolescence, I'd avoided dating by burying myself in books. Around age 21, wanting desperately to be "normal," I did start dating, but the only relationships I had were abusive. All the nice guys I drove away, quite consciously, because the thought of being kissed or stroked in a loving way was too frightening. At work, I got promotions for my calm, analytical nature, and it wasn't a facade—I was so absent from my body that I didn't feel any pain from working fifty-hour weeks. In truth, I was unable to relax. Abusing myself felt normal. I even avoided taking hot baths because as a child the hot water always made my various welts and bruises sting.

A television report on depression finally made me realize that I needed psychotherapy. I stuck with it for several years, and it helped me to come to terms with my childhood, even to forgive and authentically love my parents. But the insult had been received through my bones, muscles, and skin; my body, still so rigid and guarded, still storing its own memories of deprivation and pain and its own sense of loss, needed healing too. Fortunately, I found a skilled massage therapist who is guided by a strong sense of intuition. At first, I just endured my massages silently, checking out by occupying my mind with things I had to do, worries, and so on. But slowly and gently, she started to challenge me, asking me, "How does this feel?" as she worked on different areas. That forced me to stay present and, in time, taught me to honor my body in other ways and circumstances. It was a long process, of course, but I knew I was on the right track when one day I was caught in a summer storm and I felt the raindrops pitter-pattering on my bare skin. The gentle, loving touch of rain was new, something that I had never experienced before (Anonymous, personal communication, April 2003).

Each year in the United States there are at least one million confirmed cases of physical and sexual childhood abuse.[1] Physical child abuse is defined as *any pattern of physical discipline and punishment performed by a more powerful individual to a person younger than age 18, often resulting in physical injury, such as marks, bruises, welts, or fractures.* Sexual child abuse is defined as *any pattern of coerced sexual contact performed with a child by a more powerful individual.*

In children younger than age 2, 10% of all injuries result from abuse by adults, as do 25% of all fractures in children younger than age 3, 10% of all pediatric burn injuries, and the majority of pediatric traumatic brain injuries. An estimated 22% of children with learning disabilities acquire them as a result of abuse and neglect.[2-4] The consequences of this type of touch for children is of tremendous concern for the hands-on therapist. Abusive touch is not only the cause of tremendous suffering during childhood, it also represents an ongoing source of tactile defensiveness and tension in adult clients.

When children have been severely traumatized, from being in a natural disaster to witnessing an act of violence to being molested or beaten, they tend to have certain characteristic responses to trauma. The core reactions include hyperarousal, constriction, dissociation, and feelings of helplessness. Children may also react with hypervigilance, an extreme sensitivity to light and sound, hyperactivity, exaggerated startle responses, nightmares, abrupt mood swings, a reduced ability to deal with stress, and insomnia.[4-6] Children may not outgrow these reactions; stress can certainly have lifelong effects. It is not in the scope of this book to detail all the types of trauma that can befall a child; our focus here is on abuse that occurs through touch. For more information on this topic, see the suggested readings at the end of the chapter.

Children can be traumatized in ways that do not involve touch, such as seeing frightening images on television or movie screens, witnessing acts of violence, or being in a natural disaster or accident. Physical and sexual abuse, however, are distinguished from other forms of trauma by the element of touch and, when harm is transmitted through the hands of a powerful adult, the effects are far more complex and profound. A particularly negative effect is that children may become afraid of touch, in general or on specific areas of their bodies.

TACTILE DEFENSIVENESS CAUSED BY PAINFUL TOUCH

Examples of tactile defensiveness caused by painful touch include:

- Full-term infants who have experienced repeated heel lances for the purpose of drawing blood may associate simple skin cleansing with pain. In one study, infants of mothers with diabetes underwent 10 heel lances to test their blood within their first 24 hours. Each time, their heels were cleansed with alcohol and lanced. When the backs of their hands, which had never been cleansed or lanced before, were cleansed with alcohol prior to drawing blood samples, the infants began grimacing, moving their bodies, and crying, although no other procedure had been done. Within the first 24 hours, they were already conditioned to a certain type of touch meaning pain. They also had a more intense response to pain from blood draws than infants who had not received heel lances.[7] Another study compared infants who were circumcised soon after birth without any anesthetic with infants who received local anesthetic before circumcision. When the children who did not receive anesthetic were given vaccinations at 4 months, they had more pain and cried more than the infants who had been anesthetized.[8]

- Psychologist Thom Hartmann managed a residential treatment facility for severely emotionally disturbed children in New Hampshire. One Friday afternoon, 10-year-old Sally was left there for the weekend as an emergency placement. Nothing was known about the girl's history, only that she couldn't go home to her parents. Sally was assigned to the house of a child care worker named Linda, where the facility had an empty bed. That Friday night, Linda took Sally to the girl's bedroom and said, "Here's your bedroom, there's your bed, and there's a nightgown. You get ready for bed, and I'll be back in 10 minutes." When she returned, Sally had changed into her nightgown and was laying facedown on her bed. Linda sat on the bed next to her. Linda reached over to give Sally a gentle backrub and was just going to give the girl some words of encouragement, but she never had a chance because, just as her hand lightly touched Sally's shoulder, Sally exploded off the bed at her, screaming, clawing, biting, shouting that she was going to kill Linda, and slashing for Linda's face with her nails. Linda grabbed Sally's wrists and held her so that she couldn't hurt either of them, as Sally continued to sputter, shriek, and scream. Linda talked Sally down, saying, "It's okay, you're safe here, everything is going to be fine." After 4 or 5 minutes, an incredibly long time for such behavior to persist, Sally eventually stopped and lay quietly on the bed, panting to catch her breath. Thinking it was now a safe time to sit up, Linda let go of Sally's wrists and hoisted herself erect. She looked down at the little girl and saw that during the struggle, Sally's nightgown had worked its way up to the middle of her back. To her horror, Linda saw that Sally's back was covered with cigarette burns, both old and recent.[9]

There is a strong correlation between early physical and sexual abuse and adult health problems. Adults who were sexually or physically abused as children are more likely to be hypervigilant; to overreact to stress; to be depressed and anxious; to have chronic pain, including chronic pelvic pain and irritable bowel syndrome; and to be prone to substance abuse and sexual dysfunction.[10-15] Sexual abuse victims are also more likely to be sexually active earlier in life. A history of childhood sexual abuse increases a woman's chance of contracting AIDS by 2 1/2 times because she is more likely to have multiple sexual partners.[16]

Inappropriate and hurtful touch may lead children to abuse others.[4,17,18] Being abused or neglected as a child also increases the likelihood of arrest for a violent crime by 38%.[4] Disturbances in the capacity to accept touch can deeply affect interpersonal relationships, especially those involving intimacy, because there is often an inability to trust others. Abused children are, consequently, unlikely to receive the healthy touch they need. Psychotherapy has limited value for them, even as adults, because they carry the effects of abuse in their bodies, as well as their minds.

APPROACH AND GOALS

Many of the tactile problems seen in adults' massage sessions may stem from childhood abuse. The author worked with an adult client who could not tolerate tapotement on his back; he was reminded of the physical abuse from his brothers, who used to punch him in the back. Another adult client could not tolerate having her scalp massaged because, as a child, her grandmother braided her hair so tightly it made her cry; even the slightest pull on her hair was intolerable. Another was wary of touch in a large area around his armpits because, as a child, he had been tickled until he could not breathe. A friend of the author, who was taking a Hakomi bodywork class, lay down fully dressed upon a treatment table. When the instructor gently placed his palm on her lower abdomen, it triggered her first memories of the incest she had suffered as a small child more than 30 years before. Any hands-on therapist may inadvertently trigger memories, complete with tactile defensiveness, during a massage session. The recognition of abuse and the effects on both client and therapist during massage sessions led to "Trauma Touch," a special training for massage therapists. Therapists learn to recognize and help abuse victims in the context of massage therapy.

POINT OF INTEREST BOX 6–2
Helping Children Heal From Physical or Sexual Abuse

Ruth Rice's doctoral thesis in psychology was on the sensorimotor stimulation of premature infants. Called the Rice Sensorimotor Stimulation Technique, the technique consists of whole-body stroking and vestibular stimulation. It is extremely gentle and non-invasive and can be used with hospitalized infants, even very small or sick infants.[1] Dr. Rice worked with a 7-month-old infant who had been removed from his home because of physical abuse. He was so afraid of touch, he would shake and sweat whenever anyone touched him. Using her gentle technique, Dr. Rice massaged him for 10 minutes each day, every day for 1 week. At that time, there was a significant difference in his response to touch: He would no longer shake or sweat when touched and could relax instead (Rice R, personal communication, February 1985). A Touch Research Institute (TRI) study of sexually and physically abused children who lived in a shelter investigated the effect of massage. Children received a 15-minute Swedish massage once a day for a month; as a result, the children were less afraid of touch, more sociable, and better able to sleep.[2] Another TRI study found that massage reduced fear of touch, anxiety, depression, and blood cortisol levels of adults who were sexually abused.[3]

In Mexico, the author treated Raquelita, a 13-year-old girl with polio, in a class on massage for children who are disabled. When Raquelita was brought to the therapy room and realized she would be receiving some type of hands-on treatment, she began sobbing. She said all the physical therapy she had ever received had been painful. She was told that no one but her mother would touch her without her permission; her mother learned to do some simple Swedish massage strokes and massaged her twice in one afternoon. Raquelita was happy when she left for the day and gave her permission for students in the class to massage her. The last day of the course, she lay on the treatment table and smiled as her mother and three therapists massaged her at one time.

Suzie Klein is a massage therapist, a recreation therapist, and a foster mother to special needs children. Trained in the Trauma Touch program, she does "touch recovery work" with children. She provides them a safe environment to receive and accept healthy touch. The children are encouraged to explore her massage environment and are given many choices, including level of dress, lighting in the room, and how much touch or massage they receive, if any. Ms. Klein's emphasis is on gentle, nonthreatening touch; rather than stroking a child, she may use calming polarity therapy holds; pressure point massage; and the soothing weight of warm, rice-filled bags. Little by little, children who have been abused learn to trust her touch (Klein S, personal communication, March 1999).

References
1. Rice R: Neurophysiological development in premature infants following stimulation. *Journal of Developmental Psychology*, 13: 1977, p 69-76
2. Field T: Massage therapy for infants and children. *Developmental and Behavioral Pediatrics*, 16:108, 1995
3. Field T, Hernandez-Reif M, Hart S, et al: Massage therapy reduced aversion to touch and decreased anxiety, depression, and cortisol levels. *Journal of Bodywork and Movement Therapies*, 1:65-69, 1997

They are taught to respect the client's limits on touch and to help them accept touch without forcing it on them.[19] Hands-on therapists have also devised ways to heal the effects of abusive touch (see Point of Interest Box 6–2).

GENERAL PRINCIPLES FOR MASSAGING PHYSICALLY OR SEXUALLY ABUSED CHILDREN

When working with children who have been abused, the goal is not to practice a massage technique, but rather to provide a safe environment to receive healthy, safe touch. Technique must be secondary.

1. Parents should accompany children at all times, to support them and to help the therapist arrive at an appropriate treatment.
2. Care must be taken to honor the child's boundaries and empower him to say no to undesired touch.
3. Give them choices, such as:
   a. would they like to have their hair brushed instead of being massaged?
   b. would they like to lie on the massage table or would they prefer to sit in a chair?
   c. would they like to have a massage or would they like to just lay down under a blanket, with a hot pack on their chest or under their neck?
4. Any therapist may inadvertently do something that triggers an association with abuse; for example, one woman had experienced childhood abuse that involved having her arms tied above her head. As a result, she not only avoided lifting her arms above her head to wash her hair or hang curtains, she could not tolerate having her arms raised above her head during massage sessions.[20]
5. Avoid areas that children do not want touched. A child who has been sexually abused can fear touch in many parts of the body, but especially around the pelvis, buttocks, thighs, or abdomen. Do not massage a child unclothed until a few sessions have been performed with the child clothed.
6. Use gentle touch and do not cause pain.
7. Ask the child often for feedback; observe the child for signs of stress, such as increased heart rate, increased muscle tension, a change in their breathing pattern, sweating, or anxiety.

MASSAGE TREATMENT FOR PHYSICALLY OR SEXUALLY ABUSED CHILDREN

The first time the child comes for treatment, give the parent a short massage while the child plays. Then ask the child if she would like you to give her a massage. If she does not want you to massage her, ask if she would like her parent to give her a massage. If she is agreeable to this, have her choose where she will receive the massage and what clothing she will take off. Let her pick any massage tools or hot packs she would like used. Show the parent a few basic strokes (see Appendix A). Passive touch and other static techniques, such as polarity therapy, Jin Shin Do, Reiki, or craniosacral therapy, may be most effective at first. Swedish massage techniques may be too unpredictable; as your hands constantly change position, the child will not know exactly where your hands will move next. If she does not want massage at all, try to interest her in hot packs or massage toys she can use herself, and then continue to massage the parent. That may be all that is possible for a first session.

MASSAGE SEQUENCE FOR THE CHILD WHO WILL ACCEPT TOUCH

Positioning:

Have the child lie supine and fully clothed on the treatment table. Drape her completely, and give her a hot pack. A hot water bottle on the chest may be a comforting weight and, if the child is supine, she may place her hands on it, as well.

Step 1. Begin with the basic relaxation sequence and passive touch on the face (Figure 3–1). Keep the hands still for at least 2 minutes. This may be all that is possible during the first session. If the child jumps off the table after 5 minutes, do not try to restrain her, but return to massaging the parent.

Step 2. If the child appears comfortable, ask permission to massage the head and neck, hands, or feet. These are generally safer and less guarded areas. Use the Swedish massage strokes described in Chapter 3, but do not use tapotement. Continue to observe the child carefully and ask for her feedback. As trust is built with the child over time, more massage may be allowed. For example, after a session with just the head, neck, hands, and feet, the back may be massaged next. Gradually, all the strokes of a whole-body massage may be accepted and appreciated.

AUTOIMMUNE DEFICIENCY SYNDROME

Autoimmune deficiency syndrome (AIDS) is an infection with the human immunodeficiency virus (HIV). This virus infects and destroys the body's T helper cells, which normally kill invading bacteria and fungal cells. When enough T cells are destroyed, children develop immunodeficiency, with a poor ability to fight infection, extreme weight loss, and central nervous system problems. Although there have been major advances in treatment, AIDS is still considered a terminal illness. Each year in the United States, 1,000 new cases of AIDS are reported in children younger than 13. HIV infection is the seventh leading cause of death in children ages 1 to 4.[1] 90% of American children with HIV acquire it from their mothers, in utero, during birth, or from breast-feeding. The remaining 10% acquire it from contaminated blood products, sexual abuse or activity, and intravenous blood use.[2] Of those who acquire HIV from their mothers, 25% have serious symptoms related to infection by age 1 and die in 2 to 4 years. The others have virtually no symptoms in the first 5 years and survive, at least, until age 9.

The most common physical complaints of children with HIV/AIDS are chronic fatigue; recurring diarrhea; acute weight loss; insomnia; fungal and viral infections, leading to mouth and dental pain; and the development of serious infections, such as pneumonia, sepsis, and meningitis. These children are also more likely to have cancer, particularly lymphoma, and they can develop diseases of the heart, lungs, kidneys, or other organs. HIV may also have subtle effects on cognition and neurodevelopment, and so these children may have greater incidences of attention deficit disorder and learning disabilities. Children with HIV may also experience depression, anxiety, and adjustment reactions, which may be related to the child's reaction to the fatigue and pain of a chronic illness, to neurologic aspects of the disease, or to a general feeling of malaise from the adverse effects of medication. Children with this disease frequently have extremely high stress levels: Only 38% of children with AIDS live with their parents, and they may experience other major stresses, such as long-term hospitalization or neglect. Unfortunately, this suppresses the immune system; one study of HIV+ children showed that those with an increased number of negative life events also had more suppressed immune systems.[2]

APPROACH AND GOALS

Kathleen Weber is a pediatric nurse, massage therapist, and project coordinator for pediatric AIDS clinical trials at Children's Memorial Hospital in Chicago, Illinois. She found that massage can help children with AIDS to relieve insomnia, reduce the muscle aches and cramps common with this disease, and maintain good circulation throughout the body. Because many people fear contracting the disease, many children with AIDS have not had their needs for touch met; sensitive, gentle massage can go a long way toward meeting this need. Massage may also stimulate the child's digestion and appetite and help

make breathing easier. Most important, massage releases the tension and stress that can be caused by the guarding of specific body areas traumatized by invasive medical procedures or physical pain (Weber K, RN, LMT, personal communication, April 1992).

Researchers at the Touch Research Institute conducted three studies on children with HIV/AIDS. In two separate studies with HIV-exposed infants, the massaged infants had significantly greater weight gain and less stress behavior than the nonmassaged, control infants. Sadly, the nonmassaged infants deteriorated, showing early signs of developmental delay and failure to thrive.[3] A third study investigated the effect of massage with HIV-positive adolescents, ages 13 to 19, receiving similar drug regimens. Teens in the control group were led through 20 minutes of progressive muscle relaxation, twice a week for 12 weeks. Teens in the massage therapy group received a 20-minute seated massage, twice a week for 12 weeks. The technique included kneading, pressing, long strokes, finger pressure along the spine, and hand massage. The massage therapy group reported feeling less depressed than those in the relaxation group and showed improvement in immune function not shown in the relaxation group.[4]

MASSAGE FOR CHILDREN WITH HIV/AIDS

The basic relaxation sequence described in Chapter 3 cannot be used too often; continually remind the child to relax. Be sensitive to what the child needs and ask often for feedback. At the outset, ask the child if he or she has any areas that are sore, from needles or any other painful medical procedures, and carefully avoid touching these areas. Gentle stroking may be more appropriate than vigorous massage. At times, energy techniques, such as polarity therapy, Reiki, or craniosacral techniques, may be most effective. Simply laying your hands on a tight area, letting it be warmed by the heat of your hands, can be soothing. If the child is sick, massage only the hands and feet and gently stroke the forehead. Gently percussing the chest and upper back (Figure 3–9) may help a child expel mucus and relax the chest. Gentle, but thorough, massage of the abdomen, including thumb-stroking the stomach (Figure 5–4), may help stimulate the appetite.

1. Because even common childhood illnesses can be life threatening to children with AIDS, you should be careful that you are well and do not expose them to illness.
2. Do not massage tumors, undiagnosed lumps, or skin with open sores. Stay at least 2 inches away from any skin rash, unless the child is clothed; then gentle stroking, pressure points, or range-

of-motion exercises can be used. Certain therapists recommend staying away from the armpit and groin areas where there are large concentrations of lymph nodes; consult with the child's physician about this.

3. Wash your hands before and after massage. Gloves should always be worn if the child's skin or the skin on your hands is not smooth and intact. Weeping skin lesions or bleeding are absolute contraindications for massage of a specific area. Consult with the child's doctor about whether or not gloves should be worn at all times.

ASTHMA

Asthma, an allergic disorder compounded by emotional stress, is a chronic disease of the lungs. Children with asthma typically have airway hypersensitivity, inflammation, and occasional acute obstruction.[1,2] It is the most common chronic condition and cause for hospitalization of children. Pediatric asthma is currently occurring in epidemic proportions in the United States, affecting 5 million children. In 1980, 3.6% of children suffered from asthma, compared with 7.5% in 1995 and 9% in 2001. Incidents of acute asthma among children have increased 100% in the past decade. Black children have significantly more asthma than white children, and hospitalization rates are up to 21 times higher in poor or minority areas than in affluent communities.[3] Robert Ivker, an ear, nose, and throat physician and author of *Asthma Survival*, believes that four major factors contribute to the pediatric asthma epidemic—air pollution, immune dysfunction, allergies, and stress.[2]

When children have asthma, there is often a history of allergy in the family or they may have a parent with the disease. They may also have other allergic responses, such as hayfever. Common allergens that provoke an attack are animal fur and dander; mold; dust mites; fungi; and chemicals, such as paint fumes, car exhaust, and tobacco smoke. In cities, airborne particles of mouse and rat urine and the feces and corpses of dead cockroaches are primary indoor air pollutants that trigger pediatric asthma. Sudden vigorous exercise, viral infection (especially chest infections), or sudden changes in temperature and humidity can provoke an asthma attack, especially when children are emotionally stressed. During an attack, the muscles that surround the bronchi spasm and cause the airways to narrow. This constricts the outward passage of exhaled air; the effort of exhaling produces the characteristic wheeze. The mucous membranes become swollen and mucus is secreted in large amounts (Figure 6–2).

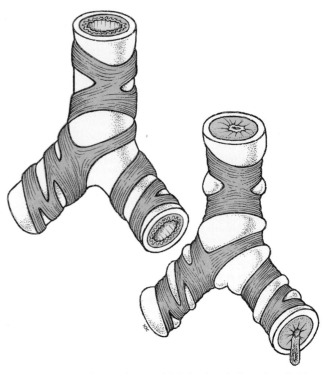

FIGURE 6–2 ■ Changes in Bronchiole During Asthma Attack. Note the constriction of the muscles surrounding the bronchioles, causing them to become narrower, and also the increased secretion of mucus. Reprinted with permission from Hardy NO: Westpoint, CT.

Pediatric asthma symptoms vary; one child may have less bronchospasm and more inflammation and swelling of the airways, another child may experience the opposite. Attacks may last minutes, hours, or even days. During this time, reduced oxygen causes alarm or panic. Usually the child needs to sit up and lean forward, which assists the accessory muscles of the chest to expand and contract. Lips and faces may become pale or bluish from lack of oxygen, if the attack is extreme. Lack of oxygen is truly a life-or-death situation, and panic can worsen an attack; the more scared a child becomes, the more the bronchial tubes spasm. The stress of asthma attacks often causes extreme tension in the respiratory muscles. Years of difficult breathing may cause a child to have extreme tension in the muscles of the back and rib cage, reduced mobility in the rib cage and spine and, possibly, a spinal curvature.[4]

Standard medical treatment for asthma consists of avoiding allergens; a daily dose of inhaled steroids; and an emergency bronchodilator, which may be used during an attack. Long term, these medications do not remove the cause of the asthma; however, inhaled corticosteroids do repair inflammatory damage to bronchial tissue without systemic adverse effects. Oral and intravenous corticosteroids, however, disrupt endocrine balance and damage a child's growth, metabolism, appearance, and muscular and nervous function.[1]

Several studies found that stress may have a major influence on the development of asthma and its clinical course. In one study, each child studied had one parent with asthma. Researchers found that parenting difficulties, such as the mother's depression, problems with infant care, and inadequate marital support significantly correlated with developing asthma early in childhood.[5] Another study found that a child's risk of having asthma attacks significantly increased in the weeks after major negative life events or stress.[6] Another study found that children in families that experienced intense levels of stress were three to four times more likely to develop asthma. The earlier stress was experienced in life, including in utero, the greater the risk of asthma.[2] A fourth study found that children hospitalized for asthma who later died of an asthma attack outside the hospital were more likely to have had psychological problems, such as depression, family dysfunction, or difficulty dealing with separation or loss.[7] Robert Ivker identified several factors as possible sources of emotional stress that may aggravate asthma in children with the condition, including grief caused by the physical or emotional loss of a parent; a lack of bonding, especially a lack of physical affection, between the child with asthma and her parents; and a lack of closeness between the child's mother and father. Ivker believes that these emotional factors should be addressed and integrated as part of asthma treatment that goes beyond managing symptoms.[2]

EFFECTIVE MIND-BODY INTERVENTIONS IN ASTHMA TREATMENT

1. Medical hypnosis can affect the status of acute episodes by decreasing anxiety and relieving wheezing. For example, a 6-year-old boy with active wheezing and a respiratory rate of 36, improved dramatically under medical hypnosis and, within minutes, had no detectable wheezing and a respiratory rate of only 16.[8] Even very young children can use hypnosis to reduce the frequency of acute episodes and the number of emergency department visits and hospitalizations. When they learn how to control their symptoms, children not only learn to stop acute episodes but also to increase their ease of breathing, which ultimately decreases medication.[8,9]

2. Relaxation training, such as biofeedback and relaxation exercises, has been successful in shortening asthma attacks, reducing severity and frequency of acute attacks, and reducing the child's need for medication.[10-14]

3. Touch may have an immediate effect on a child's breathing. Brian Athorp has been a res-

piratory therapist for 30 years and a massage therapist for 10 years. It was when working as a respiratory therapist that he became so impressed with the therapeutic power of hands-on therapy that he was inspired to study massage therapy. For example, when doing a simple chest assessment before giving medication to an individual in an acute asthma attack, the respiratory therapist's hands are gently placed on the lateral aspects of the patient's ribcage. At times, Athorp noticed an immediate and dramatic improvement in the patient's breathing and emotional state; simply placing his hands on the person in a caring way could help a patient become less anxious and reduce the severity of an attack (Athorp B, personal communication, July 2002).

Diane Charmley observed that, in a hospital setting, a child's asthma worsens when anxious. A pediatric nurse and massage therapist, she found that **therapeutic touch** was an effective way to decrease children's asthma symptoms; standing behind children, talking to them, and helping them identify their feelings. Therapeutic touch anchored them and decreased their anxiety while they identified their feelings. With the therapist standing behind them, with no one looking at their face, the children could more freely express their feelings (Charmley D, RN, personal communication, October 2002).

APPROACH AND GOALS

Massage therapy can accomplish two goals: reduce symptoms of an acute asthma attack and reduce the frequency and severity of asthma attacks over time. Athorp feels that effectively applied massage techniques can reduce the child's symptoms during an asthma attack, which may reduce use of bronchodilators and other drugs. If a child can be reassured by massage and drawn out of her panic-driven isolation, she may require less medication for the asthma attack and less sedative or antianxiety medication. "Massage can introduce comfort and serenity into a world of pain and chaos . . . mitigating the adverse effects of what can be coldly impersonal critical care in a hospital setting (Athorp B, personal communication, July 2002)."

Dr. Cesario Hossri, a clinical psychologist and professor at the State University of Santo, Brazil, has been able to eliminate asthma attacks in most of the children with whom he works by using massage during an attack to relieve muscle spasm (most common in the muscles between the ribs and those of the back, shoulders, and diaphragm), to help dilate the bronchioles and to encourage respiration. When respiratory distress is lessened and nasal breathing restored, Hossri uses hypnosis to suggest body relaxation and a sense of peace.[15]

Massage can also benefit children with asthma simply by reducing their stress levels. A Touch Research Institute study found that when parents gave daily Swedish massage to their children with asthma for 1 month, the children had fewer asthma attacks and were less anxious. The children also had improved pulmonary function, determined by daily peak airflow readings. The parents gave the children simple relaxation massages, not addressing specific patterns of tension in the children.[16]

A long-term goal of massage therapy for children with asthma is to help them become aware of how it affects them physically and to give them tools to breathe more easily, before they build up a high level of muscle tension. During an asthma attack, a child may find it easier to breathe with her torso braced and supported by her arms. However, this position, although it stabilizes the chest wall, tenses the entire body. As a result, children may have tension in the intercostal, pectoral, trapezius, sternocleidomastoid, and scalene muscles. Massage therapists working with adults with respiratory problems find deep tension in the ribcage and back muscles and, yet, the adults are not aware how stress relates to the ability to breathe easily. A pilot study of massage with adults who had chronic asthma found that, despite having asthma for many years, most did not realize that stress played a role in their illness. After 12 weeks of seated massage sessions, they reported less chest tightness, wheezing, and fatigue, and a better ability to handle stress.[17] Massage therapists Pamela Klimowitch and Patrick Malone, who work with adults with respiratory problems, observed deep tension in the chest, diaphragm, and back muscles of adults with chronic difficult breathing. After massage, these adults breathe easier and have less chest tightness.[18,19]

MASSAGE AND HYDROTHERAPY FOR ASTHMA ATTACKS

During an attack, always observe the child carefully and have the child's bronchodilator or other medication available in case her condition worsens. Most individuals with asthma cannot lie down during an attack without further compromising the ability to breathe. They usually must sit up or recline at an angle of more than 45 degrees.

DRINKING HOT LIQUID

Provide hot liquids at the onset of an attack, such as soup or green or black tea. Any warm liquid may lessen the severity of an asthma attack or quickly relieve it because warm liquids can soothe the bronchial tubes. The caffeine in green or black tea may stop initial symptoms for some individuals before the attacks escalate. Caffeine opens the airways much like the inhalers used by asthmatics. According to allergist and clinical immunologist, Eric Schenkel, MD, "Even during an attack, warm drinks can soothe it in 5 to 60 minutes. During the day of an attack, I recommend between six and eight glasses of warm water or another drink, continuing even after the attack ends."[20,21]

STEAM INHALATION

Certain children's symptoms decrease if they are in a warm, humid room (temperature, high 70°s to low 80°s). Parents may take children into a bathroom, turn the shower on, and let it run, filling the air with steam. If this helps children breathe better, parents may stay in with them as long as is needed or until the hot water is gone. Make sure the child stays warm and does not become chilled when leaving the bathroom.

MOIST HEAT APPLICATION

Apply a moist heating pad or fomentation from the back of the neck to the waist. Have the child lay on this for 30 minutes. If she cannot lay supine, have her sit down in front of a table, place a pillow on the table, have her rest her hands on a pillow, and place her head on her hands. Put the hot application on her back in that position. Cover her back with a blanket or sheet.

CHEST HEATING COMPRESS

Step 1. Put a hot fomentation or Hydrocollator pack on the chest for 10 minutes.
Step 2. Make a compress by dipping a towel in cold water, wringing it out, and covering it with another towel or other insulating material.
Step 3. Apply the heating compress around the child's chest.
Step 4. Leave it for 1 hour or more.

MASSAGE SEQUENCE FOR AN ASTHMA ATTACK

The suggestions here are from a classic article by Dr. Cesario Hossri.[15] Do not wait until a child is in the middle of an asthma attack to try massage! Learn at least some basic body massage strokes (Chapter 3), especially for the chest, stomach, and back. Do these strokes with the child, and emphasize learning to relax. When massaging the chest, stroke in between each rib with the fingertips, beginning at the sternum and stroking around to the back. This will help relax the intercostal muscles. Use abdominal effleurage (page 82) and let your hand trace along the bottom ribs while it circles the top half of the abdomen. Do not push on the xyphoid process. Practice the massage sequence in this section at least a few times before trying it during an asthmatic attack. Have the child's bronchodilator or other medication available in case massage does not eliminate the attack.

Step 1. Have the child lie prone. If not possible, place two or three large pillows on a table, seat the child on a chair in front of the table, with his hands on the pillow and his head on his hands. This exposes the back.

Step 2. Massage next to the spine, from the lower back to the base of the occiput. Put your hands on either side of the spine, beginning at the lower back. With the tips of the middle and ring fingers, use gentle pressure to rub up and down on the tissue next to each vertebra 10 times, ONLY ON EXHALATION. Do more in areas that feel tight. Then vibrate or quiver your fingers on the same area briefly, ONLY ON EXHALATION. Work up the back one vertebra at a time.

Step 3. Chest percussion (Figure 3–9) Gently percuss the spine between the shoulder blades. Continue for 30 seconds.

Step 4. Thumbstroke between the scapulae (Figure 3–18). Repeat for 1 minute.

Step 5. Thumbstroke on both sides of the neck next to the vertebrae. Repeat for 1 minute.

Step 6. Abdominal effleurage (Figure 3–36). Have the child lie on his back. If he cannot lie supine, prop him up with as many pillows as needed to be comfortable. Massage the entire abdomen, using gentle pressure. Use more pressure as the child exhales. Repeat 10 times.

Step 7. Chest friction (Figure 3–35). Repeat 10 times.

Step 8. Basic relaxation sequence, emphasizing relaxation of the feet, stomach, and chest.

MASSAGE AND HYDROTHERAPY FOR CHILDREN WITH CHRONIC ASTHMA

MOIST HEAT APPLICATION

Moist heat application. Apply moist heat packs on the chest to warm and loosen the anterior myofascia and muscles of the chest before treatment, and on the upper back to warm and loosen the posterior musculature. An ideal way to integrate moist heat is to massage another part of the child's body for 10 minutes, while he or she is supine and heat packs are warming both the chest and the upper back.

CONTRAST TREATMENT OF THE CHEST

(Figure 3–55; see directions in Chapter 5)

MASSAGE SEQUENCE

Step 1. Basic relaxation sequence with a focus on relaxed breathing. Include suggestions for relaxing the chest, upper back, and abdomen, such as "Feel your chest relax and get wider," "Feel your stomach get soft and warm," "Feel the muscles in between your shoulder blades relax," "Let your back slowly sink into the bed," and "Feel how softly and easily your ribs can move." It is also important to teach the child to breathe abdominally. Have him lie on his back, put his hands on his abdomen, and concentrate on the way his hands move during inhalation and exhalation. Ask him to see how much he can increase the movement of his hands by breathing deeply into the stomach. (Breathing should still be relaxed.) You may also have the child sit up, put one hand on the abdomen and one hand on the lower back, and increase the space between his hands by breathing into the abdomen. Another way to encourage deep, relaxed breathing is for the child to imagine his breath flowing into the lungs and pelvis as he inhales—feeling the chest and pelvis expanding—then, on the exhale, letting the chest and pelvis settle back to their original size. Repeat 10 to 20 times.

Step 2. Effleurage the back (Figure 3–2). Repeat 10 times.

Step 3. Knead the upper trapezius (Figure 3–17). Repeat for 30 seconds on each side.

Step 4. Thumbstroke between the scapulae (Figure 3–18). Repeat for 1 minute.

Step 5. Thumbstroke the lower back (Figure 3–19). Repeat for 1 minute.

Step 6. Shoulder and neck effleurage (Figures 3–26 and 3–27). Repeat 10 times.

Step 7. Chest and abdomen effleurage (Figure 3–34). Repeat for 1 minute.

Step 8. Chest friction (Figure 3–35). Repeat for 30 seconds.

Step 9. Rake between the ribs. Begin at the sternum and rake out to the sides of the chest, with each finger tracing between a different rib. Do not push on the xyphoid process. This stroke relaxes the intercostal muscles; however, the area may be ticklish, so go slowly and let the child become accustomed to the sensation. Work from the bottom to the top of the ribcage. Avoid breast tissue on a girl.

Step 10. Chest and abdomen effleurage three times.

Step 11. Passive range-of-motion exercises for the neck and shoulder joints (Figures 3–11 and 3–12).

Step 12. Basic relaxation sequence, with a focus on relaxed breathing.

COMPLEMENTARY TREATMENTS

1. Acupuncture can relieve acute attacks.
2. Movement therapies, such as Feldenkrais and Alexander technique, can improve

breathing by releasing tension and increasing mobility in the child's respiratory muscles.

3. Manipulative therapies can improve the mobility of the ribcage and spine.

ATTENTION DEFICIT DISORDER AND HYPERACTIVITY

Attention deficit disorder (ADD) is the most common neurodevelopmental disorder of childhood, affecting 3–5% of school-age children and at least four times as many boys as girls. ADD is a general term that includes a wide variety of children who may actually have different neurologic profiles and problems. ADD is characterized by a short attention span, impulsivity, and distractibility. Children display a low tolerance for frustration, a lack of motivation for all but the most stimulating activities, and a tendency to become bored easily. It is difficult for them to recognize the future consequences of their behavior and learn from their mistakes. Many have difficulty reading the nuances of social behavior and controlling their impulses, which causes social problems. Of children with ADD, 25% have a learning disability. Children with ADD are also at increased risk for depression and anxiety. Certain children with ADD are hyperactive as well; it is then termed attention deficit hyperactivity disorder (ADHD). Hyperactivity is a general restlessness or excessive level of movement; the child is in perpetual motion. ADD/ADHD can have serious and life-long effects on an individual's functioning (see Point of Interest Box 6–3). Despite these difficulties, some children with ADD/ADHD are highly successful in those areas where they devote their motivation, energy, and enthusiasm.[1]

ADD can be inherited; however, other factors known to affect brain development may predispose children to this disorder, including infections of the brain, head trauma, maternal use of alcohol or cocaine, metabolic disorders, premature birth or low birth weight, and exposure to high levels of lead and mercury in utero or afterward. (One in 12 women of childbearing age has blood mercury levels that could interfere with fetal brain development.) Complications during labor, delivery, and infancy may also be related.[2-4] Osteopath John Upledger believes that a structural problem involving malalignment of the cranial bones may be a primary factor in a significant percentage of children with ADD. He believes that head trauma, including that which occurs at birth, can cause this malalignment.[5]

Standard medical treatment for ADD includes appropriate school programs, behavior modification, counseling, and medication. As of 2002, about 4 million American children, mostly boys, were taking

POINT OF INTEREST BOX 6–3
ADD Is Serious

Diagnosis and treatment of ADD can be controversial, given the high number of children who have been diagnosed and that so many receive psychostimulant medications. Parents and professionals worry that children who have other problems are being diagnosed with ADD; for example, a child who is inattentive in a classroom may have a hearing problem, learning disability, or other problem that is not ADD. Despite these legitimate concerns, it is wrong to think that ADD is a minor disorder. The consequences of untreated ADD are: 52% will have drug and/or alcohol abuse as adults; 43% of untreated, aggressive boys who are hyperactive will be arrested for a felony by age 16; 35% never finish high school. A study of new inmates to one of the largest prisons in California reported 75% had a childhood history of ADD or learning disabilities.[1]

Reference

1. Amen D: *ADD: A Guide for Primary Care Physicians.* Fairfield, CA: The Amen Clinic for Behavioral Medicine, 1999, p 51

methylphenidate (Ritalin).[6] Psychostimulant medications, such as Ritalin and Cyclert, stimulate the parts of the brain associated with attention, arousal, and inhibition, but the effect lasts only as long as the drug is in the child's system. These drugs do nothing to treat neurologic dysfunction. Adverse effects may include loss of appetite, insomnia, and nervousness. According to child psychiatrist Elizabeth Guthrie, "Whenever I write a prescription for a child or a teenager, I am concerned not just about the possible adverse effects, but also the unknown. What about the subtle changes impacting the child's personality development? Are they all for the good? Do we know what they are?"[7]

There is an ongoing concern, within the medical community and among parents, that Ritalin may be overprescribed. Children with such problems as inattentiveness associated with a learning disability or a hearing impairment or simply very active and alert children, may be receiving Ritalin inappropriately.[6,8]

Parents seeking additional therapies for their children have tried nutritional approaches, treatment of food allergies, craniosacral therapy, **neurofeedback,** and neurodevelopmental therapies. Each treatment appears to be effective for some children but not for all, probably reflecting the fact that ADD is a general term which covers a variety of conditions. Medical understanding of ADD is still evolving, and brain scans and other technology may soon alter how this disorder is perceived. For example, psychiatrist Daniel Amen now asserts that there are six basic types of ADD, each with a different treatment.[9]

Parents of children with ADD may also experience a great deal of stress. They may be exhausted from years of chasing a hyperactive child; fielding complaints from neighbors, teachers, and peers about the child's behavior; trying various types of therapies; and worrying about their child. Even those parents with excellent parenting skills can be worn down by the constant demands of a child with ADD.

APPROACH AND GOALS

ADD is stressful for children, who often struggle academically and receive negative attention at school, in social situations, and at home. Certain therapies do not treat the cause of ADD but help the child deal with stress. Medical hypnosis, although not a primary treatment for attentional problems, can help the child be less anxious, sleep better, and develop strategies for controlling emotional outbursts. Relaxation training with biofeedback machines is also effective for controlling symptoms of ADD and hyperactivity.[10] Massage therapy may fit in this category; although not treating the cause of ADD, it helps children reduce stress and be calmer. In one study, adolescent boys with ADD received 15-minute Swedish massage sessions on the back and neck. Massages were given every day after school for 10 consecutive school days. At the end of the study, the boys were less fidgety, rated themselves as happier, and were able to stay on a task longer in the classroom.[11] Acupressure has helped some children reduce or eliminate medication.[12] *High-Tech Touch* (Academic Therapy Publications, 1987) cites hyperactive children treated with acupressure massage. One 9-year-old girl not only began to act in a calm, poised manner, but also followed more complex directions and improved in fine- and gross-motor skills. Her medication (Ritalin) was withdrawn after three massage sessions. A 17-year-old boy with chronic behavior problems was resistant to massage at first, and it was several months before he showed improvement; with time, he became more relaxed, better able to focus, and more interested in his environment. Other children had less frequent and less intense temper tantrums.[13] One hyperactive young boy received a few minutes of polarity therapy from his therapist whenever his behavior became hysterical; he would then fall asleep for an hour or two and awaken relaxed and able to interact normally with others.[14] Other forms of touch have been used to treat hyperactive children. An approach developed by Jean Ayres treats hyperactive and touch-phobic children by gradually introducing them to touch. For example, a technique that incorporates the calming effects of deep pressure, warmth, and slow stroking is to wrap the child snugly in a blanket and roll a ball slowly and firmly down her back for about 3 minutes.[15]

MASSAGE TREATMENT FOR ADD

Massage therapy, using the techniques described in this book, will help children reduce their tension levels and give them a true sense of what it means to be relaxed. Teaching children to manage their tension levels is as important as the physical benefit of massage. Use massage first to give the child the experience of relaxation and then spend more time teaching relaxation exercises. It may require considerable ingenuity on your part to get the child to lie relatively still during the first few massages. A short massage, rather than the time required for a full-body massage, will be necessary at first. It may be necessary to follow the children around to massage them, rather than expect them to lie still. Begin with the massage of the back described in Chapter 3; however, be prepared to use strokes from other parts of the body if the child is moving around. Do not restrain the child. If strokes for the back are well accepted, try to follow the entire sequence described in Chapter 3.

Be certain that there are no distractions in your office, such as clutter or loud noises. If children have specific music that they find relaxing, have the parent bring it along. A few simple toys may help keep the child occupied. You may wish to teach parents one or two simple massage strokes and the basic relaxation sequence, which can be done at naptime or bedtime when children are more likely to lay still. If parents practice them for just a short time every day, it will reinforce the learning of relaxation. Many such short repetitions can help the child learn to relax. Over time, children with ADD/ADHD can learn to relax and enjoy all the strokes of a full-body massage.

AUTISM

In order to receive pleasure from physical touch, it ought always to have been initiated by me and I ought, at the very least, to have been given a choice . . . When people didn't touch me, I never experienced this as neglect. I experienced it as love and understanding.[1]

—*Donna Williams, adult with autism*

Autism is a biochemical brain disorder or dysfunction of the central nervous system, possibly caused by a neurochemical abnormality or a metabolic problem (see Point of Interest Box 6–4). About one in 1,000 children have autism; however, since

POINT OF INTEREST BOX 6–4
Autism and Sensory Input

There are three particular aspects of the decoding of sensory information that tend to be abnormal among people with autism. The registration of sensory information, controlled, in part, by the brain stem, is chronically often dramatically, faulty; common visual stimuli such as bright lights or moving objects often seem to go unnoticed, unobserved, while seemingly trivial objects—a loose thread on a jacket, a crumb on a patterned carpet—receive rapt attention.

The ability to modulate sensory input similarly appears to be flawed, leaving many people with autism unable to hear a focused conversation in a busy restaurant, for example, instead hearing each voice and every voice in a loud, confused, and congested jumble. In much the same manner, a hand placed on a shoulder or a forearm can seem like a stranglehold; a grape's slight acidity is little less than poison; an unfamiliar object—a chair, a doll, a ball—invades a bedroom, an otherwise safe environment, and holds the person horridly captive.

The ability to integrate information from the senses and to make that information meaningful similarly seems compromised, of course . . . the inability to use the senses to help locate one's body in space can impart something that you and I can only imagine as a kind of constant dizziness, making it difficult to plan and organize the series of muscle movements that lead a spoon to an open mouth, or that result in shoelaces successfully tied into bows—the senses getting in the way in those cases and in dozens more analogous to them.[1]

—Russell Martin

Reference

1. Martin R: *Out of Silence: A Journey into Autism.* New York, NY: Henry Holt, 1994

sitive to touch that they avoid it altogether. Repetitive behaviors, such as hand-flapping, biting themselves, or rocking, are common. Many years ago, psychiatrist Nik Waal observed that children with autism tend to have stiff shoulders, tightly clenched jaws and mouths, and shallow breathing.[3]

It is often difficult for health professionals to distinguish the autistic child's health problems from the odd behavior. For example, a 5-year-old boy with autism had not slept regularly for 3 years; he had chronic diarrhea, screamed repeatedly, and often lay on the sofa rubbing his stomach. Numerous pediatricians were unable to find an organic basis for his diarrhea, and psychiatrists told his parents that the screaming, sleep problems, and stomach rubbing were autistic behaviors. When the boy's family sought treatment from gastroenterologists in another country, it was found that the diarrhea was overflow from persistent constipation. A radiograph showed a fecal mass the size of a small cantaloupe. After treatment with laxatives, the boy was no longer in physical agony and his screaming, stomach rubbing, and sleep problems ceased.[4]

A child with autism is stressful for a family because these children have difficult behaviors, need a great deal of supervision, and give no emotional reward to their families as a result of their social disorder. Parents may feel isolated and need a great deal of both practical and emotional support.

Treatment should focus on promoting development and learning and reducing rigidity and stereotypical mannerisms. Standard treatment consists of behavior modification, teaching social and communication skills, speech-language therapy, medication, and family support.[5] New approaches show promise, including biochemical approaches, such as the use of supplements and special diets, and therapies to improve sensory processing, such as the **HANDLE** approach.[6,7]

APPROACH AND GOALS

Contrary to popular belief, children with autism can learn to relax, although it may require repeated training. In 1963, a group for children with autism began at a child development center. It consisted of four children with autism; three boys, ages 5, 6, and 9, and a girl, age 6. These children had lifelong patterns of extreme aloneness, no speech, and feeding problems; only one was toilet trained. At home, they were totally aloof or uncontrollably wild, with frequent, prolonged, and violent tantrums. After 2 years of behavior modification techniques, the children learned some speech and were able to interact with others. The staff had successfully reduced the length and intensity of the tantrums through mild physical restraint and repetition of rules; however, the children were still tense

the late 1980s the prevalence is increasing—it may currently be as high as 1 in 500.[2] For each girl with autism, there are three to four autistic boys. Children with autism typically have little ability to process social cues, emotional information, and language, meaning that they are unable to understand the feelings of others. About one-third has some type of visual dysfunction, one-half are nonverbal or have severely impaired speech, and three-fourths are mentally retarded. They often have sleep problems, short attention spans, phobias, rapid mood changes, and hyperactivity. Children with autism commonly have insensitivity or hypersensitivity to pain, heat, noise, smell, or touch. Many children with autism are so hypersen-

and volatile. At this point, relaxation training became part of the daily routine. In each session, the children were told "Okay, now it's relax time." Lights were turned out and the children were told to put away their toys and relax on a mat. The children were then told to pretend they were lying in bed "where it is nice and comfortable," to breathe easily and to be calm, settled, and relaxed. The staff gently manipulated the children's arms, legs, and necks, while reminding them to relax. Any response approaching relaxed behavior was given immediate praise. Relaxation sessions were held every school day for 8 months. The first session lasted only 2 minutes before one child walked away but, as the children became more comfortable, the sessions increased to about 12 minutes. The children learned to become quiet and relaxed, clearly enjoying the sessions and spontaneously practicing relaxation at the program and at home. Their violent outbursts virtually disappeared, as well.[8] When massaging children with autism, repeatedly coaching them in the basic relaxation sequence can help them learn to relax in much the same way.

There is a delicate balance between breaking through the isolation of a child with autism and overtreating the child. Donna Williams feels that it is important to persist even when the child appears to reject touch or other stimulation. She says, "I must, against my own feelings, suggest a strongly persistent, sensitive, although impersonal, approach to teach the child that 'the world' will not give up on [him]; that it will relentlessly make demands of the child. Otherwise, 'the world' will remain closed out."[1] Massage accustoms children to touch, helps them relax, and increases body awareness. Massage can help the child sleep better and reduce self-stimulatory behaviors, such as hand-biting or head-banging. According to psychologist Marian Meyed, by trial and error, the parents of some children with autism have realized that their child is physically and psychologically tenser than their other children and that they must help him relax so that sleep is possible. Although most children with autism do not want to be held at bedtime, other physical contact, such as patting, massaging the child's body, and sitting or lying down beside the child, is often successful.[9]

Psychiatrist Nik Waal used massage with a boy with autism and found that it released his muscle tension and created deeper breathing and better emotional adjustment. Waal had the boy sit on her lap and she began very gentle stroking to soothe him. Later, she used deeper pressure on the areas carrying the most tension.[3] Two Touch Research Institute studies investigated the effects of stroking on autistic children. In the first study, each received touch therapy 15 minutes a day, 2 days per week, for 4 weeks. The children were fully clothed, but barefoot, and their bodies were rubbed using moderate pressure and smooth stroking movements. When tested at the end of the study, touch aversion, stereotypic behaviors, and inattentiveness decreased.[10] The second study compared two groups of autistic children; one group received a 15-minute massage before bedtime every night for 1 month, and the other group was read to. The children in the massage group showed fewer sleep problems at home, less stereotypic behavior, and were more attentive at school.[11]

Several special education teachers used acupressure with children with autism and discovered that the children become more outgoing and responsive.[12] Osteopath John Upledger has successfully treated many autistic children with craniosacral therapy.[13] In teaching massage classes for parents of children with disabilities, the author found that many of the simple Swedish massage strokes of a full-body massage must be modified to accommodate children with autism. Adjusting the environment or time of day may help a child be more accepting of massage. Parents usually know when their child will be most responsive to massage and what strokes will be most acceptable. Parents can massage the child at bedtime who will not lie still for a massage during the day. Larry Burns-Vidlak, a massage therapist and the father of three children with autism, combines wrestling or playing with massage. Rolling around on a bed or trampoline, he has his children put their arms around his neck while he uses his hands to rub their backs (Burns-Vidlak L, personal communication, April 1989).

MASSAGE FOR THE CHILD WITH AUTISM

Before beginning your first session with an autistic child, talk in detail with the parents to learn what is too little tactile stimulation and what is too much. Then, the extent of massage should be gauged by what the child can tolerate. Ask the parents to give the child a brief massage at least twice daily for a week before she is brought in for a session; this will give her some comfort with the idea of massage.

Swedish massage strokes are ideal and generally safe. The feet and hands may be a less defended area to begin with. Children should not disrobe unless they are comfortable with the idea, which may only come after a few sessions. If the child is only able to tolerate a short massage, she can be massaged for a few minutes, then the parent can be massaged, and then the child again. Showing the child how to do the strokes on her body may increase acceptance of massage.

Experiment with pressure; for example, try light stroking for children who tend to reject touch and deep pressure for children who are self-abusive (see self-abusive behavior in the Developmental Delay section). Use what works well for the child. Gentle, slow massage to the wrist, elbow, shoulder, ankle, knee, and hip joints can be calming. Parents should learn massage strokes to give their child at bedtime or in the bathtub, where they can use soap lather instead of massage oil.

CATASTROPHIC ILLNESS

Catastrophic illnesses are those conditions in which children are gravely ill, whether from an acquired health problem, such as AIDS or cancer, or from a hereditary condition, such as cystic fibrosis. Catastrophic illness is both a major stress and a major challenge to children, including physical discomfort or pain, prolonged immobilization, and a loss of the sense of body intactness caused by disability. Medical regimens, such as dietary restrictions, limitation of activities, medication side effects, and painful or invasive medical procedures, may cause additional stress. Insomnia, anxiety, and depression are common manifestations of stress. Family members are under enormous strain, as well; they must do extensive caretaking at the same time that they are experiencing feelings of fear, helplessness, guilt, and anger.

In chronic diseases such as cystic fibrosis, children may have repeated hospitalizations, during times when they are too ill to remain at home. Should medical treatment fail and the illness become terminal, they may return to the hospital or remain at home under hospice care.

APPROACH AND GOALS

Gentle, individualized Swedish massage can address the needs of gravely ill children. It can help with the specific discomforts of each illness, as well as the major stress and discomfort noted above. Field et al. studied the effects of massage on 20 children with acute lymphoblastic leukemia. Children were given 15-minute whole body massages by their parents every day for 30 days. When compared with a standard treatment control group, they were less anxious and depressed and their white blood cell count increased significantly.[1] Hernandez-Reif et al. found that after 30 days of Swedish massage at bedtime from a parent, children with cystic fibrosis were less anxious, their mood was better, and their breathing was improved, as measured by peak airflow readings.[2] Similar findings were found when massages were given to teenagers with AIDS (see AIDS section).

Massage therapist Lyse Lussier has treated children with grave illnesses (Chapter 3) and finds that massage can relieve physical distress, such as pain, nausea, and discomfort from being immobilized, and psy-chological distress, such as anxiety, lack of stimulation, insomnia, and feelings of isolation.

Massage therapist and former social worker Helen Campbell has worked with many gravely ill children, many with terminal illnesses, and has taught their families how to massage them. She has found that, in addition to the benefits to the previously mentioned child, massage has great gifts for the family, as well. Having something concrete and positive to do eases the feeling of helplessness and allows the family to express their love in a way beyond words. Massage can reduce the likelihood of parents becoming isolated from each other and grieving separately. Ms. Campbell also taught children to massage their siblings who were dying and found that they felt included as part of the health care team and had an opportunity to communicate their love and tenderness (Campbell H, personal communication, January 1989).

Receive permission from the child's physician before giving massage to the gravely ill child. It is usually feasible, even if there are surgical wounds, tubes, wires, ventilators, or other items to avoid. Helen Campbell worked with one girl with advanced aplastic anemia, which precluded massage. Instead, the girl was held gently, which was comforting to her. Permission should always be obtained from children themselves, who are already experiencing many medical procedures about which they have no choice. Before the first massage, the family could say, "A back rub might help you sleep better. Would you like to try it?"

SPECIFIC POINTS

- Identify all areas that should be avoided, especially intravenous sites, sores, dressings, catheter sites, and any painful areas. No matter how much of the child's body has cancer, or how many medical devices have to be worked around, there is usually at least one area of the body not affected by the cancer that the hands-on therapist can give comforting touch.

- Relief of edema is temporary, but comforting. The child often experiences relief for hours, with greater ease of movement, a more normal local temperature, and a more alive feeling due to the stimulation. The limb should be elevated, then massage distal to proximal (toward the heart) with a repeated gentle Swedish effleurage. The proximal part of the limb should be done first to open the lymph vessels for edema drainage.

- Children with cancer may have skin problems from medication, chemotherapy, or radiation. Problems areas should not be massaged unless there is a specific reason; the physician's permission must be obtained.

- No massage should be performed on or near an incision until 6 weeks after surgery, and then the child's physician should be consulted (see Scar Tissue, Chapter 4).
- Ask if children feel stiff or sore from lying in bed. Have them lay in novel positions and use range-of-motion exercises to relieve the effects of immobilization by increasing joint movement and circulation and giving them a three-dimensional experience of their bodies.
- Treat constipation with the techniques in Chapter 5; perform the strokes gently.

MASSAGE FOR CHILDREN WITH CATASTROPHIC ILLNESS

Positioning: Make sure the child is comfortably positioned, with extra pillows if needed. If the child is unable to talk, begin with a little massage, watching for such nonverbal signs of discomfort as tension in the face or changes in breathing.

Use the basic Swedish strokes of effleurage, petrissage, kneading, and raking described in Chapter 3, but be very gentle. Do not use vigorous muscle kneading or tapotement. Strokes should be long, even, and slow rather than short, fast, or choppy. For an emaciated child, use very light stroking from the head down toward the feet. The hands and feet can be massaged thoroughly, but gently. Head, neck, and shoulder massage may help relieve headaches. Gently stroking the forehead can release tension. If possible, help children breathe more freely by using the basic relaxation sequence. Energy techniques such as Polarity therapy, Reiki, and craniosacral therapy may also be appropriate because they use little or no pressure. Do not tire children by long sessions; even a few minutes of massage can be powerful and can be the nicest minutes of their day. If they want only a few minutes of massage, you may give massages to other family members as well. You may teach other family members how to massage children.

It cannot be stressed enough that children should not be exposed to germs. If you are ill, or even suspect that you are catching a cold or other minor illness, do not have any contact with gravely ill children.

COMPLEMENTARY THERAPY

Medical hypnosis has been successful for children as young as age 4 to treat the pain of their disease; reduce anxiety and pain caused by invasive medical procedures (such as spinal taps and bone marrow aspirates); and alleviate depression, insomnia, behavioral difficulties, and fear of death. Hypnosis for pain management has allowed children to reduce use of pain medication. Self-hypnosis has also been taught to children; those who practice regularly, get the most consistent pain relief.[3]

CEREBRAL PALSY

Matthew, 4, had cerebral palsy and was both blind and quadriplegic. His mother told me she didn't think it was possible to become any closer to her son than she already was. But after learning to massage him, she said, with tears in her eyes, 'It's like he can cuddle back when I hold him now, the massage relaxes him so. When I massage him before bedtime he is able to sleep with his arms straight and not flexed like they always had been. When I don't have time for a complete massage, I will massage his arms, his hands, and his legs that are always so tight. He holds his thumb inside his fist, but since I've been massaging his hand, it is relaxing more and more.'[1]

About one in 300 children is born with or develops cerebral palsy, a developmental disability that originates when the parts of the brain that control movement are damaged before or during birth or during infancy. This damage can result from certain infections during pregnancy, an Rh incompatibility, bleeding in the brain, and lack of oxygen or trauma during birth. After birth, prematurity and infections, such as meningitis, are causative. Damage may occur simultaneously to other areas of the brain; therefore, at least 25% of children with cerebral palsy have seizure disorders; at least 30% have visual, hearing, speech, and language impairments; and about 50% have mental retardation.[2]

Children with cerebral palsy have impaired voluntary movement. The effect of this varies, depending on the severity of the brain damage, the location of the damage, and if any other parts of the brain are damaged. There are three main types of cerebral palsy:

- Spastic cerebral palsy, the most common type, in which the voluntary muscles are stiff and contracted.
- Athetoid cerebral palsy. The child's muscles make involuntary writhing or stiffening movements.
- Ataxic cerebral palsy. The child has poor balance, difficulty using his or her hands, and difficulty beginning to sit or stand.

Hemiplegia, diplegia, and **quadriplegia** describe how much of the child's body is affected by the cerebral palsy (Figure 6–4). In addition to hypertonic musculature, children often become fixed in a tense position.

Standard medical treatment usually involves various types of therapy. Physical therapy works to increase gross motor activities and functional movement and to decrease tone. Occupational therapy

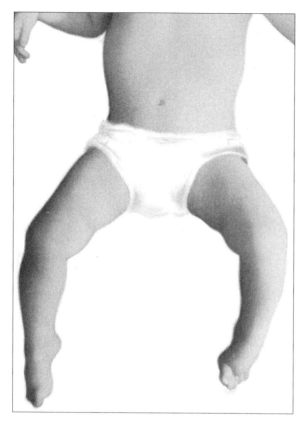
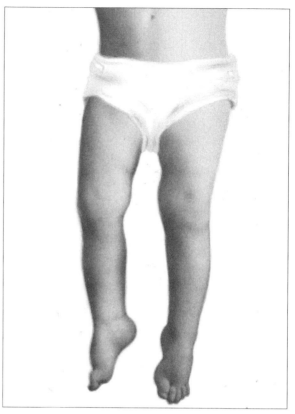

FIGURE 6–3 ■ Infant With Cerebral Palsy; **A,** Before, and **B,** After 10 Rolfing Sessions. Reprinted with permission from Robert Toporek.

helps the child with fine motor activities and activities of daily living. Orthopedic treatment may include surgery, braces, crutches, or splints, depending on the type and severity of cerebral palsy.

Massage has a number of benefits for children with cerebral palsy (see Case Study 6–1).Whether their condition is mild or severe, regular massage can make a significant improvement in the quality of their day-to-day life. As with all children with disabilities, stimulation, relaxation, greater acceptance of touch, deeper sleep, and improved body image are typical benefits. Swedish massage has helped children with cerebral palsy in the following ways:

- Alleviates constipation, which can be caused by hypotonic or hypertonic abdominal muscles (see Constipation Treatment, page 124).[3]
- Because spasticity is an ongoing problem for those with cerebral palsy, there is constant danger of contractures. Massage helps normalize muscle tone, can prevent contractures, and helps prevent existing contractures from worsening (Figure 6–5).
- Encourages deep breathing.
- Children with spastic cerebral palsy have learned to relax during treatments to consciously calm muscle spasms.

- By putting their bodies in different positions during therapy, releasing muscle tension and moving their joints in unaccustomed ways, massage can increase children's range of motion.
- Malocclusions are common as a result of the uncoordinated movements of the jaw, lip, and tongue muscles.[2] Massage can stimulate tone and/or release tension in the facial muscles and help decrease hypersensitivity around the mouth.

Researchers at the Touch Research Institute compared two groups of young children with cerebral palsy. The massage group received 30 minutes of massage, twice weekly for 12 weeks; the control group was read to for the same time. At the end of the study, the children who were massaged had reduced spasticity, less rigid muscle tone in the upper limbs, and improved gross and fine motor functioning.[4] Other forms of massage and bodywork may also be effective for cerebral palsy.[5] Myofascial techniques, such as Rolfing, can release restrictions and improve alignment (Figure 6–3). Regular acupressure massage helped several children with cerebral palsy advance in sensory-motor skills and improve relaxation and behavior.[6] Swedish massage has been successfully combined with acupressure, as well as with trigger point therapy (Horden L, LMT, personal communica-

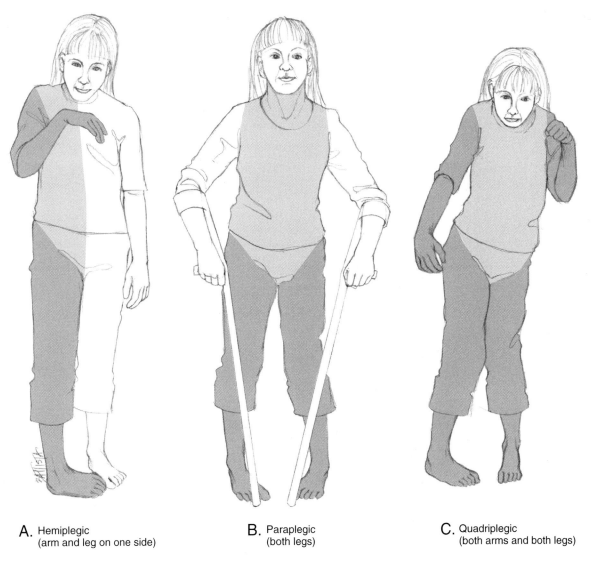

A. Hemiplegic
(arm and leg on one side)

B. Paraplegic
(both legs)

C. Quadriplegic
(both arms and both legs)

FIGURE 6–4 ■ Patterns of Involvement in Cerebral Palsy. **A,** Hemiplegia (arm and leg on one side); **B,** Paraplegia (both legs); and **C,** Quadriplegia (both arms and both legs).

tion, April 1991) and Thai massage.[7] Craniosacral therapy has helped children with cerebral palsy with improved motor skills, increased range of motion in all joints, and decreased spasticity.[8]

MASSAGE FOR CEREBRAL PALSY

Because many children with cerebral palsy are hypersensitive to light or sound, begin with natural or low lighting and either soothing music or no music at all. The environment should be quiet and calm. Begin with the basic massage techniques in Chapter 3. In general, a whole-body massage once a week and 15 minutes daily on problem areas is recommended. If you teach parents how to do the daily massage, you can do the whole-body massage every week.

Pressure point massage, such as for neck and shoulder tension may also be effective (see Figures 5–6 and

5–7). Good positioning is important; consult with your physical therapist. The legs and back are good places to begin. Often, the feet may be hypersensitive to touch and massage may cause a reflex tightening of the leg. If this happens, use slow, deep pressure on the top of the foot first and, if the child can accept it without tensing, do the same on the bottom of the foot.

Facial massage can be valuable, especially if children have deep tension around the mouth or any feeding problems. Use the face massage techniques described in Chapter 3 and spend extra time on the face. Intraoral massage may be performed for deep tension inside the mouth, but you should receive extra training before doing this technique.

On any area that is sensitive to touch, begin with just a stroke or two until the child is more accepting of massage. As range of motion is increased after massage, this is an excellent time to do passive range-

CASE STUDY 6–1

TINA

Background

Tina is a 5-year-old girl who has floppy/ataxic cerebral palsy. Her development was normal until she was age 2, when she contracted an infection accompanied by a very high fever. She has been at a clinic for children with disabilities for 1¹/₂ years. The staff member caring for her is a kind, motherly, elderly woman. She has given Tina good care but is too busy to spend a great deal of time with her; therefore, Tina has spent a lot of time in a crib.

Tina is able to sit up but cannot roll over or crawl. She opens and closes her mouth and wrings her hands constantly. Her face is completely expressionless. In general, her muscles are low in tone, but her left hip rotators, right hip adductors, calf muscles, upper back and neck, and jaw are very tight. She is unable to lie flat on her stomach, but props herself up on her elbows.

Impression

Floppy/ataxic cerebral palsy, accompanied by boredom and lack of stimulation.

Treatment

Tina's initial treatment was a 30-minute whole-body Swedish massage. She showed no signs of hypersensitivity or tactile defensiveness. Massage sessions two through 10 included Swedish massage of the whole body. Extra time was spent on the tightest areas, and more stimulating strokes, such as tapotement, were done on hypotonic areas. Tina received a massage every day for 2 weeks. During the time she received the massages, she not only interacted with the author, she also had contact with the other people in the therapy room—patients, observers, and other new people. Out of the crib where she was accustomed to spending most of the day and night, she received far more stimulation than usual.

Response

During her third session, Tina rolled over for the first time since her illness. She also was able to lay flat on her stomach for the first time. After her fourth massage, she became animated and smiled for the first time. Tina received deep petrissage on her hands, which she showed signs of enjoying; she even stopped wringing her hands for a few minutes. After her fifth massage, she rolled over twice. When she was picked up and set down in a prone position, Tina put herself

on all fours and stayed up for a few seconds, for the first time since her illness. She then rolled over three times while her "grandmother" was changing her diaper and stopped wringing her hands. Each session found Tina slightly more animated and communicative and, by her tenth session, she looked like a different child. Tina also showed a dramatic improvement in her ability to move after a relatively small number of treatments. Not all children with cerebral palsy would show such fast improvement. Tina had the advantage of 2 years of normal brain development before contracting cerebral palsy, rather than having it at birth.

A visiting physical therapist recommended physical therapy to achieve these specific goals:

1. Exercises to strengthen and stretch the sides of her trunk and lateral neck muscles, to enable her to consistently rotate her trunk and roll over.
2. Exercises to strengthen her arm muscles to help her begin to crawl.
3. Exercises to stretch the gastrocnemius muscles so that they didn't interfere with her learning to walk. Tina habitually pointed her toes, and the muscles were tight and shortened.
4. Exercises to stretch the neck and shoulder muscles to help her as she began to crawl.

The author recommended that Tina continue to receive massage in combination with the physical therapy, because she needed to continue releasing tension in tight muscle groups and receiving the physical and social stimulation of the massage. The exercises to strengthen her muscles could be tiring and, by alternating a few minutes of exercises with a few minutes of massage, her exercise goals could be met without undue stress or physical discomfort.

Discussion Questions

1. Which tissues were affected by Tina's cerebral palsy?
2. What symptoms were present?
3. What changed features of Tina's daily life could have been related to her progress during the time she received massage?

---

of-motion exercises. An excellent shoulder range of motion, prescribed by physical therapist Deborah Bowes, is as follows: As you move the arm to rotate the shoulder, bring the child's hand around to touch her body, first the face, then the chest, arms, and legs

and back to the face. Using the child's hand to touch herself during range-of-motion exercises helps with joint motion and increases her awareness of the connection between the different parts of the body (Bowes D, personal communication, June 1990).

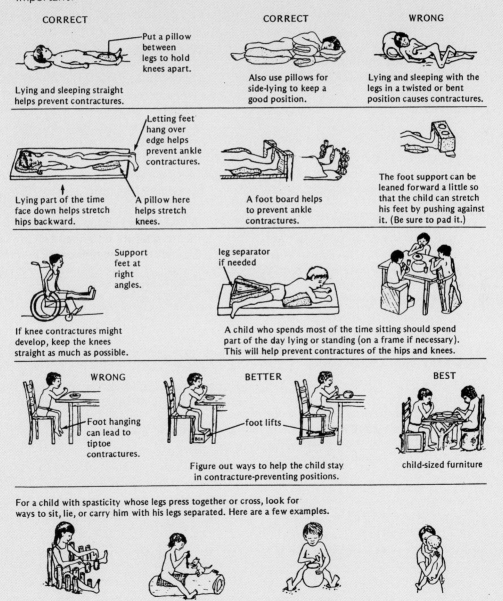

PREVENTION AND EARLY MANAGEMENT OF CONTRACTURES

Contractures can often be prevented by (1) positioning, and (2) range-of-motion exercises.

POSITIONING

If a child is likely to develop contractures or has begun to develop them, try to position her to stretch the affected joints. Look for ways to do this during day-to-day activities: lying, sitting, being carried, playing, studying, bathing, and moving about.

During a severe illness (such as acute polio), or a recent spinal cord injury, contractures can develop quickly. Therefore, early preventive positioning is very important:

FIGURE 6–5 ■ Prevention and Early Management of Contractures. Reprinted with permission from Werner D: *Disabled Village Children*. Palo Alto, CA: Hesperian Foundation, 1987, p 196-198.

THE HYPOTONIC CHILD

Active voluntary movement and body awareness are increased following massage. Use bouncier, more rapid strokes. Experiment with different pressures to see what is most effective. Try using the pressure point massage techniques described in Chapter 3. Hydrotherapy may be combined with massage to stimulate muscle contraction (see Muscle Weakness, Chapter 5). Changing the texture of the surface on which the children are lying may also stimulate muscle tone. A pilot study of young, hypotonic children, some with Down syndrome, found that the simple act of lying prone on surfaces of different textures produced measurable increases in muscle tone. A surface with more texture, such as plush, velvet bathmats or rough, rubber doormats covered with cotton sheets, increased muscle tone more than a neutral surface, such as slick, uncovered vinyl.[9] Wait until after massage to have the child do exercises that develop muscle tone.

THE HYPERTONIC CHILD

Massage will help reduce tone. Use slow, even rhythmic strokes. Experiment with different pressures to see which is most relaxing. Observe the child carefully; if there seems to be an increase in spasticity, delete the stroke that causes it. If any stroke causes spasticity or if the child's positioning during the stroke causes spasticity, try doing it in different ways until you find a way that reduces muscle tension. Facial massage can be valuable; consult with the child's occupational or speech therapist for a specific program.

If the child has a seizure disorder, be observant for signs of petit mal or eye muscle seizures that could lead to a larger seizure. Consult the physician or therapist if seizure activity occurs during massage sessions; deep relaxation may help reduce seizures that occur. Things that normally trigger seizures (such as loud noises or urination) may not do so when the child is deeply relaxed. Massage therapist Kathy Knowles worked with a child who consistently experienced seizures during massage. When he learned to relax and breathe easily while she massaged areas that were tight, his seizures stopped during the massage session (Knowles K, personal communication, June 1989).

> ❗ A person with flaccid (limp) paralysis could be injured if a joint is moved or forced beyond its existing range of motion. The muscles could be stretched and joints dislocated without the individual's awareness. If muscle spasticity occurs during passive range of motion, stop the movement temporarily but continue to apply slow, gentle pressure on the part until the muscle relaxes, then proceed with the motion.[10]

COMPLEMENTARY THERAPIES

1. Aquatic pool therapy is excellent for children with cerebral palsy to relieve spasticity/muscle spasm, stretch tight areas, increase range of motion, learn how to relax, and encourage deeper breathing and greater body awareness.[11]
2. *Yoga for the Special Child* is a program of hatha yoga adapted for children with disabilities by yoga teacher, Sonia Sumar. A physical therapist documented positive changes in a boy who received yoga therapy for 4 months in addition to his regular physical therapy. There was decreased muscle tone of his upper extremities; increased passive range of motion of his hamstrings, hip adductor, and hip rotator muscles; and overall quieting of his central nervous system. The boy's tendency to thrust his body into total body extension, hold his breath during efforts to move, and extend his jaw severely decreased. He was also better able to concentrate, was less distractible, made more eye contact, breathed more slowly and deeply, and was more able to relax his muscles.[12]
3. Poor fine-motor control in children with cerebral palsy has been successfully treated with relaxation training through biofeedback.[13]
4. Children with cerebral palsy have made major improvements in both fine- and gross-motor skills with the Feldenkrais Method.[14,15]
5. HANDLE neurodevelopmental therapy has helped children with cerebral palsy make major advances.[16]

CHRONIC PAIN

This section briefly discusses three conditions that cause chronic pediatric pain and the use of massage therapy to help relieve stress and pain. Rather than discuss all conditions that cause chronic pain in children, the goal of this section is to help you understand the potential that massage has in dealing with painful conditions in general. Conditions causing chronic pain should only be treated with massage therapy after consulting with a child's physician.

HEMOPHILIA

Hemophilia is an inherited flaw in the blood clotting system and occurs only in males. Because the blood is deficient in an essential blood clotting protein, the body is not able to clot at the site of a wound. The boy has a permanent tendency toward spontaneous and traumatic hemorrhages. Hemophilia can be mild, moderate, or severe, depending on the amount of clotting protein the body makes. Most boys have severe hemophilia. Boys with mild hemophilia have 5–50% of the normal clotting factor level. They don't bleed into their joints, but surgical or dental procedures can cause serious bleeding. In severe hemophilia, boys have no clotting factor. Bleeding into their muscles and joints can occur spontaneously, and any type of trauma or surgical procedure can be dangerous. Broken bones must be immediately immobilized so that soft tissue around the bone does not begin to bleed.

At the present, hemophiliacs regularly receive clotting factor. By infusing themselves with clotting factor, they can now prevent many bleeds and adverse effects before they occur. However, there are still many hardships with this disorder. Physical limitations, limited mobility, and hospitalization are stressful and disruptive. Pain is also a constant part of life. Joint bleeds are painful; as blood pools in the synovial membrane and stretches it, severe pain may result. Boys will also feel stiffness and swelling and refuse to move their joints because of the pain, often holding them in flexion. This leads to muscular atrophy and contractures. Contractures may even be seen in preschoolers, if hemophilia is severe. As one joint becomes less flexible, boys start to move differently and muscular compensations can occur in other parts of the body. Repeated bleeding into a joint will cause synovitis, arthritis, and degeneration.[1]

Most boys with hemophilia have had negative experiences with touch from an early age. As even slight injuries cause bleeds, parents may have been afraid to touch them for fear of causing a bleed, resulting in touch deprivation and a lack of bonding. Boys may come to feel that they are "untouchables." In addition, painful medical experiences, such as injection of clotting factor (either intravenously or intramuscularly), heel sticks, and Port-A-Caths may have led them to think of touch as a negative experience. Many men with hemophilia say they have never had a day in their life without pain.

JUVENILE RHEUMATOID ARTHRITIS

Juvenile rheumatoid arthritis (JRA) is defined as *the presence of arthritis lasting 6 weeks or longer in a child under 16 years of age.* This disease of chronic joint inflammation and pain is suspected to be an immune system disorder. Some children are more severely affected than others, but everyone with JRA has chronic pain. The most commonly affected joints are the knees, hips, ankles, wrists, fingers, and the cervical spine. These joints can be swollen and painful, making movement difficult. Contractures are likely if children do not move their joints through the maximum range of motion every day. Standard medical treatment for juvenile rheumatoid arthritis consists of anti-inflammatory medications, gentle exercise, and devices such as hand splints.[2]

Chronic pain and the loss of free movement invariably lead to some degree of depression in both these children and their families. Uncertainty about the future, feeling different from other children, and dependency on health care providers and significant others make it challenging for the child to cope.[3]

FIBROMYALGIA

Fibromyalgia is a syndrome of chronic widespread musculoskeletal pain. It occurs in about 10,000 American children, 90% of them adolescents.[4] One study of 338 schoolchildren found that 6% of the children, some as young as age 10, met the American College of Rheumatology criteria for fibromyalgia (see below).[5] Physicians who are expert in diagnosing fibromyalgia have identified it developing in toddlers.[6]

Fibromyalgia has two defining symptoms. The first is a widespread aching that has lasted at least 3 months and feels like the achiness of influenza. The second symptom is severe pain when specific points are pressed, including pain on both sides of the body, both above and below the waist, with point tenderness in at least 11 of 18 specified sites (see Figure 6–6). These tender points are not trigger points, and they do not refer pain like a trigger point. Children with fibromyalgia not only have chronic pain in their muscles and joints but they are stiff, sleep poorly, and are chronically tired. They are also more prone to headaches, swelling of the hands and feet, rigidity of the myofascia, numbness and tingling in the arms and legs, and sensitivity to cold. Fibromyalgia can affect a child's functioning as severely as juvenile rheumatoid arthritis.

Devin Starlanyl, a physician and fibromyalgia researcher who has fibromyalgia, believes that fibromyalgia is a systemic, nondegenerative, noninflammatory, nonprogressive disease of the brain's neurotransmitters.[6] Fibromyalgia may be hereditary, as 40% of people with it have a close relative with similar symptoms. True fibromyalgia in a child often begins with an injury or a flulike illness. Traumatic events in childhood may also predispose a child to fibromyalgia; 47% of adults with fibromyalgia in one study had suffered physical or sexual abuse as children.[7] Children may easily become depressed as they cope with constant physical discomfort; fatigue; restrictions on their activity; and an invisible, poorly understood condition. Children with widespread pain are significantly more likely to have emotional and behavioral problems.[8]

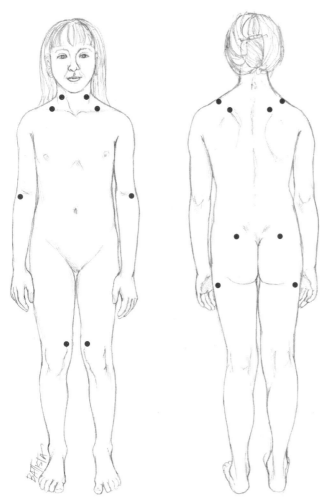

FIGURE 6–6 ■ The Tender Points of Fibromyalgia

reduce pain, release stress and tension, and increase range of motion and nutrition to their joints. It is possible they may have fewer spontaneous bleeds. These effects, particularly the reduction in pain, have already been seen in adults.[10] Massage therapist Renee Weaver specializes in working with people with hemophilia. When receiving massages at summer camp, boys with hemophilia slept better and needed less pain medication (Weaver R, LMT, personal communication, August 2002).

Massage helps children with rheumatoid arthritis release emotional tension, relieve pain and stiffness, and prevent contractures. It has an advantage over muscle relaxants, which relax muscles all over the body and cause drowsiness.[11] A Touch Research Institute study found that children with JRA between the ages of 5 and 14 experienced both short-term and long-term pain relief from massage. Parents gave the child a 15-minute Swedish massage every day for 30 days. At the end of the study, the children had less pain and morning stiffness, were less anxious, and had lower levels of the stress hormone cortisol.[12] The most substantial pain relief the author has observed in a child with this condition was in a 4-year-old boy whose parents learned massage, purchased a hot tub, and regularly massaged him and did range-of-motion exercises in the tub.

Massage therapy can also be extremely effective for fibromyalgia. It is reported to alleviate musculoskeletal aching and stiffness in children and adolescents.[9] A Touch Research Institute study found that adults with fibromyalgia who received two massages a week for 5 weeks felt major improvements in their condition. They slept better and had less pain, fatigue, anxiety, and depression and their blood cortisol levels were lower. The massages consisted of 30 minutes of Swedish type stroking on the head, neck, shoulders, back, arms, legs, and feet.[13] Unfortunately, no such research has yet been done with children.

MASSAGE AND HYDROTHERAPY FOR CHILDREN WITH CHRONIC PAIN

MOIST HEAT APPLICATIONS

1. Hot moist packs, such as an electric moist heating pad or Hydrocollator pack, help relax muscles and soothe the area before massage.
2. Warm baths with Epsom salts for 20 minutes can relax muscles before massage. For an adult, 1 cup Epsom salts would be used in a tub of warm water. Adjust the amount of Epsom salts to the size of the child; for example, use 1 cup for a 150-pound adult, ½ cup for a 75-pound child, and ⅓ cup for a 50-pound child. The temperature should be 100° to 105° F, whatever is comfortably warm to the child.

Standard medical treatment for fibromyalgia in children includes regular physical therapy (including stretching and conditioning), muscle relaxants and/or steroid medication, and emotional support. A new treatment includes prescribing the medication guaifenesin to correct a metabolic defect.[8] Children often are urged to exercise, but may suffer pain flare-ups if they exercise too hard. Warm water swimming can keep muscles conditioned without causing fatigue.

Children should be treated early and consistently to prevent their pain from developing into a full-blown condition.[8,9] Their prognosis is better than that of adults: If therapy is aggressively pursued, 80% of young people have substantial resolution of the syndrome within 2 to 3 years.[9] An untreated child may have lifelong fibromyalgia.

APPROACH AND GOALS

Massage therapy can help boys with hemophilia become accustomed to positive nurturing touch,

MASSAGE

Step 1. Begin with the basic Swedish massage techniques in Chapter 3, treating any muscle or muscle groups that are causing or adding to sleep problems. For example, if children have areas that hurt and wake them up when they roll over at night, this can interfere with their sleep. Treat the areas causing the greatest pain or the greatest restriction of movement.

Step 2. Begin with very light pressure. If children find deeper pressure helpful, you may gradually use more. Progressing from light to deep pressure may take many sessions. Children should not experience any flare-ups from the massage, and they may never be able to tolerate deep pressure. Overdoing massage can lead to a flare-up of pain and fatigue. Children should not return for another session if they are experiencing any flare-up of pain from the first session.

Step 3. The therapist should err on the side of caution and be careful not to use too much pressure. Possibly supplement the techniques in this book with lighter pressure techniques, such as energetic techniques or craniosacral therapy.

CONTRACTURES

A contracture is the lack of complete active or passive range of motion due to limitation of joint, muscle, or soft tissue. Whenever joints are not regularly moved through their normal range of motion, contractures may develop. For children who are immobilized, it is vitally important that attention be paid to joint range of motion.

APPROACH AND GOALS

To prevent contractures, it is important to regularly position children in a way that stretches their affected joints. After massaging an area, stretch the affected part and do full range of motion. Doing massage first will loosen the area so that you will be able to stretch the soft tissue farther and move the joint much more. This should be done gently, to children's tolerance. Overstretching leads to pain, injury, and scar formation. It should feel great to the child to feel a stiff area loosening up!

MASSAGE AND HYDROTHERAPY FOR CONTRACTURES

HYDROTHERAPY: MOIST HEAT APPLICATION

Prior to massage, apply a hot pack, hydrocollator pack, or towels that have been wrung out in hot water, around the joint. Leave it on for 15 minutes.

MASSAGE AND STRETCHING SEQUENCE

Along with casts, braces, or special equipment to stretch contractures, steady, gentle, firm stretching can be done.

Step 1. Effleurage the entire limb for 2 minutes.

Step 2. Perform gentle range-of-motion exercises, even if you feel little or no movement in the joint, for 2 minutes.

Step 3. Hold the limb in a steady, stretched position for 30 seconds.

Step 4. Stretch the joint a little more and again hold the limb in a stretched position for 30 seconds.

Step 5. Continue increasing the stretch this way for 5 to 10 minutes. Do this at least several times a day. Do not overstretch. It is okay if the stretching hurts slightly, but it should not be very painful.[1]

For the effects of prolonged spasticity, the elongated or stretched position must be held for at least 4 of every 24 hours.[2]

DEVELOPMENTAL DELAY

Developmental delay is defined as *slowness in a child's mental or neurologic development.* As children mature, milestones, such as sitting, walking, and speaking, usually occur in a typical order. With developmental delay, these milestones may be achieved much later or may not be achieved at all; children learn more slowly than other children their age. For example, because the processes governing eye motion, alignment, visual acuity, and visual perception may mature slowly or abnormally, more than half of children with developmental delay have significant ocular disorders.[1] Children who are significantly delayed in all developmental areas are usually diagnosed with mental retardation. Emotional, behavioral, and psychiatric disorders are also three to four times more common in people with developmental delay than in the general public.[2] The leading cause of developmental delay is fetal alcohol syndrome, followed by cerebral palsy, Down syndrome, and spina bifida. Mothers who are alcoholics have a 30–40% chance of having a child with fetal alcohol syndrome.[1] Other known causes of developmental delay are brain damage during or after birth, **meningitis** in early childhood, head injuries, and maternal malnutrition. Prematurity is a major risk factor for developmental delay (see Point of Interest Box 6–5). Many times, however, the cause of developmental delay is never known.

APPROACH AND GOALS

Peggy Jones Farlow is a speech/language pathologist and massage therapist with 20 years of professional experience with developmentally delayed children.

POINT OF INTEREST BOX 6–5
Prematurity and Developmental Delay

Premature infants are those born before 37 weeks of gestation or who weigh under 5 $1/2$ pounds at birth. Because their bodies are not fully developed at birth, they may face major challenges, including jaundice; brain damage due to hemorrhage; problems with the digestive system, kidneys or lungs; an inability to control heat loss; and a greater susceptibility to the effects of stress and infection.[1] In the long-term, premature children have an increased incidence of developmental delay, cerebral palsy, hydrocephalus, blindness, deafness, or seizure disorders. Even without these obvious neurologic problems, subtle abnormalities may occur. Children born prematurely are also more likely to have ADHD, lower cognitive test scores, and be enrolled in special education classes. They are also more prone to behavior problems and psychiatric disorders. It is not possible to separate the damage to the child's brain from being underdeveloped at birth from the negative effects of early stress that are so common in premature infants, such as illness, maternal separation for long periods, and multiple painful procedures. Both are known to be harmful to the brain.[2,3] It is has only recently been recognized that many babies with brain-damage need follow-up for their lifetime. Although there may be little deficit at age 2, problems may arise later. Pilot studies show that just as catch-up growth may occur in the physical structure of the body, early intervention with educational and other therapies that help the development of the nervous system may be of considerable use.[1]

A 1987 analysis of 19 studies of the effects of tactile/kinesthetic stimulation on premature infants showed that 72% of the infants receiving some form of tactile stimulation received positive benefits, such as better weight gain, more mature motor development, signs of less distress, or better sleep.[4] Since that time,

other studies have substantiated those results, including studies at the Touch Research Institute that show benefits for premature babies with the additional challenges of exposure to cocaine or HIV in utero.[5-7] Generally, the infants were gently stroked from head-to-toe on both sides of the body. No attempt was made to massage the muscles to release tension or eliminate knots.

When massaging a child who was premature, the massage techniques discussed in Chapter 3 may be used. If the child has not been massaged before, great care should be taken to notice any areas of tactile defensiveness, and they should be avoided until the child can be massaged with less fear. Stimulation and relaxation are important benefits from Swedish massage, but deep massage is probably not called for. Regular full-body massage is important for the child's neurologic and social development throughout childhood.

References

1. Nathanielsz P: *Life in the Womb—The Origins of Health and Disease.* Ithaca, NY: Promethean Press, 1999, p 211, 212
2. Bhutta AL, et al: Cognitive and behavioral outcomes of school-aged children who were born preterm: A meta-analysis. *Journal of the American Medical Association,* 288:728-737, 2002
3. Porter FL, et al: Long-term effects of pain in infants. *Journal of Developmental Behavioral Pediatrics,* 20:253-261, 1999
4. Ottenbacher KJ, et al: The effectiveness of tactile stimulation as a form of early intervention: A quantitative evaluation. *Journal of Developmental Behavioral Pediatrics,* 8:68-76, 1987
5. Acolet D, et al: Changes in plasma cortisol and catecholamine concentrations in response to massage in preterm infants. *Archive of Diseases of the Child,* 68:29-31, 1993
6. Hayes J: TAC-TIC therapy: A nonpharmocologic stroking intervention for premature infants. *Complementary Therapies in Nursing and Midwifery,* 4:25-27, 1998
7. Field T: *Touch Therapy.* London, England: Churchill Livingstone, 2000, p 3-21

She teaches parents and other caregivers a 10-minute routine of acupressure and Swedish massage strokes combined with specific words and sounds (see Point of Interest Box 6–6) She has observed significant increases in interchanges of language, speech, and vocalization, as children respond to the pleasure and fun of a massage routine. As an additional benefit, parents have reported that their children relax more readily and have improvement with problems such as constipation, hyperactivity, insomnia, and acceptance of touch.[3]

Pamela Marshalla-Rosenwinkle, also a speech-language pathologist, uses massage as part of oral sensorimotor therapy to help developmentally delayed children have normal oral-tactile sensitivity, improve tongue and jaw movements to enhance feeding and speech, and treat drooling and lip retraction (Rosenwinkle P, personal communication, December

1993).[4] A simple, yet still sophisticated, use of massage is part of the *Yoga for the Special Child* approach of Sonia Sumar. Sumar has incorporated massage into her yoga program for developmentally disabled children to reduce constipation, relax and stimulate circulation in the muscles after strengthening exercises, and help children lie quietly during relaxation time.[5]

The authors of *Aromatherapy and Massage for People with Learning Disabilities* (Hands-On Press, 1991) advocate simple massage strokes to help people who are multihandicapped feel reassured, supported, and recognized by another person, as well as to increase body awareness. Those with multiple, severe disabilities may go through several stages before they can accept this massage. The stages typically progress from initially resisting touch to tolerating it to cooperating passively to actively enjoying the massage. The

POINT OF INTEREST BOX 6–6
Acupressure and Swedish Massage for Developmental Disability

Kathy Knowles, a massage therapist, worked for 10 years at the Pearl Buck Center in Eugene, Oregon. For many years this facility had an acupressure treatment program for adults and children who were developmentally disabled. Ms. Knowles's work was primarily with profoundly retarded teenagers; some had additional handicaps, such as cerebral palsy or autism. The teenagers tended to have poorly developed speech, delayed motor and self-help skills, and behavior problems. Many had experienced other stresses, such as deprivation or abuse. As a rule, they had not been touched and were afraid of it. Ms. Knowles did one or two sessions of massage per week with each child. She generally used acupressure, with some Swedish massage similar to the techniques described in Chapter 3. The children she worked with showed great improvement in four areas: (1) They showed more willingness to be touched. Some children who had shunned massage began to ask for it. This indicated increased trust of others, which was especially important for the children who had been deprived or abused. (2) They relaxed a great deal, which made them feel better and helped reduce inappropriate social behavior. Not able to lie still during the first sessions, some were able to after weeks or months of treatment. One more advanced teenage girl learned to consciously relax her back to stop muscle spasms. (3) They gained greater body awareness, which contributed to a more definite and more positive body image. (4) The teenagers became increasingly aware and present in relating to others, shown by less whining, the ability to make eye contact, and a greater willingness to communicate (Knowles K, personal communication, June 1989 and September 2002).

A 1986 Michigan State Department of Education study investigated the possibility that massage could reduce self-abusive behavior in teenagers and young adults who were severely mentally impaired. Self-abuse, such as repetitive head-banging, hand-biting, and body-slapping, had not responded to conventional approaches. For 16 weeks, each person was given two or three 45-minute treatments per week by a massage therapist. Although not successful for everyone, massage helped in many cases; benefits noted were a reduction of agitated and self-abusive behavior, relief from chronic insomnia, and a more relaxed appearance.[7] According to three separate case reports from psychiatrists and occupational therapists, massage or a combination of massage and vestibular stimulation (such as rocking) has had great success in reducing self-abusive behavior in difficult cases in which no other approach had been successful.[8-10]

Massage is a rich source of not only relaxation, but also of stimulation. Researchers at the Touch Research Institute investigated the effect of massage on two groups of young children with Down syndrome. One group received 30-minute massages twice weekly for 2 months, while the other group was read to. The children in the massage group improved in fine- and gross-motor functioning and decreased in hypotonicity, while the children in the other group did not.[11] The author has observed a significant increase in muscle tone after beginning massage in several children with Down syndrome. Exercise to increase their muscle strength will be more effective if massage is given first.

As a result of inadequate fluid and fiber intake, uncoordinated muscle contractions, and poor rectal sphincter control, constipation is a long-term problem for most children with severe developmental disabilities. Stool may be retained for long periods and become progressively harder and more immobile. If given regularly, the strokes for constipation discussed in Chapter 5 can help reduce it significantly.

MASSAGE FOR CHILDREN WITH DEVELOPMENTAL DELAY

The basic long-term goal for children with developmental delay is to accept and enjoy a full-body massage (Chapter 3). This may be possible only after a period of shorter massages. Begin by massaging the hands and feet, and observe children carefully. If they do not show signs of resistance or overstimulation, try massaging the back. If the back is well accepted, then proceed with the rest of the body. The head and abdomen are often guarded, so do not work with them until the children are accustomed to massage, and then you may use the neck and shoulder tension and constipation treatments discussed in Chapter 5.

authors cite the story of a blind, severely spastic, and profoundly retarded 8-year-old girl. Massage was selected to help her increase body awareness and respond to touch and offer her more opportunities for close nonverbal communication and sensory learning. Initially, she was given only a 20-minute back massage at each session, which gradually progressed to include the entire body. She tended to sleep through massage at first; this may have been resistance or simply an adjustment to profound new feelings of relaxation. Gradually, she began to stay awake more, vocalize more, and show signs of pleasure by moving her body. Soon she began to show anticipation after simply smelling the scent of the massage oil and cooed and gurgled at the beginning of a session.[6]

Varying types of sensory stimulation strokes (Chapter 3) should be used when children can tolerate them. The extra forms of sensory stimulation on the section on tactile defensiveness (see page 189) may be used, but always follow the children's lead and do not force massage.

To teach conscious relaxation, have the child exhale all the way. Model this by making loud sighs when you exhale during the basic relaxation sequence.

> Consult the child's physician and physical therapist before massaging the neck of any child with Down syndrome. Of children with Down syndrome, 15% have **atlantoaxial instability,** and forward flexion of the head could contribute to subluxation or spinal cord injury.

FETAL DRUG OR ALCOHOL EXPOSURE

Cocaine is a major assault on the children in the uterus. An assault far worse than hitting a small child with the palm of your hand in a fit of anger… They have been beaten and battered just as surely as if their parents had taken a stick to them after birth.[1]
—*Peter Nathanielsz, obstetrician*

My son is adopted and was born drug affected and was abused in his first 5 years. He bit, spit, kicked, and hit often. Tantrums were huge and long. I used his blanket to roll him in some times and hold, snuggled and safe. We had a 60-minute bedtime routine. I'd sit close to him and read bedtime stories, firmly rub his back, and sing to him. . .When he was older and I started massage, he came to my 'office' (home practice room) and would let me do some massage… When I became licensed, we scheduled actual appointments for him at my real office. He determined how the massage would go, what was massaged and for how long, his level of dress, and the lotion. He would flip several times on the table as he put his massage together. He's 14 today and still asks to be massaged. It has been a huge part of our life.
—*Suzie Klein, massage therapist (Klein S, personal communication, September 2002)*

In the United States, 11% of newborns are born to mothers who use illicit drugs; 10% use marijuana, 1% use cocaine, and 0.5% use opiates.[2] It is impossible to estimate the number of babies affected by one substance alone because maternal substance abuse often includes multiple drugs, alcohol, and nicotine. For example, women who are trying to reduce the withdrawal crash after using cocaine often take alcohol, marijuana, opiates, tranquilizers, or barbiturates.[2] These women are also less likely to nourish their babies by eating a nutritious diet.

Babies with a history of maternal substance abuse face many challenges. They not only have physical problems caused by the drug, but also must go through drug withdrawal. The pattern of withdrawal varies according to what the abused drug was, how much and for how long the mother had been using the drug, and when it was last taken.[2] Cocaine causes decreased blood flow to the placenta, predisposing the fetus to brain injury and stunted growth before birth. Cocaine-affected infants are often extremely irritable and hypertonic (stiff), and esophageal reflux and severe gas pain are common because of weak or underdeveloped digestive systems. They respond poorly to attempts to comfort them and have difficulty receiving tactile stimulation. Because something as simple as a diaper change can cause inconsolable crying, nursing staff in the hospital may leave them alone for fear of irritating them; however, this deprives the infants of the touching and bonding needed to develop normally.

It may be extremely difficult for a parent, especially one recovering from drug use or still actively using drugs, to bond with an irritable, stiff, and difficult-to-calm baby, and this may further deprive the baby of the loving touch he or she needs to develop. Almost one-third of children whose mothers used cocaine, opiates, heroin, or methadone are removed from their parents and placed in foster homes.[2] As drug-affected children grow, they are at risk of having developmental delays, learning disabilities, hyperactivity, hearing deficits, and visual impairments.

Five to ten percent of pregnant American women drink enough alcohol to put their children at risk of having fetal alcohol syndrome (FAS), damage resulting from repeated exposure to alcohol in utero. Of every 1,000 American children, one to two are born with FAS each year.[2] Infants with FAS are jittery, irritable, have low muscle tone (including a weak suck), and may have tremors and abnormal sleep patterns. Most have severe feeding problems and grow slowly, even when given excellent nutrition.[2] At birth, their joint range of motion is restricted, especially in the hands and feet and, occasionally, they have contractures. Hypersensitivity of the hands and feet is common. They may have motor problems and seizures, heart defects, and craniofacial abnormalities, such as a thin upper lip, no groove below the nose, and small eyes[3] (Figure 6–7). They are at risk of central nervous system abnormalities, such as hyperactivity and developmental delays and language difficulties; the majority will be mildly mentally retarded. FAS is the leading cause of mental retardation in the United States.

Because they are so irritable, they, like the drug-exposed infants, may be deprived of the loving touch they need to develop normally. Painful or invasive procedures may also cause trauma and tactile defensiveness.[4] Infants may also develop trigger points as a result

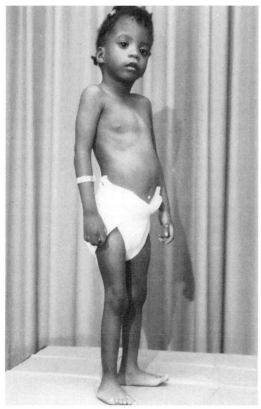

FIGURE 6–7 ■ Three-Year-Old Girl With Fetal Alcohol Syndrome. She has characteristic facial features and is small for her age. Reprinted with permission from Morrissy R: *Lovell and Winter's Pediatric Orthopaedics.* Vol. 1. Baltimore, MD: Lippincott Williams & Wilkins, 2001, p 310.

of the effects of drugs on their systems. For example, gastroesophageal reflux may be associated with abnormal torticollislike head and neck positioning as the baby reacts to discomfort.[5] As infants tense in reaction to pain, they may activate trigger points in the sternocleidomastoid muscles.[6] Gastroesophageal reflux is also known to initiate trigger points in the abdominal muscles.[7]

APPROACH AND GOALS

Because they begin life with such major challenges, infants of substance-abusing mothers have a tremendous need for any methods that enhance growth and development. Studies at the Touch Research Institute show that premature infants who were prenatally exposed to cocaine benefitted from daily massage and passive exercise. In one study, the infants received three 15-minute Swedish massages and passive exercise of the arms and legs every day. After 10 days, they had gained more weight and had more advanced motor development, fewer postnatal complications, and fewer stress behaviors than a control group of infants who were exposed to cocaine but did not receive massage.[8] Gentle massage given over time can release tension and encourage acceptance of touch.[9]

Massage therapist Robin Gregory, who has given massages to drug-affected babies in a neonatal intensive care unit, uses strokes tailored to their needs. These may include gentle cradling with the hands enclosing the head and buttocks; gentle rolling and pulling of the hands and fingers; slow flexion and extension of the limbs; and gentle strokes over the tops of the feet, toes, hands, and fingers. In the beginning, an entire touch session might consist of simply cradling the infant's body for a few minutes. At the first sign of infant stress, the therapist should stop stroking and use simple passive touch. Often, after two or three touch interactions, the drug-exposed babies begin to release and seek social interaction. There is an increase of oxygen to the bloodstream and their heart rates slow down. The infants sleep better, their appetites are stimulated, and they gradually become more interactive when massaged.[10]

Occupational therapists Pat Joyce and Cindy Clark use craniosacral therapy to treat gastroesophageal reflex in infants. They suspect that craniosacral therapy is effective because many cases of gastroesophageal reflux may be related to impingement on the vagus nerve where it passes through the jugular foramen and at the cranial base.[11] Massage therapist Kathy Knowles uses massage and **Watsu** to encourage deep relaxation in children with FAS, whom she has found have very rigid bodies, extremely malaligned cranial bones, and an impaired cranial rhythm (Knowles K, personal communication, September 2002).

Massage therapist Suzy Klein has worked with troubled children in many different settings; she has also been a foster parent for 17 children and has adopted a special needs child. For drug-affected children, she suggests doing gentle stretching along with massage, using water to reduce stress, and making as much skin contact as possible. She urges therapists not to fear handling children with severe problems. For tactile defensiveness, she believes that light stroking may actually irritate rather than soothe. Deeper touch; pressure point massage as opposed to stroking; and myofascial, craniosacral, and polarity therapy can be effective. Flaxseed-filled bags of different sizes can be used as calming devices for children with tactile defensiveness. The weight of the bags is soothing when warmed and placed on the back or abdomen (Klein S, personal communication, March 1999). Because one-third of children who have stomachaches in response to stress will continue this pattern as adults, helping children learn to release tension in the abdomen may help avoid chronic abdominal pain or problems.[12]

Different forms of vestibular stimulation are especially important for drug-affected infants and children. Drugs and alcohol can interfere with vestibular development during fetal life and, if the children were hospitalized as infants, they may have been deprived of vestibular stimulation at that time as well. Small children normally receive this stimulation from being rocked, picked up and put down, and from their own body movements. If they are sick enough to be hospitalized as infants, they are not likely to get that stimulation. With the physical therapist's or physician's approval, vestibular stimulation such as rocking, swinging, or having them spin in a swivel chair may be incorporated into a massage session.

MASSAGE FOR THE DRUG-EXPOSED CHILD

As the drug-exposed infant grows, the basic techniques discussed in Chapter 3 will be beneficial. Frequent warm baths help reduce stress, and massage may be done in the bathtub using soap lather instead of oil. A gentle, sensitive full-body massage on a regular basis would be ideal. Be careful to do massage at the child's pace. It will be more effective to give the child frequent massages for shorter periods (two 30-minute massages rather than one 60-minute massage). Have the child do the basic relaxation sequence as often as possible.

Areas that have been traumatized should be given special attention to prevent the child from developing lifelong habits of guarding. For example, guarding around feeding tubes, monitors, and feet lances is common. Even when the child is older and does not have a feeding tube, there may be tension and restriction around the scar. If the child was on a ventilator, there may be tremendous tension in the mouth, jaw, and throat. Abdominal massage to the child's tolerance level will help release tension from the pain of esophageal reflux or gas.

HYDROCEPHALUS

Hydrocephalus is a condition in which a disruption in the flow of cerebrospinal fluid causes an accumulation in the ventricles of the brain. When the fluid backs up, the ventricles become enlarged, resulting in increased intracranial pressure, enlargement of the cranium, and compression and subsequent damage of nerve tissue. Many different signs and symptoms may result, including seizures, headaches, **strabismus,** swallowing difficulties, and atrophy of the brain. About one in 1,000 children has hydrocephalus.

Hydrocephalus has various causes, including maternal infection (with rubella or cytomegalovirus) during pregnancy, meningitis, head trauma (including birth trauma), brain hemorrhage, tumors, or cysts. This condition is also associated with other birth defects; the majority of children with spina bifida

(incomplete closure of the spine) also have hydrocephalus.[1]

To treat hydrocephalus, a shunt is inserted that diverts the cerebrospinal fluid to the child's abdominal cavity. A small hole is drilled in the child's skull and a tube is inserted and threaded subcutaneously from small incisions at the ventricular and peritoneal insertion site (Figure 6–8). Unfortunately, shunts can become blocked by scar tissue or infection of the surrounding tissue; then the shunt is no longer able to divert the cerebrospinal fluid. If this occurs, the child will begin to have symptoms of increased intracranial pressure, including severe pain, lethargy, headache, vomiting, irritability, and visual problems. Blocked shunts must be replaced; unfortunately, each time another tube is inserted, brain matter is damaged or destroyed.

APPROACH AND GOALS

Massage can be a significant source of comfort for children with hydrocephalus (see Point of Interest Box 6–7). Basic Swedish massage (Chapter 3) can offer relaxation and relief from aches and pains and provide much-needed stimulation when the children's activities are limited or if immobilized. As the Keenes have done, other massage therapy techniques may be combined with the basic techniques described in Chapter 3.

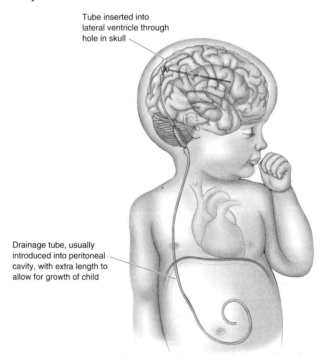

Tube inserted into lateral ventricle through hole in skull

Drainage tube, usually introduced into peritoneal cavity, with extra length to allow for growth of child

FIGURE 6–8 ■ Boy With a Ventriculoperitoneal Shunt. The shunt removes excess cerebrospinal fluid from the ventricles and shunts it to the peritoneum. A one-way valve is present in the tubing behind the ear. From Bear MF, Connors BW, and Parasido MA: *Neuroscience—Exploring the Brain*. 2nd ed. Philadelphia, PA: Lippincott Williams & Wilkins, 2001.

POINT OF INTEREST BOX 6–7
Tim Keene's Story

Tim Keene, now 21, was born with hydrocephalus of unknown cause. His first shunt was inserted when he was 6 days old. Tim's childhood was normal and fully active; he excelled in sports and traveled with his family. Then, in 1997 at age 16, with no warning, his shunt failed. Tim immediately had neurosurgery to insert a new shunt. The original valve had deteriorated so much that, during surgery, it simply crumbled in the neurosurgeon's hand. The new shunt malfunctioned repeatedly as a result of scar tissue in Tim's brain; he remained hospitalized for 4 months.

Rich and Diane Keene, Tim's parents, are both professional massage therapists. At first, they used Swedish massage and reflexology to rouse him after surgery and to ease his discomfort. When his skull sutures were healed weeks later, they used craniosacral therapy to reduce the swelling and improve circulation. Aromatherapy was used to elevate his mood and help him relax. With massage, Tim required less pain medication than normal. Although he was discharged from the hospital after 4 months, he continued to have moderate to severe headaches daily and a slight motor weakness on the right side of his body.

When Tim's headache pain is a 1–7 on a 1–10 scale, his mother and father treat him with energy balancing, reflexology, and acupressure. Any pain greater than seven is probably a shunt failure and requires an immediate trip to the hospital. The pain is so severe, Tim says it is "like someone hitting your head with a hammer. The pain and the pressure are so bad you can't even think. The only thing on your mind is making it stop." Generally, for a headache he is massaged for about 30 minutes. "Sometimes I'll have a pounding headache

and my mom will work on me, doing some energy work and reflexology. Relief usually comes between 15 and 30 minutes and sometimes I fall asleep for hours." His father uses one particular technique when Tim has an optical headache. He presses inward with both thumbs near the bridge of Tim's nose and holds that point for at least 2 minutes. This takes the pressure off, and the pain diminishes in 5 to 30 minutes.[1]

As of September of 2002, Tim had endured 92 shunt revisions, for which 22 holes had been drilled in his skull. The resulting damage, including scar tissue on his skull and brain, eventually caused seizures. Tim and his parents have thus spent long periods in the intensive care unit because Tim has experienced strokes, cardiac arrests, and other major medical problems as a result of the seizures. His parents continue to massage Tim every day. His mother says they do not always use the same techniques; they will try different types of massage and will not quit until they find something that makes him comfortable (Keene D, personal communication, September 2002). For example, sometimes they use myofascial release and light cross-fiber friction to strengthen and unwind Tim's tight muscles. Foot reflexology is helpful just to get him to relax. After 15 to 20 minutes of trigger point therapy, Tim's cognitive level is better, his speech is clearer, and his pain is greatly relieved. Alternating hot and cold packs on different parts of his body stimulate his circulation and help him feel more alive.

Reference
1. George T: With his parents' touch. *Massage Magazine*, January/February:44-48, 2000

MASSAGE FOR CHILDREN WITH HYDROCEPHALUS

Children with hydrocephalus are not all the same. There may be varying degrees of pain, restriction of activities, and other discomforts. A careful medical history should be taken to find out what is most bothersome to the child.

Positioning: Children may lie in any preferred position; even prone with the head turned to one side is safe.

All full-body massage technique strokes described in Chapter 3 may be used and adapted to the individual child's concerns. Observe the following cautions carefully and the massage will be safe.

1. Stay at least 4 inches away from the operative site, where the tube comes out of the skull.

2. Move the head slowly and gently so as not to traction the tube any time the child's neck needs to be moved or repositioned.

3. Do not use deep-tissue massage techniques that put pressure on the drainage tube; anything that yanks on the tube could disconnect it!

4. Craniosacral therapy has proven effective for Tim. Diane Keene cautions, however, that it could be dangerous because craniosacral therapy may affect the cerebrospinal fluid, and hydrocephalus is a disruption of the cerebrospinal fluid. She knows her son and his cranial rhythm well and does not want anyone working on him who does not know him just as well. Craniosacral therapy has been helpful in other cases of hydrocephalus, especially when the condition is due to improper pressure from

the occipital bone.[2] However, it should only be attempted if you have received advanced training with an expert in craniosacral therapy.

MUSCULAR DYSTROPHY

When I volunteered to bring massage to Muscular Dystrophy Camp in St. Louis, Missouri, I was overwhelmed by the youngsters' responses. They all wanted to get on the table, the response was incredible. When we couldn't get them up on the table, I worked on them in their wheelchairs. I let them tell me where they wanted me to work. Every one of them had a different ache or pain and some had numb places they wanted to feel again. These kids desperately wanted to be touched.[1]

—*Terrie Yardley-Nohr, massage therapist*

Muscular dystrophy (MD) is an inherited muscle disease that affects about 1 in 3,000 males. Because their bodies do not produce dystropin, a protein that stabilizes the muscle membrane during muscle contraction, the muscle fibers gradually deteriorate and are replaced by fat and fibrous tissue. This muscle deterioration causes a gradual loss of muscular strength. The pelvic and leg muscles are affected first, followed by the muscles of the upper extremities. The involuntary muscles of the heart and diaphragm also deteriorate, eventually leading to respiratory and heart failure. Many boys require a wheelchair by age 10, and scoliosis often develops at approximately this age. Contractures are almost inevitable, and are caused by an imbalance of agonist and antagonist muscles, bad posture resulting from trying to stabilize the limbs when standing, or loss of range of motion from sitting in a wheelchair. Because the muscular tension that normally stimulates bone growth is deficient, MD can also lead to osteoporosis. Then, because their muscles are

weak, boys with this condition are prone to severe falls that can easily break their porous bones. Fractures are most common in the diaphyses of the femur and upper humerus.[2] Boys with this condition also tend to have learning disabilities and cognitive impairments.[3]

Standard medical therapy for muscular dystrophy includes physical therapy to delay or prevent contractures through daily passive stretching, and splinting and exercises to maximize muscle strength. Pool exercise encourages stamina and endurance, without the stress of fighting gravity, and enhances breathing. Orthopedic surgery may be used to release shortened tissue, lengthen contracted tendons, or transfer tendons to different locations. Corticosteroids are often prescribed. As boys and their families face his increasing disability and impending death, depression is common and counseling is often suggested. Despite medical therapy, the current prognosis for boys with muscular dystrophy is respiratory failure leading to death before adulthood.[3]

APPROACH AND GOALS

The massage techniques described in Chapter 3, combined with a routine of strengthening exercises and passive stretching, can help prevent or delay the onset of contracture, keep connective tissue supple, and dramatically increase comfort (Figure 6–9). When massage is introduced into a regular routine, strengthening and stretching can be less tedious and more enjoyable. Because boys with MD experience chronic high levels of stress, massage is especially appropriate for relaxation. The progressive relaxation sequence described in Chapter 3 is excellent for both relaxation and for strengthening muscles.

Dr. Meir Schneider has developed a special program to treat muscular dystrophy that includes a

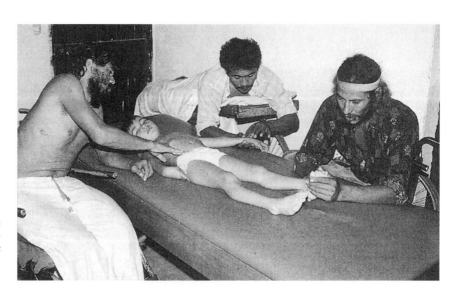

FIGURE 6–9 ■ Massage for a Boy With Muscular Dystrophy. Reprinted with permission from Werner D: *Nothing About Us Without Us*. Palo Alto, CA: HealthWrights, 1998, p 270.

POINT OF INTEREST BOX 6–8
Massage for a Boy With Muscular Dystrophy

In 1991, the author showed a video of Meir Schneider's techniques for muscular dystrophy to the staff and patients of a clinic for children with disabilities in Ajoya, Mexico. The clinic staff, with no instruction, began intensive treatment of Angel, a 6-year-old boy with muscular dystrophy (MD) who was visiting the clinic with his mother. Three young men with spinal-cord injuries, with no massage training other than receiving massage therapy from the author, formed the core of those treating the boy. Angel was insecure, fretful, uncooperative, and feared everyone but his mother; he was judged impossible to treat by a visiting physical therapist. The boy received an intense program of daily massage sessions, followed by exercise to build muscle strength. Exercises were playful and designed to encourage full muscle use without fatigue. Angel was treated for several hours daily for 2 weeks. At this time, his gait was visibly improved, and he had made gains in his capacity to lift and move different parts of his body. He had also changed from a fearful, whiny boy to a much happier one. His mother was so happy with the results that she continued his massage and exercises at home and, when the boy returned to the clinic 3 months later, his walking had improved even more.[1]

Reference

1. Werner D: *Nothing About Us Without Us—Innovative Technology By, For, and With Disabled Persons.* Palo Alto, CA: HealthWrights, 1998, p 109-111, 269-273

unique form of massage (Point of Interest Box 6–8). Consisting of gentle circular motions with the fingertips over the entire body and concentrating on the most important and affected muscles, it is designed to regenerate weak muscle. The massage is combined with movement, visualization, and relaxation exercises. Dr. Schneider, whose doctoral thesis was on movement therapy for muscular dystrophy, has helped many affected individuals regain normal muscle strength, but this is not a "cure" for MD—therapy must be ongoing.[4,5]

MASSAGE AND HYDROTHERAPY FOR CHILDREN WITH MUSCULAR DYSTROPHY

Hydrotherapy:

1. Moist heat applications, such as hydrocollator packs, may be used before massage to improve circulation to the tissue and aid relaxation.

2. Hydrotherapy may be combined with massage to stimulate weak muscles (see page 142).

MASSAGE THERAPY FOR MUSCULAR DYSTROPHY

Step 1. Use the basic relaxation sequence to encourage deep, relaxed breathing. The progressive relaxation sequence can also be used but, if the child appears to be fatigued by the muscle contractions, stop immediately.

Step 2. Use the full-body Swedish massage strokes described in Chapter 3. Be especially careful to not apply too much pressure. A few minutes of strengthening exercises and passive stretching may be alternated with a few minutes of massage.

- The tissue around the joints can be tight and fibrous; spend extra time performing effleurage and petrissage around the joints, moving at right angles to the muscle fibers. Use light to medium pressure.
- When massaging the chest and stomach, stroke between the ribs and along the bottom ribs (see the section on asthma, page 162). Do not push on the xyphoid process.
- It is important to massage the feet and hands. Include gentle range-of-motion exercises on the ankles, toes, wrist, and fingers and include passive stretching as prescribed by the physical therapist.
- If constipation is a problem, see page 124.

SCOLIOSIS

About one in 100 children younger than age 8 has scoliosis, which is defined as *an abnormal lateral and rotational curvature of the spine* (see Figure 6–10). More simply, scoliosis is not only a sideways deviation of the spine, but also a spiral twisting of the vertebrae. In children ages 7 to 16, one in 50 has scoliosis; however, less than 10% have curves large enough to require treatment. Of the more serious cases that do require treatment, there are six girls to each boy.[1]

Scoliosis has several causes. It can be caused by a congenital defect in the bones of the spine, such as two or more vertebrae being fused together or a vertebrae having missing or poorly formed parts. It can also develop from a neurologic or muscular disorder. For example, a child with athetotic cerebral palsy who has spasticity on only one side of the trunk muscles can develop scoliosis. It can also be caused by the way children use their bodies. For example, a **leg-length discrepancy** can be a cause of functional, not anatomic scoliosis.[2] Other causes of functional scoliosis include habitual sitting or standing in an improper position, tilting of the head caused by some type of

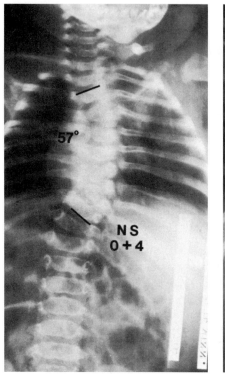

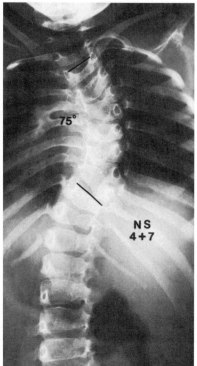

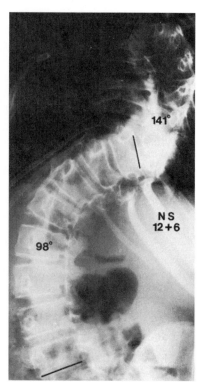

A. Four months of age   B. Four years of age   C. Twelve years of age

FIGURE 6–10 ■ A Girl's Skeleton Radically Deformed by Untreated Congenital Scoliosis. Reprinted with permission from Morrissy R: *Lovell and Winter's Pediatric Orthopaedics.* Vol. 1. Baltimore, MD: Lippincott Williams & Wilkins, 2001, p 728.

visual dysfunction, and paralysis of spinal muscles. During an attack of sciatica, muscles on the painful side can contract and cause a temporary lateral curvature.[3] Many times the cause of scoliosis is not known. Functional scoliosis can become anatomic; if the scoliosis is left untreated long enough, the vertebrae eventually remodel to reflect the imbalances and permanently imprint a postural pattern. In many cases, muscle tension both causes and accompanies scoliosis. Muscles may pull the spine out of alignment, and the malalignment may activate trigger points. For example, scoliosis is known to activate trigger points in the rhomboid and serratus posterior muscles.[2]

Scoliosis can have serious consequences. Adults with untreated scoliosis, aged 40 to 60, have about twice the mortality rate as control groups with no scoliosis; those with thoracic curves can have significant cardiac and respiratory complications. Adults may also have major cosmetic deformities, significant back pain, and difficulty breathing.[1]

Standard medical treatment for scoliosis consists of postural exercises, such as gluteal and abdominal muscle strengthening, stretching of the muscles of the chest and lower extremities, braces, and surgery for severe curvature. Spinal fusion, which involves inserting rods that straighten and fuse the affected verte-

brae, is the most common surgical procedure for scoliosis.

APPROACH AND GOALS

Massage alone cannot heal scoliosis. The child's physician or physical therapist should be consulted about the cause. If some congenital problem requires surgery or another underlying cause has not been addressed, this should be done first. For example, inefficient postural habits can be retrained, a short leg may be treated with a lift in the shoe, or a poorly fitted wheelchair can be adjusted. After the cause is addressed, massage may help with chronic muscular tension and imbalance.

Excess muscle tension can be treated with whole-body Swedish massage strokes (Chapter 3) and with other types of massage and bodywork. Extra time should be spent massaging the muscles of the back but, because scoliosis affects the entire body, the entire body should be treated. A great deal of time should be devoted to passive range-of-motion exercises. A whole-body massage once a week, along with daily massage to the entire back, would be ideal. Parents can learn to do the daily massage.

Massage therapist and educator Meir Schneider has had excellent results reducing or correcting scoliosis with a program combining massage and passive and active movement. He believes that massage is needed before exercise can be effective because many back muscles may be too tight to allow any movement. Gentle touch is used to stimulate and warm weakened muscles; deep tissue massage is recommended in only those areas where strong muscles have become rigid.[4]

MASSAGE FOR CHILDREN WITH SCOLIOSIS

Positioning: Children should be put in unusual positions that stretch their muscles and put their bones in a different relationship to each other during massage. For example, as they lie supine on the treatment table, have them twist the spine by rotating both legs to one side and turning the head and upper body to the opposite side. This stretches the midback. Positions should always be comfortable; use pillows or bolsters for support, if necessary. Parents can help hold children in these positions. Another novel position is with children laying prone over a large pillow or padded stool that is at waist level, so that they are almost on all fours. This gives you the opportunity to move their hip joints in internal and external rotation in a way that they will not normally do themselves, and to have greater access to the muscles around the hip joint and the muscles on the sides of the torso. They may also be lying on their sides, with one arm overhead and twisted to the back, with the hips rolled forward. Massage strokes should be modified for these different positions. For example, if the child is lying on his side, back effleurage, which is described in Chapter 3, will need to be done on the half of the back that is uppermost, then when the child rolls over, back effleurage can be done on the other side of the back, which will now be uppermost.

WHOLE-BODY MASSAGE

The ideal regimen for this condition is a whole-body massage, with concentration on the muscles of the back. Back muscles that are especially tight should be massaged for a longer time, with as much pressure as can be well tolerated. Any stretching or strengthening exercises prescribed by the child's physical therapist can also be incorporated into the massage.

TACTILE DEFENSIVENESS

One thing I couldn't learn was how to feel. Robyn's mom would always hug her before she went off to school, and she insisted on doing this to me, too . . . So every morning, like a rock, I learned to tolerate get-

ting hugged. I told my friend's mother that being hugged hurt me and that it felt like I was being burned. She insisted that this was nonsense, but it didn't make the feeling go away. At first my head would spin, I felt like I was going to faint. I would only hug her when routine called for it.[1]

—Donna Williams, who is autistic

Tactile defensiveness is defined as *the fear and dislike of most touch sensations.* There are two types of tactile defensiveness. The first is caused by negative experiences with touch, such as child abuse (page 158). The other is caused by an irregularity in the nervous system, often seen in children with learning disabilities and other, more serious, conditions. This irregularity causes certain sensory information to be overwhelming. Its cause is not known, although one suspected cause is oxygen deprivation during birth, which could damage cells that process tactile stimuli. Another suspected cause is environmental toxins that affect genetically predisposed children.[2] Examples of tactile defensiveness include:

- Avoiding having hands in sand, mud, or finger paints, or having bare feet in mud, sand, or grass.
- Stiffening the body when being picked up and struggling against being held, cuddled, hugged, patted, or stroked; being resistant to being dressed; having dental work or having hair cut.
- Difficulty concentrating or learning when there is a minor tactile distraction that most other children could tolerate, such as a loose thread in a sock or a breeze that blows the hairs on the skin.
- Removing clothes more often than most children to get rid of annoying sensations caused by the tags in a shirt or socks on the feet. Conversely, wearing long-sleeved shirts or sweaters even when it is warm.

Tactile defensiveness can have profound effects on development. Children may be unable to develop a good body image and spatial awareness; they may have a tendency to retreat from interpersonal contact and communication with others; and they may not want to use their hands for grasping, feeding themselves, and reaching out to explore their environment. Some children may react with irritation, anxiety, restlessness, fear, or emotional stress to ordinary touch sensations. This response may severely limit their activities; tactile defensiveness often results in tactile deprivation. Tension or stress may make the child even more tactile defensive.

Relaxation training can effectively reduce tactile defensiveness in certain children. In a study of children ages 4 to 11, both progressive relaxation and autogenic training increased tactile perception and decreased tactile defensiveness.[3]

APPROACH AND GOALS

The massage therapist will rarely see a child for tactile defensiveness alone, but may see children with neurodevelopmental differences who are touch phobic. The authors of *Aromatherapy and Massage for People With Learning Disabilities* use an approach they call "Multisensory Massage." This approach is used to increase tolerance of touch. This approach uses fabrics of different textures, massage tools, water, soft brushes, massage oils and lotions, and oils scented with essential oils. A foot massage may begin by gently rubbing the feet with a piece of velvet, then with a soft brush and, finally, with silky material. This could be followed by a few minutes of soaking the feet in a portable foot spa with essential oils in the water, drying the feet with a soft towel, and giving a foot massage. After the massage, the lotion or oil could be wiped off with flannel, a soft towel, or another soft cloth. All this touch would certainly not be easily accepted in a first session; it may require many sessions of only one type of touch sensation, such as fabric alone or water in a foot bath, before a child could accept all these forms of tactile stimulation on the feet.[4]

The author taught the mother of a 2-year-old child with **Behr syndrome (**a condition in which the child has mental retardation, visual deficits, ataxia, and spasticity) to stimulate and massage her daughter's hands using a variety of tactile sensations. The girl's hands were so sensitive that she had not progressed to grasping objects. Her mother let her play with bathtub toys in a pan of warm water, then in a pan of cold water with new toys. The little girl loved water and was so distracted that she barely noticed her mother massaging one hand at a time with soap lather. Later, her mother used Epsom salts and rubbed one hand at a time. Gradually, as she could tolerate more stimulation, her hands could be massaged out of the water with lotion or oil. This was done daily by the mother. After 2 weeks, her occupational therapist reported that the little girl was finally able to tolerate holding a spoon and could now begin learning to feed herself.

MASSAGE FOR CHILDREN WITH TACTILE DEFENSIVENESS

With some children it may seem that they will never be able to tolerate receiving massage. The key is to find one, small type of tactile stimulation that is acceptable and, from that, gradually build their tolerance. Great patience is required. Parents are often aware of what tactile stimulation is acceptable to their child. Massage therapist Larry Burns-Vidlak has three autistic children. He began by wrestling playfully with them when that was the only physical contact they could tolerate (see Autism, page 167). You may need to try every massage stroke you know and do each one in different ways; you may need to invent a touch game using toys or music; you may need to try many types of sensory stimulation. Parents often know a toy or game that appeals to the child, and that one small thing can be a bridge to helping the child accept more touch.

Often if the child can hold or play with an item, he or she will feel more comfortable with it. For example, let the child roll a textured massage tool on someone else's hand or leg, play with a piece of fake fur, or put a warm flaxseed bag on his body. Massage techniques in which your hands remain still, such as passive touch and pressure point massage, may be more acceptable. Energetic techniques such as Polarity therapy and Reiki may also work well.

When stroking, move slowly and soothingly so that your actions are predictable. Always proceed at the child's pace and do not overwhelm her. Explain what you are about to do, and do not give touch in a way the child does not like. Other forms of sensory stimulation that can be incorporated into a massage session include:

- Warm water, heat applications, or linens. Washcloths can be wrung out in warm water and put on the hands and feet. The child can be washed off with warm water after a massage. Bathtub toys can be placed in a container of warm water with a towel underneath. Hot water bottles, heating pads, or microwaveable flaxseed- or rice-filled bags can be used. Warmed towels, blankets, or clothing may persuade a reluctant child to lie still. It also feels great to be wrapped in warmed linens after a massage.
- Cold water. Washcloths can be wrung out in cold water and put on the hands or feet on a hot day. The child can also be washed off with cool water after a massage. Bathtub toys can be placed in a container of cold water with a towel underneath.
- Soap lather. Soap lather may be used to massage a hand when a child is playing with toys in a container of water. Parents may try doing massage in the bathtub, using soap lather instead of massage oil.
- Epsom salts. One part of the body at a time may be rubbed with salt. This is great for decreasing tactile sensitivity in the hands. A good way to begin with a child with sensitive hands is to have him or her play with toys in a tub of warm or cold water, then slip one hand out and rub gently with salt, and replace in the water. The child will have her hand in salt water, and when her hands come out they should be washed with clean water or rubbed with oil or lotion.

- Different fabric textures. Make a glove and stroke the child with it during the massage for another tactile sensation. Give the child a piece of fake fur to play with. Coarse or soft towels can be used. Rubbing can be done slowly or briskly.
- Brushes of different textures. Try different brushes. If you cover the skin with a sheet, this makes the tactile stimulation easier to absorb. Soft baby brushes are easier for some children to accept.
- Balls (see page 68, Chapter 3). Large balls may work better for some children because they are less specific. Cover the child with a blanket and roll a large ball slowly down the back to the feet and back up.
- Flaxseed-filled fabric bags of different sizes. When placed on the back or abdomen, many children find the weight of the bag soothing. They can be warmed in a microwave, as well.

WHEELCHAIR RIDERS

Like prostheses, exercise equipment, or massage tables, wheelchairs are tools. They are a tremendous help in making children who are disabled more independent and should not be viewed as prisons by the children or the world at large. From a musculoskeletal point of view, however, they do have certain disadvantages (Figure 6–11). These include:

- Prolonged sitting can lead to habitually slumping forward, with constriction of the abdomen, a loss of cervical and lumbar curve, and increased thoracic **kyphosis.** In a sitting position, many joints are in constant flexion and contractures are more likely, particularly if there is spasticity or muscle weakness.
- Using a manual wheelchair is an excellent way to get physical exercise and keep the arm muscles strong, but the constant pushing while leaning forward can create upper body strain and thoracic kyphosis. The chest and upper back muscles can become chronically tightened. Overuse of the arms can cause pain in the shoulders, arms, and hands.
- Pressure ulcers are an ever-present danger for wheelchair riders because their weight is constantly pressing down on the hips, buttocks, and coccyx (Point of Interest Box 6–9). To prevent pressure ulcers, children need to take their weight completely off the buttocks for 1 full minute, at least once every 15 minutes. When they begin to use a wheelchair, children need careful supervision to help learn this habit. Their entire skin surface should also be checked for sores daily. Checking can be done by an adult or,

if they are old enough, children can learn to do this themselves with a mirror.[1]
- Whether or not their wheelchairs fit them originally, children grow out of them. It is vital that wheelchairs continue to fit well, providing proper support and trunk and pelvic symmetry. As children grow, their wheelchairs should be checked frequently. Children can develop back pain, contractures, or scoliosis if their chairs are not well fitted.
- Being in a sitting position most of the time means decreased circulation to the legs, and less sensory stimulation to the rest of the body. Minor cuts may heal slowly, and the legs may be pale and cold to the touch.

APPROACH AND GOALS

Hydrotherapy can be helpful in conjunction with massage: moist heat applications may be used for muscular relaxation, salt glows of the legs and contrast treatments of the lower legs and feet may be used to dramatically improve the circulation in the legs, and cold water immersion can stimulate muscle contraction. All of these treatments are also an excellent source of sensory stimulation. Contrast treatments for developing or existing pressure ulcers can temporarily increase circulation to an area 70–100%, and exposure to a heat lamp helps pressure ulcers heal.

Massage therapy can address local problems, which are discussed below. However, when we look at the child's body as a whole, we can see that perhaps the greatest value of a massage session in this case is for wheelchair riders to experience their bodies in different configurations, not just the one or two positions they are normally in. This widens their body experience and enhances their body image. Local problems that can be addressed with massage include:

1. Upper body massage can counteract the chronic tightness of the pectoral muscles and the upper back if the child uses a manual wheelchair.
2. Massage can increase circulation to the legs, which is often very poor because the leg muscles are not contracting.
3. Lack of body awareness and contractures. Using passive movement can help a child reconnect the information from the joint proprioceptors to the brain, move fluid through the joints, and prevent contractures by combining passive movement with stretching. Passive movement is also very important to maintain joint motion following operative release or injury.
4. Pressure ulcers. Massage may prevent the development of pressure ulcers because poor

Healthy, comfortable, and functional positions

Whether or not a chair has wheels, **the position in which it allows a child to sit is very important.**

For most children, the chair should help them to sit more or less like this:

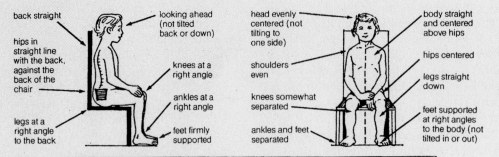

back straight

hips in straight line with the back, against the back of the chair

legs at a right angle to the back

looking ahead (not tilted back or down)

knees at a right angle

ankles at a right angle

feet firmly supported

head evenly centered (not tilting to one side)

shoulders even

knees somewhat separated

ankles and feet separated

body straight and centered above hips

hips centered

legs straight down

feet supported at right angles to the body (not tilted in or out)

CAUTION: **The seat should be wide enough to allow some free movement and narrow enough to give needed support**

Common seating problems and possible solutions

Problem: **Hips tilt back**

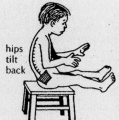

hips tilt back

In children with spastic cerebral palsy the hips often stiffen backward. This triggers spasms that straighten the legs and cause other muscle tightness with loss of control.

Also, children with weak hips or back, from *spinal cord* injury, spina bifida, or severe polio, often sit slumped with their hips tilted back and the back severely curved. This can lead to permanent deformity.

One of the most common causes of backward tilting hips is **a chair like this one that is too big** for the child.

Other causes of backward tilt and bad position are:

a chair back that tilts far back

and a cloth back that sags.

These let the child lean back and cause the hips to slip forward. **Also, footrests that are far forward** so that knees do not bend enough can increase *spasticity* that tilts hips back.

BAD

A good position can often be gained through:

a fairly **stiff, upright back** at a right angle to the seat,

a chair that fits the child so that his hips reach the chair back,

the knees at right angles, and **feet firmly supported.**

GOOD

BETTER

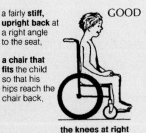

Most children, and especially a child who tends to fall forward in his seat, will sit better and more comfortably if the whole chair tilts back a little. But be sure to keep right angles at hips, knees, and ankles.

FIGURE 6–11 ■ A healthy, comfortable and functional sitting position is essential. Reprinted with permission from Werner D: *Disabled Village Children*. Palo Alto, CA: Hesperian Foundation, 1987, p 591.

POINT OF INTEREST BOX 6–9
Pressure Ulcers

Pressure ulcers, or decubitus ulcers, are skin lesions resulting from loss of tissue. They develop when the weight of one limb or the entire body puts pressure on the tissues overlying bony prominences or protuberances, which cuts off circulation to the area. Without oxygen and the nutrients that are carried in the blood, the skin and underlying tissue begin to die. Pressure ulcers, if not carefully treated, can worsen from a skin lesion to a deeper ulcer that can destroy the epidermis, the dermis, and the superficial fascia, as well as erode tissue down to the bone. The sore can become infected by bacteria, and then secondary infection of an open wound can occur, causing blood poisoning and even death if the bacteria gets into the general circulation. Potential sites of pressure ulcers include the heels, ankles, hips, buttocks, coccyx, elbows, and shoulders.

Those most likely to develop pressures ulcers include children who are so ill, weak, or disabled that they cannot roll over by themselves (caregivers need to turn them frequently and lay them on soft surfaces that reduce pressure on bony areas) and certain children with no sensation in parts of their body, such as those with spinal cord injury or spina bifida. Other factors that contribute to pressure ulcer development are protein or iron deficiency, vitamin C deficiency, incontinence, and poor local blood supply.[1,2]

References

1. Taylor RV, et al: Ascorbic acid supplementation in the treatment of pressure sores. *Lancet*, 2:544-546, 1974
2. Bergstrom N, et al: *Pressure Ulcer Treatment. Clinical Practice Guidelines*. Quick Reference Guide for Clinicians, No. 15. Rockville, MD: Department of Health and Human Services, Public Health Service, Agency for Health Care Policy and Research. AHCPR Publication. No. 95-0653, December 1994, p 7

local blood supply contributes to their development. Massage can enhance the circulation of the general area where a pressure ulcer is developing, indirectly treating the ulcer.[2,3]

HYDROTHERAPY AND MASSAGE FOR WHEELCHAIR RIDERS

Hydrotherapy treatments. Choose one to perform before massage:

MOIST HEAT APPLICATION

Apply a moist heating pad or Hydrocollator pack to areas of muscular tension or soreness for 3 minutes. Give cooler applications to any areas with decreased sensation and monitor the child's skin more carefully than usual.

CONTRAST TREATMENT OF THE FEET

See Growing Pains section in Chapter 5 but, if possible, use taller containers of water that will immerse the feet and the entire lower legs.

COLD WATER IMMERSION FOLLOWED BY EXERCISE FOR MUSCLE WEAKNESS

See Muscle Weakness, page 142.

SALT GLOW OF THE LEGS

A salt glow of the back is pictured in Figures 3–53 and 3–54. See Chapter 3 for directions.

MASSAGE

1. Regular whole-body Swedish massage with extra time spent on passive range-of-motion exercises to all joints is recommended.
2. Follow the specific instructions in the section on each disability such as spinal cord injury or cerebral palsy.
3. During massage, children should be out of their wheelchairs and in different positions than they are normally accustomed to. Massage strokes can be adapted to these different positions, such as sidelying, prone, with the torso or legs rotating to one side or the other, or in a partial spinal twist. Do not put the child in any position that they find truly uncomfortable, but encourage them to try a position they would not normally be in. Extra bolsters or pillows will be helpful.
4. If children are in manual wheelchairs, their upper bodies should be thoroughly massaged, and the pectoral muscles should be stretched. Spend more time on passive range-of-motion exercises for the shoulder joints. Strengthening exercises to move the shoulders back may be necessary as well.
5. If children's legs are cold, white, or appear to have poor circulation, perform the basic effleurage strokes for the front and back of the legs (see Figures 3–21 and 3–49) many more times than in the basic full-body massage. For very poor circulation, continues these two strokes for 5 to 10 minutes.
6. If children have had problems with pressure sores in the past, massage of the buttocks can be helpful to increase the local circulation. Parents and other caregivers can be taught how to perform kneading of the buttocks for a few minutes each day. It should never be performed if there is a developing pressure sore.

7. If children are on a physical therapy program of stretching and strengthening exercises, these can be incorporated into a session. They can receive massage for a few minutes, they can do their exercises for a time, and when they become tired, they can rest and receive massage for a few minutes, and repeat. This can prevent fatigue and make their sessions more interesting. Stretching exercises are beneficial for muscles that are usually in a shortened position while sitting; these include the flexors of the shoulders, elbows, hips, knees, and ankles.

 Passive movement to a paralyzed limb before it is massaged and massage of the paralyzed limb should be done carefully, especially if the child has reduced sensation.

MASSAGE AND HYDROTHERAPY FOR PRESSURE ULCERS

CONTRAST TREATMENT

Step 1. Cover the pressure ulcer with a sterile dressing.

Step 2. Apply washcloths or small towels that have been wrung out in hot water around the covered pressure ulcer. Cover the towels with a layer of plastic and then a towel to keep in the heat. Leave on for 3 minutes. Several small hot packs may be used instead of towels. Be sure to monitor the skin underneath the heat so the child's skin does not get burned.

Step 3. Remove the towels and do ice massage over the same area—around the ulcer, not on it—for 1 minute. See page 91.

Step 4. Repeat Steps 2 and 3 twice, for a total of three changes. The skin around the pressure ulcer will now be red, indicating that more blood has flowed into the area.

HEAT EXPOSURE

Use a 60-watt lightbulb in a goosenecked lamp. The light should be about 2 feet away from the ulcer. Shine the light on the ulcer to expose it to the heat from the bulb three times a day for 15 minutes. Because the child's skin must be monitored carefully for burning, do not leave the child unattended.[2]

MASSAGE

The first sign of a developing pressure ulcer is red skin that blanches or whitens when pressed firmly with a finger. At this point, pressure ulcer development may be halted by treatment with massage. Gently wash and dry the reddened area. Then gently massage the general area, but not the reddened portion. Stay at least 12 inches away from the reddened area; you are addressing the bloodflow in the general area, not the ulcer itself. Any circulation-enhancing techniques, including effleurage toward the heart, gentle kneading, and petrissage, will be effective. Manual lymph drainage techniques may be indicated as well.[3]

SUMMARY

Massage therapy can be safely applied to children with many different special needs and situations. Many of the benefits that children with different disabilities receive from massage also highlight the powerful effects massage can have on different systems of the body. It is important for the therapist to consult with the child's physician or physical therapist and to observe contraindications; however, with proper information, you should never be afraid to handle a child. The information presented in Chapter 6 gives you the tools to touch children with special needs. Massage has tremendous potential to help children physically, emotionally, and mentally and to make a significant contribution to their well-being and quality of life.

REVIEW QUESTIONS

1. Explain the difference between a disability present at birth (birth defect) and an acquired disability. Give three examples of each.

2. Discuss the causes of some common problems faced by children who are disabled.

3. Name both the primary and secondary effects of cerebral palsy, hemophilia, premature birth, and visual impairment.

4. Name three conditions discussed in Chapter 6 in which hydrotherapy is used in conjunction with massage therapy and explain what effects the hydrotherapy produces.

5. Name one disability in which the most important effect of massage therapy is sensory stimulation, one in which mental relaxation is the most important effect, one in which relief of pain is the most important effect, and one in which increased joint circulation is the most important effect.

6. Give four examples from Chapter 6 of why a child might not wish to receive massage, and discuss how the therapist might make massage more acceptable to the child.

7. Explain how the full-body massage techniques described in Chapter 3 may be tailored to meet the needs of children with different conditions. Give examples.

Introduction

1. Mikita S: Voice of the client. *Professional Bodyworker's Journal,* Spring:88, 1998
2. The Risk and Prevention of Maltreatment for Children with Disabilities. Available at: www.nccanch.calib.com. Accessed May 2003

Problems Common to Children With Disabilities

1. Simon J, Calhoun J: *A Child's Eyes: A Guide to Pediatric Primary Care.* Gainesville, FL: Triad Publishing, 1998, p 186
2. Batshaw M: *Children With Disabilities.* Baltimore, MD: Paul Brookes Publishing, 1997, p 269
3. Scott E, Jan J, Freeman R: *Can't the Child See? A Guide for Parents and Professionals About Young Children Who Are Visually Impaired.* Ed. 3, Austin, TX: Pro-Ed, 1995, p 36
4. Wallender R, et al: Disability parameters: Chronic strain and adaptation of physically handicapped children and their mothers. *Journal of Pediatric Psychology,* 14:23, 1989
5. Jones H, quoted in Exley H, ed: *What It's Like to Be Me.* Cincinnati, OH: Friendship Press, 1984, p 81
6. Hastorf A, et al: Acknowledgment of handicap as a tactic in social interaction. *Journal of Personality and Social Psychology,* 37:1790-1797, 1979
7. Riddle I: Nursing intervention to promote body image integrity in children. *Nursing Clinics of North America,* 7:655, 1972
8. McDonald E: A healing in the theater of life. *Canadian Holistic Healing Association,* 7:9, 1986
9. Rowe H: Massage the handicapped child. *Tender Loving Care. The Newsletter of the International Association of Infant Massage Instructors,* 4:2, 1988
10. Benedict RB, et al: Reported maltreatment in children with multiple disabilities. *Child Abuse and Neglect,* 14:207, 1990
11. Sullivan PM, et al: Patterns of physical and sexual abuse of communicatively handicapped children. *Annals of Otolaryngology, Rhinology, & Laryngology, 100:*188, 1991
12. Llewellyn A: The abuse of children with disabilities in mainstream schooling. *Developmental Medicine & Child Neurology,* 37:740-743, 1995
13. Sinclair M, Von Weller A: Don't let the well run dry: The importance of water to your child's health. *Exceptional Parent Magazine, May:*66, 2001
14. Werner D: *Disabled Village Children.* Palo Alto, CA: Hesperian, 1988, p 77

General Principles of Massage for Children With Disabilities

1. Edwards D, Bruce G: For cerebral palsy patients, massage makes life better. *Massage Magazine,* July/August:106, 2001

Physical and Sexual Abuse

1. Burg F, Wald E, Ingelfinger J, Polin R: *Gellis and Kagan's Current Pediatric Therapy.* Philadelphia, PA: W.B. Saunders, 1999, p 406

2. Ogden J: *Skeletal Injury in the Child.* Philadelphia, PA: Lea and Febiger, 1982, p 198
3. Long T, Toscano K: *Handbook of Pediatric Physical Therapy.* Philadelphia, PA: Lippincott Williams & Wilkins, 2002, p 75
4. Karr-Morse R, Wiley M: *Ghosts from the Nursery—Tracing the Roots of Violence.* New York, NY: Atlantic Monthly Press, 1997, p 262
5. Levine P: *Healing the Tiger: The Innate Capacity to Transform Overwhelming Experiences.* Berkeley, CA: North Atlantic Books, 1997, p 11
6. Terr L: *Too Scared to Cry: How Trauma Affects Our Children. . .and Ultimately Us All.* New York, NY: Basic Books, 1990
7. Taddio A, et al: Conditioning and hyperalgesia in newborns exposed to repeated heel lances. *Journal of the American Medical Association,* August 21:857-861, 2002
8. Taddio A, et al: Effect of neonatal circumcision in pain response during subsequent routine vaccination. *Lancet,* 34:599-603, 1997
9. Hartmann T: *Thom Hartmann's Complete Guide to ADD.* Grass Valley, CA: Underwood Books, 1997, p 30
10. Walling M, et al: Abuse history and chronic pain in women: I. Prevalences of sexual abuse and physical abuse. II. A multivariate analysis of abuse and psychological morbidity. *Obstetrics and Gynecology,* 84:193-199, 200-206, 1994
11. Barsky A, et al: Histories of childhood trauma in adult hypochondriacal patients. *American Journal of Psychiatry,* 151:397, 1994
12. Thakkar R, McCanne T: The effect of daily stressors on physical health in women with and without a childhood history of sexual abuse. *Child Abuse and Neglect,* 24:209-222, 2000
13. Kendall-Tackett K: Physiological correlates of childhood abuse: Chronic hyperarousal in PTSD, depression, and irritable bowel syndrome. *Child Abuse and Neglect,* 24:799-809, 2000
14. Finestone H, et al: Chronic pain and health care utilization in women with a history of childhood sexual abuse. *Child Abuse and Neglect,* 4:547-555, 2000
15. Goldberg R, et al: Relationship between traumatic events in childhood and chronic pain. *Disability and Rehabilitation,* 21:23-30, 1999
16. Mines S: Chakra Man: AIDS, bodywork and inspiration. *Massage and Bodywork,* October/November:37, 2000
17. Lewis DO, et al: Toward a theory of the genesis of violence. *Journal of American Academy of Child Psychiatry,* 28:431-436,1989
18. Magid K, McElvey C: *High Risk: Children Without a Conscience.* New York, NY: Bantam Books, 1987
19. Mowen K: Traumatouch therapy, an interdisciplinary approach to trauma. *Massage and Bodywork Magazine,* October/November:27-31, 2001
20. Edwards T: One trauma survivor's experience of massage. *The Journal of Soft Tissue Manipulation,* August/September:4-8, 1994

Autoimmune Deficiency Syndrome

1. Batshaw M: *Children With Disabilities.* Baltimore, MD: Paul Brookes Publishing, 1997, p 166-167

2. Plana LC, et al: Negative life events affect immune status in HIV+ children and adolescents. *Pediatrics*, 106:540-546, 2000
3. Scafadi F: HIV-exposed newborns show inferior orienting and abnormal reflexes on the Brazelton scale. *Journal of Pediatric Psychology*, 22:105-112, 1997
4. Field T: HIV adolescents show improved immune function following massage therapy. *International Journal of Neuroscience*, 106:35-45, 2001

Asthma

1. Duncan A: *Your Healthy Child*. New York, NY: J.P. Tarcher, 1990, p 65, 67
2. Ivker R, Nelson T: *Asthma Survival. The Holistic Medical Treatment Program for Asthma*. New York, NY: Putnam, 2001, p 2, 27-38
3. America's Children and the Environment. Available at: www.epa.gov/envirohealth/children/ace_2003.pdf. Accessed April 2003
4. Van Stratten M: *Complete Natural Health Consultant*. Northride, England: Angus and Robertson, 1987, p 119
5. Klinnert MD, et al: Onset and persistence of childhood asthma: Predictors from infancy. *Pediatrics*, 108:E69, 2001
6. Sandberg S, et al: The role of acute and chronic stress in asthma attacks in children. *Lancet*, 6356:1932, 2000
7. Strunk RC: Physiologic and psychological characteristics associated with deaths due to asthma in childhood. *Journal of the American Medical Association*, 254:1193-1198, 1985
8. Olness K: *Hypnosis and Hypnotherapy with Chldren*. New York: Guilford Press, 1996, p 215, 219
9. Spiegel D: *Living Beyond Limits: New Help for Facing Life-Threatening Illness*. New York: Times Books, 1993, p 66
10. Erskine-Milliss M, Schonell P: Relaxation therapy in asthma: A critical review. *Psychosomatic Medicine*, August:365-370, 1981
11. Kotses H, Harver A, Segreto J, et al: Long-term effects of biofeedback-induced facial relaxation on measures of asthma severity in children. *Biofeedback Self Reg*, 16:1-21, 1991
12. Lehrer PM: Emotionally triggered asthma: A review of research literature and some hypotheses for self-regulation therapies. *Applied Psychophysiology Biofeedback*, 23:13-41, 1998
13. Vazquez I, Buceta J: Relaxation therapy in the treatment of bronchial asthma: effects on basal spirometric values. *Psychotherapy and Psychosomatics*, 60:106-12, 1993
14. Schwobel G: Psychosomaticsche therapies des asthma bronchiale. *Anzeim Fortsch*, 24:481-488, 1948
15. Hossri C: The treatment of asthma in children through acupuncture massage. *Journal of American Society of Psychosomatic Dentistry and Medicine*, 23:14-19, 1976
16. Field T, et al: Children with asthma have improved pulmonary functions after massage therapy. *Journal of Pediatrics*, 132:854-858, 1998
17. Malinski M, et al: The effect of massage on improving the quality of life for adult chronic asthma patients. *Journal of Allergy and Immunology Abstracts*, 95(part 2):182, 1995
18. Klimowitch P: Massage for respiratory problems. *Massage Therapy Journal*, Spring:42, 1993
19. Malone P: Comfort and benefits of massage for the emphysema patient. *Massage Therapy Journal*, Spring:39, 1990
20. Schenkel E, quoted in *High Speed Healing. The Fastest, Easiest, and Most Effective Shortcuts to Lasting Relief*. Emmaus, PA: Rodale Press, 1991, p 38
21. Natchetelo M: Ease your asthma. *Natural Health*, November/December:81, 2000

Attention Deficit Disorder

1. Batshaw M: *Children With Disabilities*. Baltimore, MD: Paul Brookes Publishing, 1997, p 450-451
2. Steingraber S: *Having Faith: An Ecologist's Journey to Motherhood*. Cambridge, MA: Perseus Publishing, 2001, p 115, 271
3. America's Children and the Environment. Available at: www.epa.gov/envirohealth/children/ace_2003.pdf. Accessed April 2003
4. Hartsough CS, et al: Medical factors in hyperactive and normal children: Prenatal developmental, and health history findings. *American Journal of Orthopsychiatry*, 55:190-210, 1985
5. Upledger J: Craniosacral therapy and attention deficit disorder. *Massage Today*, August:12, 2001
6. Hill R, Castro E: *Getting Rid of Ritalin: How Neurofeedback Can Successfully Treat Attention Deficit Disorder Without Drugs*. Charlottesville, VA: Hampton Roads Publishing, 2002, p xii, 15
7. Guthrie E: *The Trouble With Perfect: How Parents Can Avoid the Overachievement Trap and Still Raise Successful Children*. New York: Broadway Books, 2002, p 94
8. Safer D: Survey of medication treatment for hyperactive/inattentive students. *Journal of the American Medical Association*, 260:26, 1988
9. Amen D: *Healing ADD From the Inside Out*. Fairfield, CA: Institute for Behavioral Healthcare, 1999
10. Connoly D, et al: Electromyography biofeedback on hyperkinetic children. *Journal of Biofeedback*, 12:24-30, 1974
11. Field T: *Touch Therapy*. London, England: Churchill Livingstone, 2000, p 103
12. Zibart R: Acupressure study may pinpoint kids' needs. *Sage Magazine*, September:11, 2000
13. St. John J: *High-Tech Touch—Acupressure in the Schools*. Novato, CA: Academic Therapy Publications, 1987, p 56-58
14. Gordon R: *Your Healing Hands*. Oakland, CA: Wingbow Press, 1984, p 13
15. Ayres J: *Sensory Integration and the Child*. Los Angeles, CA: Western Pyschological Services, 1981, p 115

Autism

1. Williams D: *Nobody Nowhere: The Extraordinary Biography of an Autistic*. New York: Doubleday, 1992, p 217
2. Batshaw M: *Children With Disabilities*. Baltimore, MD: Paul Brookes Publishing, 1997, p 436

3. Waal N: A special technique. In: Caplan G, ed. *Emotional Problems of Early Childhood.* New York: Basic Books, 1955, p 431-49
4. Birt L, Lopez M: Don't give up: Matthew's story. *Mothering Magazine,* May/June:53, 2000
5. Batshaw M: *Children With Disabilities.* Baltimore, MD: Paul Brookes Publishing, 1997, p 436
6. Rimland B: Promising approaches. What the experts are finding. *Mothering Magazine,* May/June:51-52, 2000
7. About HANDLE. Available at: www.handle.org. Accessed December 15, 2002
8. Graziano AM, Kean JE: Programmed relaxation and reciprocal inhibition with psychotic children. *Behavior Research and Therapy,* 6:433-437, 1968
9. Meyed M: *Parents and Children in Autism.* Washington, DC: V.H. Winston, 1979
10. Field T: *Touch Therapy.* London, England: Churchill Livingston, 2000, p 97
11. Escalona A, et al: Brief report: Improvements in the behavior of children with autism following massage therapy. *Journal of Autism and Developmental Disorders,* 31:513, 2001
12. St. John J: *High-Tech Touch—Acupressure in the Schools.* Novato, CA: Academic Therapy Publications, 1987, p 57
13. Upledger J, Vredevoogd J: *Craniosacral Therapy,* Seattle, WA: Eastland Press, 1983, p 123

Catastrophic Illness

1. Field T, et al: Leukemia immune changes following massage therapy. *Journal of Bodywork and Movement Therapies,* p 271-274, 2001
2. Hernandez-Reif M, et al: Cystic fibrosis symptoms are reduced with massage therapy intervention. *Journal of Pediatric Psychology,* 24:183-189, 1999
3. Olness K: *Hypnosis and Hypnotherapy with Children.* New York: Guilford Press, 1996, p 294-297

Cerebral Palsy

1. Farlow P: Touch to teach: Massage helps special needs children. *Massage Magazine,* November/December:111, 2000
2. Batshaw M: *Children With Disabilities.* Baltimore, MD: Paul Brookes Publishing, 1997, p 511, 653
3. Stewart K: Massage for children with cerebral palsy. *Nursing Times,* 96:50-51, 2000
4. Hernandez-Reif M, et al: Cerebral palsy symptoms in children decreased following massage therapy. *Journal of Early Intervention* (In Review)
5. Edwards D, Bruce G: For cerebral palsy patients, massage makes life better. *Massage Magazine,* July/August:93-109, 2001
6. St. John J: *High-Tech Touch—Acupressure in the Schools.* Novato, CA: Academic Therapy Publications, 1987
7. Johnson V: My healing journey. *Massage Magazine,* July/August:97-101, 2001
8. Upledger J: *Craniospinal Therapy.* Seattle, WA: Eastland Press, 1983, p 116, 262
9. Bourne R: To Omar, with love. *Massage Therapy Journal,* Spring:68-76, 1996

10. Linkous L, Stutts RM: Passive stimulation effects on the muscle tone of hypotonic, developmentally delayed young children. *Perceptual Motor Skills,* 71:951-954, 1990
11. Campion M: *Hydrotherapy in Pediatrics.* Rockville, MD: Aspen Systems, 1985, p 215
12. Sumar S: *Yoga for the Special Child: A Therapeutic Approach for Infants and Children With Down Syndrome, Cerebral Palsy and Learning Disabilities.* Evanston, IL: Special Child Publications, 1998, p 41
13. Volpe R: Feedback facilitated relaxation training in school counseling. *Canadian Counselor,* 9:117, 1975
14. Kramer L: A second chance for Seth: One family battles cerebral palsy. *Family Circle,* March:114-118, 1990
15. Silberbush C: *The Feldenkrais Method With Cerebral Palsy Children.* Berkeley, CA: Advanced Feldenkrais Seminars, 1988
16. Bluestone J, ed: *The Churkendoose Anthology.* Seattle, WA: HANDLE Institute, 2002

Chronic Pain

1. Anderson A, Hotzan T, Masley J: *Physical Therapy in Bleeding Disorders.* New York: National Hemophilia Foundation, 2000, p 9
2. Long T, Toscano K: *Pediatric Physical Therapy,* Baltimore: Lippincott Williams & Wilkins, 2002 p 58
3. Sallfors C: Chronic pain in children suffering from juvenile chronic arthritis. *Developmental Medicine and Child Neurology,* 48:44, 2001 (suppl 89)
4. Wallace D: *Making Sense of Fibromyalgia: A Guide for Patients and Their Families.* Oxford, England: Oxford University Press, 1999, p 110
5. Backstrom G: *When Muscle Pain Won't Go Away.* Dallas, TX: Taylor Publishing, 1995, p 2
6. Starlanyl D: *Fibromyalgia and Chronic Myofascial Pain.* Oakland, CA: New Harbringer Publications, 1996, p 8, 144
7. Goldberg R, et al: Relationship between traumatic events in childhood and chronic pain. *Disability and Rehabilitation,* 21:23-30, 1999
8. Mikkelson Marja, et al: Psychiatric symptoms in preadolescents with musculoskeletal pain and fibromyalgia. *Pediatrics,* 100:113, 114, 1997
9. Calabro J: Fibromyalgia (fibrositis) in children. *The American Journal of Medicine,* 81:57-59, 1986 (suppl 3A)
10. Mowen K: Turning hurt into relief: Touching the hemophilia community. *Massage and Bodywork Magazine,* October/November:31-32, 1999
11. Qaiyumi S, quoted in Hunter TC: Massage therapy—Who kneads it? *Arthritis Today,* March/April:11, 1991
12. Field T, et al: Juvenile rheumatoid arthritis: benefits from massage therapy. *Journal of Pediatric Psychology,* 22:607-617, 1997
13. Sunshine, et al: Fibromyalgia benefits from massage therapy and transcutaneous electrical stimulation. *Journal of Clinical Rheumatology,* 2:18-22, 1996

Contractures

1. Werner D: *Disabled Village Children.* Palo Alto, CA: Hesperian, 1987, p 77-86

2. Sanell L: *Fundamentals of Pediatric Orthopedics.* Philadelphia, PA: Lippincott Raven, 1998

Developmental Delay

1. Batshaw M: *Children With Disabilities.* Baltimore, MD: Paul Brookes Publishing, 1997, p 146, 215
2. Voelker R: Putting mental retardation and mental illness on health care professionals' radar screen. *Journal of the American Medical Association,* 288:433, 2002
3. Farlow P: Touch to teach—Massage helps special-needs children. *Massage Magazine,* November/December:107-116, 2000
4. Marshalla-Rosenwinkle P: Oral-Motor Techniques in Articulation Therapy. Video available from Innovative Concepts, Seattle, WA
5. Sumar S: *Yoga for the Special Child. A Therapeutic Approach for Infants and Children With Down Syndrome, Cerebral Palsy, and Learning Disabilities.* Chicago, IL: Special Yoga Publications, 1998
6. Sanderson H, Harrison J, Price S: *Aromatherapy and Massage for People With Learning Disabilities.* Birmingham, England: Hands-On Press, 1991, p 156
7. The Use of Massage Therapy in the Treatment of Self-Injurious Behavior. Wayne County Intermediate School District, Special Projects Department, Allen Park, MI, 1986
8. Bright T: Reduction of self-injurious behavior using sensory-integrative techniques. *American Journal of Occupational Therapy,* 1981, 35:167-172
9. Wells ME: Reduction of self-injurious behavior of mentally retarded persons using sensory-integrative techniques. *American Journal of Mental Deficiency,* 87:664-666, 1983
10. Dosseter DR: Massage for very self-injurious behavior in a girl with Cornelia de Lange Syndrome. *Developmental Medicine and Child Neurology,* 33:636-640, 1991
11. Hernandez-Reif M, et al: Children with Down syndrome improved in motor function and muscle tone. *Journal of Early Intervention* (In Review)

Fetal Drug or Alcohol Exposure

1. Nathanielsz P: *Life in the Womb: The Origin of Health and Disease.* Ithaca, NY: Promethean Press, 1999, p 185
2. Batshaw M: *Children With Disabilities.* Baltimore, MD: Paul Brookes Publishing, 1997, p 109, 143, 146, 150, 153
3. Long T, Toscano K: *Handbook of Pediatric Physical Therapy.* Baltimore, MD: Lippincott Williams & Wilkins, 2002, p 49
4. Taddio A, et al: Conditioning and hyperalgesia in newborns exposed to repeated heel lances. *Journal of the American Medical Association,* August:857-866, 2002
5. Meir R: Torticollis. In: Burg F, et al: *Gellis and Kagan's Current Pediatric Physical Therapy.* Philadelphia, PA: W.B. Saunders, 1999, p 945
6. Simons D, Travell J: *Myofascial Pain and Dysfunction: The Triggerpoint Manual.* Vol. 1, ed. 2. Baltimore, MD: Lippincott Williams & Wilkins, 1999, 319

7. Simons D, Travell JG: *Myofascial Pain and Dysfunction: The Triggerpoint Manual.* Vol. 2. Baltimore, MD: Lippincott Williams &Wilkins, 1999
8. Field T: *Touch Therapy.* London, England: Churchill Livingston, 2000, p 17
9. Weber K: Massage for drug exposed infants. *Massage Therapy Journal,* 30:62, 1991
10. Gregory R: Massage for drug-exposed newborns. *Massage Magazine,* 45:44-54, 1993
11. Joyce P, Clark C: The use of craniosacral therapy to treat gastroesophageal reflux in infants. *Infants and Young Children,* 9:51-57, 1996
12. Wasserman AL, et al: Psychogenic basis for abdominal pain in children and adolescents. *Journal of the American Academy of Child and Adolescent Psychiatry,* 27:179, 1988

Hydrocephalus

1. Batshaw M: *Children With Disabilities.* Baltimore, MD: Paul Brookes Publishing, 1997, p 101, 535
2. Dodson J: *Baby Beautiful: A Handbook of Baby Head Shaping.* Eugene, OR: Heirs Press, 1994, p 193

Muscular Dystrophy

1. Schneider M, Gallup C: That person in the wheelchair needs your touch. *Massage Magazine,* 64:26, 1996
2. Ogden J: *Skeletal Injury in the Child.* Philadelphia, PA: Lea and Febiger, 1982, p 187
3. Batshaw M: *Children With Disabilities.* Baltimore, MD: Paul Brookes Publishing, 1997, p 325, 327
4. Schneider M: *Handbook of Self-Healing.* New York: Penguin Putnam, 2004, p 315-329
5. Schneider M, Gallup C: That person in the wheelchair needs your touch. *Massage Magazine,* 64:26-28, 1996

Scoliosis

1. Campbell S, Vander Linden D, Palisano R: *Physical Therapy for Children.* W.B. Saunders, 2000, p 263, 271
2. Travell J: *Myofascial Pain and Dysfunction: The Trigger Point Manual.* Vol. 1. Philadelphia, PA: Lippincott Williams & Wilkins, 1983, p 104, 616, 903
3. Pugh M, ed: *Stedman's Medical Dictionary.* 2000, Baltimore, MD: Lippincott Williams & Wilkins, p 1606
4. Schneider M: *Handbook of Self-Healing.* New York: Penguin Putnam, 2004, p 314

Tactile Defensiveness

1. Williams D: *Nobody Nowhere: The Extraordinary Biography of an Autistic.* New York, NY:Doubleday, 1992, p 72
2. Ayres J: *Sensory Integration and the Child.* Los Angeles, CA: Western Psychological Services, 1981, p 54, 107
3. Anneberg L: A Study of the Different Relaxation Techniques in Tactile Deficient and Tactile Defensive Children. Master's Thesis, University of Kansas, 1973
4. Sanderson H, Harrison J, Price S: *Aromatherapy and Massage for People with Learning Difficulties.* Birmingham, England: Hands-On Publishing, 1991, p 86

Wheelchair Riders

1. Werner D: *Disabled Village Children*. Palo Alto, CA: Hesperian Foundation, 1987, p 196-198
2. Parker P, Dietz LR: *Nursing at Home—A Practical Guide to the Care of the Sick and the Invalid in the Home, Plus Self-Help Instructions for the Patient*. New York, NY: Crown Publishers, 1989, p 95
3. Harris R: Manual lymph drainage. *Massage Therapy Journal*, Winter:61-65, 1992

SUGGESTED READINGS

1. Batshaw M: *Children With Disabilities*. Baltimore, MD: Paul Brookes Publishing, 1997
2. Cautela J, Groden J: *Relaxation: A Comprehensive Manual for Adults, Children, and Children with Special Needs*. Champaign, IL: Research Press, 1978
3. Fuhr M, Drehbohl K: *Pediatric Massage for the Child With Special Needs*. Tucson, AZ: Therapy Skill Builders, 2000
4. Krementz J: *How It Feels to Fight for Your Life*. Boston, MA: Little, Brown, 1989
5. Krementz J: *How It Feels to Live With a Physical Disability*. New York, NY: Simon and Schuster, 1992
6. Levine P: *Healing the Tiger. The Innate Capacity to Transform Overwhelming Experiences*. Berkeley, CA: North Atlantic Books, 1997
7. Terr L: *Too Scared to Cry: How Trauma Affects Our Children. . . and Ultimately Us All*. New York: Basic Books, 1990
8. Werner D: *Disabled Village Children*. Palo Alto, CA: Hesperian Foundation, 1988

TEACHING MASSAGE TO PARENTS

Parenthood is a tremendous challenge and opportunity and a long-term investment of time, patience, energy, money, worry, and affection. To meet a child's needs, parents must be nurses, chefs, psychotherapists, cheerleaders, chauffeurs, teachers, and disciplinarians. There are no easy parenting formulas that are successful for every child; strategies that are successful with one child may not work at all with another. Strategies that worked at one stage of a child's development may totally fail at the next stage. In addition to these challenges, parenthood in America is significantly more stressful than in many other countries because there is less support from the extended family. When the nuclear family has no support network to help—grandparents, aunts, uncles, and cousins—a greater share of the family burden falls on the mother and father. If a child is born with, or develops, any major problem, such as a disability, a difficult temperament, or a serious illness, parents are confronted with greater challenges and need even more inner and outer resources. It is important for any health care provider working with children to understand that parents are often under a great deal of stress, and that they, as well as their children, should be treated with respect and understanding.

Parents are empowered when they are medically informed and have a say in the child's care. Learning massage will help parents be strong and effective parents. Examples of parents who used massage therapy to help their children have been given in this book, including Rich and Diane Keene and Mary Polk. They not only changed their children's lives for the better, they became active, rather than passive, advocates for their children.

GUIDELINES

Parents should be taught massage to help in the following situations:

- *First-aid massage.* When a child has any discomfort, ache, or pain that occurs frequently, it will probably be the parents who are with them when this occurs, and it is unlikely that the child will be taken to a therapist for massage. The child who wakes up at night with gas pain or growing pains, who has a headache late in the day or muscle soreness after sports, or who needs help going to sleep should have a parent on the spot able to help.
- *Need for frequent massage.* Children often need massage more frequently than it is convenient to be seen by a professional or than the family can afford. A child who is chronically constipated should receive massage every day, or a child who is fighting a serious illness may need a short back massage every night to help him sleep. A child with a disability, such as cerebral palsy, profits by receiving 10 to 15 minutes of parental massage a day, in addition to regular weekly treatments with a massage therapist. Barry, a 50-year-old man with hemophilia, grew up at a time when most persons with hemophilia were immobilized after a joint bleed, and stretching was not advised. His father, a physician, believed in stretching the muscles and tendons after a bleed, instead of immobilizing the joint. Although it hurt and, at the time, Barry resented his father, stretching was done many times a day. Now, however, Barry does not have the severe arthritis of most men his age who have hemophilia; he says they envy his flexibility.[1]
- *Improved bonding between parent and child.* Massage can enhance the parent-child relationship by providing more physical contact and quality time. A special education teacher explained how an acupressure class helped her relationship with her son: "My 13-year-old son was the subject of three acupressure sessions during a 4-day period. In the evening, we would turn on a favorite TV program and *S.* would sit in front of me on the couch with his legs on a footstool. I would give him a neck and shoulder release, in addition to using other upper body pressure points. Each session continued for about 30 minutes. The results were that *S.* immediately relaxed and continued to relax deeply throughout the session. Each session ended with mother and son cuddling and watching TV. The results were somewhat a surprise to me because my son had refused physical affection from me for about 6 months, stating that he was too old. Apparently he still craved affection of this

nature and acupressure was an acceptable form to receive; *S.* requested more sessions in the future. Another related result is an increase of communication between us. Sometime after his second session, he asked me to sit down and talk with him, saying, "We need to talk more together." The acupressure sessions have aided our relationship to become closer."[2]

PRINCIPLES

Massage therapists should keep in mind the following principles:

- Parents bring their children for massage therapy out of love and concern and should always be honored for this.
- Ask the parents how much time they have available to massage their children. If they do not have a lot of time, help them find a way to incorporate massage into the normal family routine. It is important not to overload the family with an expectation they are unable to meet. Never make the family feel guilty. Perhaps, if the parents are normally present during the child's bath time, massage can be done in the bathtub using soap lather. Or, children could receive massage at bedtime when the parents usually read to them.
- Listen carefully to what parents and children tell you; however, do not give parenting advice. The parent is the expert on their child, and the hands-on therapist is the expert on massage.
- Find out what the family knows about massage. Many parents already use small massage treatments to help their children. They may have massaged a newborn baby's tear duct to unblock it, rubbed tender gums to relieve painful swelling in a teething baby, or rubbed an injection site after an immunization to keep it from bruising. Many parents instinctively rub their children's backs to help them relax or sleep and massage them when they have pain at night, such as leg cramps or a stomachache.
- Keep instructions simple; do not overload the parents. Four strokes may be all they can absorb at one session. Anatomic terminology and technical information is not necessary. The 4-Stroke handout was created to help parents to go home and remember what was taught. Remembering four simple strokes at home is better than being taught many additional strokes and not remembering any strokes well.
- If possible, give parents a short massage session each time they come in with their child. Do not

force massage on them; if they would like to be massaged for just a short time, they do not need to disrobe or have massage oil applied to their skin. A simple massage may consist of kneading the neck and shoulders, petrissage of the palms or scalp, or using a ball to massage the back. Even 5 minutes of massage is enjoyable; this helps parents understand how the strokes feel and can motivate them to continue massage with their children.

- Always find something both honest and positive to tell parents about their parenting. This may be only something small, such as how they help the child do something, or how they relate to the child during massage. Build on the parent's strengths.

HOW TO TEACH MASSAGE TO PARENTS

Therapists can teach parents effective massage by using the following steps:

1. Use the 4-Stroke Massage handout as the basic teaching tool. Give the parents the handout and explain that you will teach them four different strokes that can be used on any part of the body.
2. With the child on the table and the parents watching, do all four strokes on the same part of the body. Then, as the parents try each stroke, offer any needed corrections. For example, if they want to learn how to massage the back, demonstrate warming (effleurage), thumbstroking (petrissage), kneading, and raking on different parts of the back. Then watch as they do each stroke and offer suggestions.
3. Demonstrate the basic relaxation sequence.
4. Write any special tips on the parent's 4-Stroke Massage instruction sheet (e.g., how many times to do a certain stroke or the best time of day to do massage).
5. Explain the contraindications on the instruction sheet.
6. Discuss the Troubleshooting and the Screening for Stress handouts.
7. Tell the parents that you are available to answer any questions.

REFERENCES

1. Finston P: *Parenting Plus—Raising Children With Special Health Needs.* New York: Dutton, 1990, p 98
2. San Benito County Special Teacher Education, quoted in Project PRES Newsletter, Capitola, CA, Winter:6:1986

MASSAGE STROKES

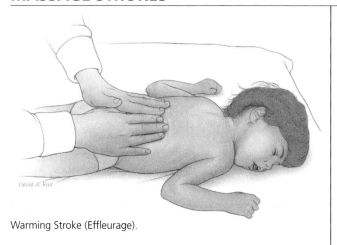

Warming Stroke (Effleurage).

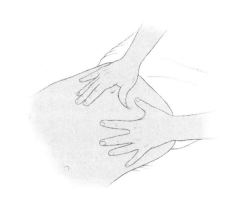

Thumbstroking.

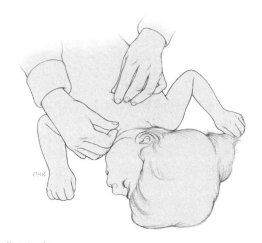

Kneading Stroke.

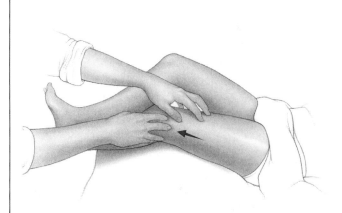

Raking Stroke.

Perform the basic relaxation sequence to help teach your child to relax.

Special tips or instructions:

_____

_____

_____

_____

_____

_____

_____

_____

.

 CAUTION: Do not massage skin with sores, cuts, burns, boils, or infectious rashes, such as scabies. Do not massage inflamed joints, tumors, or any undiagnosed lumps. In the event of injuries, such as severe bruises, joint sprains, broken bones or dislocations, or chronic medical conditions, consult with your child's physician before beginning massage

TROUBLESHOOTING

The more you massage your child, the easier it will be for the child to release tension. However, everyone responds differently to massage each day, depending on their mood, tension level, need for closeness, exercise, and other factors. When massage does not seem to be working, for whatever reason, here are some ideas to help your child relax during the massage.

PROBLEM: MY CHILD FLINCHES OR WITHDRAWS WHEN A SPECIFIC AREA IS TOUCHED.

Possible solutions:

1. Ask your child how the area feels. Then ask if it is all right to massage there.
2. Place your palms on the area gently and slowly. Have the child do the basic relaxation sequence and then try massage again.
3. Continue massaging, but use very light pressure.
4. Move to an area where massage *is* comfortable, such as the back, and return to the first area when your child is relaxed.

PROBLEM: MY CHILD IS EXTREMELY TENSE AND CANNOT RELAX.

Possible solutions:

1. Do the basic relaxation sequence a few times.
2. Massage the area where the child feels most comfortable (often, the back).
3. Suggest a 20-minute warm bath. Try massage again.
4. Talk to your child about what is causing the tension.
5. Give your child a book to read during the massage.
6. Play soft music.
7. Wrap your child in a warm sheet or towel or give your child a hot pack or hot water bottle.

PROBLEM: MY CHILD CANNOT LIE STILL.

Possible solutions:

1. Do the basic relaxation sequence a few times.
2. Don't restrain your child! Try doing just a little massage each time. Doing less massage now often means you can do more later, as tolerance for touch increases.
3. Pick a time when your child is very relaxed, such as nap time or bedtime.
4. Use soap lather and massage the child's upper body when he or she is in the bathtub.
5. Follow the child around and do massage as he or she plays.
6. Tell a story or sing; this may hold a small child's attention.

PROBLEM: MY CHILD IS TICKLISH (TOO MUCH TICKLING CAN ALSO CAUSE THIS)

Possible solutions:

1. Do not persist or try to make the child ignore the tickles. This drives tension inward.
2. Try heavy pressure with your palms. Light pressure makes tickles worse.
3. Hold your hands over the area and let the child feel the warmth of your hands.
4. Massage the ticklish area when your child is just about to fall asleep.

PROBLEM: MY CHILD IS ANXIOUS ABOUT BEING UNDRESSED.

Possible solutions:

1. Respect your child's privacy. Use a sheet or towel to cover the entire body, except for the part being massaged.
2. Let your child remain clothed; massage head, neck and shoulders, hands, and feet.
3. Do pressure points through clothes (ask your therapist for instructions).

SCREENING FOR STRESS

Everyone experiences stress in a unique way; however, there are many indications when a child is stressed. No single symptom is an indicator of stress or underlying emotional disturbance. Many emotional problems can be reflected by the same symptoms. Look for clusters of symptoms that endure for extended periods.

It is difficult to compile a list of all the red-flag behaviors your child might display. The following list attempts to provide a comprehensive reference. This is a good start.

EMOTIONAL SIGNS:

- Worked up, excited
- Worried, anxious
- Crying spells
- At loose ends
- Forgetful, confused
- Memory loss or lapses
- Difficulty concentrating, inattentive, distractible
- Sleeps too much or can not sleep, nightmares, fitful sleep
- Overeating, not eating
- Excessive snacking
- Depression, apathy
- Not responsive to nurturing efforts or comments
- Persistent fatigue
- Lowered level of achievement or performance
- Complains of being dizzy and disoriented
- Grouchy, irritable
- Makes excessive demands
- Bed-wetting, daytime wetting, or soiling
- Nervous
- Paces about, cannot sit still
- Excessive or irrational fear
- Panic or anxiety
- Clinging or overly dependent on caregiver
- Obsessive, repetitive, or ritualistic behavior
- Finger-tapping, foot-tapping, pencil-tapping, or leg tremors
- Frowning or scowling
- Anger outbursts, temper tantrums, aggressive acting out

BODY SIGNS:

- Upset stomach, nausea, churning sensation
- Heartburn, acid indigestion
- Intestinal upset or cramps
- Fast or irregular heartbeat
- Clammy, cold, or clenched hands
- Light-headedness or faintness
- Hot or cold spells
- Increased blood pressure
- Loss of breath or uneven breathing pattern
- Feels "tight" all over
- Tingling sensations on skin
- Cold sores in mouth or lips
- Feeling sick, with no observable symptoms
- Grinding teeth, jaw clenching
- Headaches
- Backaches and other muscular aches
- Low-grade infections
- Generalized body pain
- Hives
- Rash or acne
- Increased asthma or allergies
- Constipation or diarrhea
- Coughing, habitual throat clearing or vocalizations
- Dry mouth or throat
- Tight and stiff muscles
- Muscle twitching, facial tics
- Stuttering or stammering
- Inability to stand still or stay in one place
- Shaky hands
- Onset of poor vision
- Increased perspiration

When more than three or four of these signs are demonstrated within a week or so, there is a strong possibility your child is experiencing high stress levels. Emotional problems could also be part of the picture.

Adapted from Martin G: *Help! My Child Isn't Learning*. Colorado Springs, CO: Focus on the Family Publishing, p 41-43.

GLOSSARY

Affect: State of mind or emotional response.

Amblyopia: Also called *lazy eye.* Amblyopia occurs when one eye rolls in a different direction from the other: nothing is wrong with the optic equipment. The eye sends a poorly focused image to the brain, which can cause the loss of vision-related brain cells. Because the brain cannot fuse the two images into one image, it suppresses one image. The child with amblyopia has poor vision because the visual areas of the brain did not correctly develop before age 6.

Anomaly: A deviation from the general rule. In anatomy, an anomaly is any anatomic difference from the norm. For example, vertebrae that are differently shaped than normal are vertebral anomalies.

Anorexia nervosa: Literally means "without desire." A mental disorder characterized by an intense fear of gaining weight or becoming fat; a disturbance in the way an individual experiences weight, size, or shape; a low or life-threatening body weight; denial of the seriousness of the current low body weight; and, in girls, loss of menstruation. At least 25% of those who are anorexic eventually die of this disorder.

Astigmatism: Near and far vision are blurred as a result of a misshapen cornea or lens of the eye.

Ataxia: The inability to coordinate voluntary muscle activity during voluntary movement.

Atlantoaxial instability: The laxity of the transverse ligaments that hold the odontoid process of the second cervical vertebrae close to the anterior arch of the first cervical vertebrae. To prevent subluxation and spinal cord injury, individuals with this condition should avoid exercises that place pressure on the neck muscles or any activity that causes extreme forward flexion of the neck.

Behr syndrome: A syndrome characterized by mental retardation, visual deficits, ataxia, and spasticity. Although the cause is unknown, it is thought to be genetic.

Bulimia: [Greek, *hunger of an ox*] A chronic disorder characterized by repeat episodes of binge eating (rapidly eating large quantities of food), followed by self-induced vomiting. Self-evaluation is unduly influenced by body shape and weight. Despite a lack of outcome studies on bulimia nervosa, many clinicians believe that it will be shown that patients who are bulimic have a higher mortality rate than anorexics.

Cataract: Clouding of the lens of the eye, causing blurred vision and, in severe cases, white pupils.

Catatonia: A syndrome characterized by stupor or temporary loss of feeling and consciousness. Often found in schizophrenia.

Chorea: Irregular, spasmodic, involuntary movement of the limbs or facial muscles, often accompanied by hypotonia. Caused by a cerebral lesion of an unknown definition.

Conversion reaction: An unconscious defense mechanism in which anxiety that is caused by an unconscious conflict is converted and expressed symbolically as a physical symptom; an emotion is transformed into a physical manifestation. For example, cases have been reported such as a child who cannot walk although no pathology is found, or a child who has extreme pain with no organic cause. Rather than a major psychiatric disorder, a conversion reaction represents a form of body language— a plea for help from a child with no alternative method of communicating stress.

Cortisol: A steroidal hormone secreted by the adrenal cortex in response to stressors, such as extreme temperatures, rage, or fear. Cortisol is the most potent, naturally occurring, anti-inflammatory glucocorticoid hormone.

Craniosacral therapy: A gentle, hands-on therapy that addresses distortions in the bone and connective tissue of the skull, spine, and sacrum. Craniosacral therapy balances the flow of the cerebrospinal fluid and relieves tissue restriction throughout the body.

Cutaneous: Pertaining to the skin.

Danceability: A dance form, based on contact improvisation, that helps all children, with and without disabilities, discover the joy of self-expression through movement. Helps break down barriers between those with and without disabilities.

Debridement: Removal of dead tissue and foreign matter from a wound, often with a brush. Debridement is often painful.

Developmental delay: A delay or slowness in a child's development. A term often used interchangeably with mental retardation; however, a child can be delayed in some areas of his or her development without the IQ being affected.

Diplegia: Paralysis of corresponding parts on both sides of the body.

Encopresis: Persistent fecal soiling with no organic cause. A child is not considered to have encopresis until he is at least 4 years old because most toilet training is not complete until age 2¹/₂ years and a margin of error is allowed.

Endorphin: An opioid peptide hormone that may alter pain perception; thought to be analgesic (pain-killing) in action.

Eustachian tube: A tube that runs from each middle ear to the throat. Also called the pharyngotympanic tube because it connects the tympanic cavity to the nasopharynx.

Exocrine gland: A gland that secretes externally, either directly or through a duct. A sweat gland is an example of an exocrine gland.

Feldenkrais technique: A system of movement therapy pioneered by Moshe Feldenkrais. Based on gentle movements and performed with focused awareness, the technique improves ease of movement.

Growth hormone: A hormone produced by the pituitary gland that promotes body growth and fat mobilization.

HANDLE: Holistic Approach to NeuroDevelopment and Learning Efficiency. An integrative approach to identify and treat neurodevelopment disorders in children and adults that includes principles and perspectives from medicine, rehabilitation, psychology, education, and nutrition. The program focuses on the weaknesses in the child's neurologic system that are causing learning and social problems. Attention deficit disorder, autism, head injury, cerebral palsy, motor problems, hypersensitivity, obsessive-compulsive disorder, and other behavioral challenges may improve by addressing these basic weaknesses. Children are given a comprehensive neurodevelopmental assessment and a daily exercise program to strengthen the nervous system.

Hemiplegia: Paralysis of one side of the body.

Hydrocephalus: Excess fluid between the brain and the skull (see Hydrocephalus, Chapter 6).

Hydrochloric acid: An acid secreted by the stomach; part of the gastric juices that help digest proteins.

Hypermobility: Excessive range of motion in a joint, commonly caused by slack or relaxed ligaments around the joint. Diagnosis of whole-body hypermobility may be made if three of the following signs are present: (1) Opposition of the thumb to the flexor aspect of the forearm; (2) Excessive dorsiflexion of the ankle and eversion of the foot; (3) Hyperextension of the elbows or knees by more than 10 degrees; and (4) Hyperextension of the fingers parallel to the extensor aspect of the forearm.

Hyperopia: Blurred near vision. Also called *farsightedness*.

Hypopituitarism: Inadequate secretion of pituitary hormones, with deficiencies in adrenocorticotropic hormone (ACTH) and somatotrophic growth hormone.

Ischemia: A lack of blood flow in a specific area, usually a result of constriction or damage to the arterial blood supply.

Jin Shin Do: A synthesis of traditional Oriental acupressure/acupuncture theory and technique with Taoist philosophy and modern psychology. Jin Shin Do releases muscular tension and stress through application of gradually deeper finger pressure to specific acupressure points on the body.

Kyphosis: An overdeveloped curve of the thoracic spine.

Leg-length discrepancy: When one leg is shorter than the other. The leg bone may actually be anatomically shorter, but instead the child may have muscle spasm, bad postural habits, or other factors that contribute to a functional discrepancy.

Malocclusion: A condition caused when the upper and lower teeth do not properly fit together.

Meconium: The first intestinal discharge of the newborn infant, consisting of mucus, bile, and epithelial cells. If meconium is aspirated by the newborn, it can cause aspiration pneumonia.

Medical hypnosis: Hypnosis administered by a physician.

Melatonin: A hormone, manufactured by the pineal gland, that is linked to sleep-wake cycles. Ordinarily, melatonin levels in the blood increase 10-fold just before sleep and peak around midnight.

Meningitis: An inflammation of the brain and meninges (spinal cord membranes), often caused by a bacterial infection. Meningitis most seriously affects children between ages 6 to 12 months. It can be fatal; in survivors, it can cause paralysis and mental retardation.

Mental retardation: A slowness or limitation in mental development. Often used interchangeably with the term *developmental delay*. Some individuals with developmental delay have normal IQs that may only become clear when those delays are treated.

Metastasize: To pass or invade; for example, dissemination of tumor cells by the lymphatics or blood cells.

Myopia: Blurred distance vision. Also called *near-sightedness*.

Neurofeedback: A nondrug therapy for attention deficit hyperactivity disorder (ADHD) and epilepsy. Electroencephalogram (EEG) sensors are placed on a child's head, and the brain waves are displayed on a video screen in an interactive game format. With practice, the child learns to change his or her brainwaves in order to score points on the game. Over time, neurofeedback teaches the child with ADHD to control his activity level and concentration and the child with epilepsy to decrease the number of seizures he or she has.

Norepinephrine: A vasoconstrictor stress hormone, secreted by the adrenals.

Occlusion: The act of closing. In dentistry, it refers to the way the upper and lower teeth contact. A normal occlusion occurs when the upper and lower teeth on both sides of the mouth come together at the same time. A malocclusion is when the teeth come together in an abnormal way, such as when the upper and lower teeth meet on one side before the other.

Ossification: The formation of osseous (bone) tissue by replacing cartilage with calcium phosphate, a mineral salt. Calcium phosphate occupies about 65% of the bone mass and gives it strength. The remainder of the bone mass is a collagen matrix that gives the bone elasticity.

Osteotomy: [*oste*, Latin for bone; *tomy*, Latin for incision] Cutting a bone.

Periodontal: Literally "around the teeth." It usually refers to the tissues around the teeth—the gums and bony tissues. Periodontal disease is most often an inflammation or infection of the gums.

Poliomyelitis: [*polio*, gray matter; *myelos*, marrow; *itis*, inflammation] Caused by the polio virus, this inflammation of the spinal cord leads to death or irreversible damage to nerve cells.

Polydipsia: Extreme thirst.

Prolotherapy: A therapy for torn ligaments, in which the ligament is injected with a sclerosing agent that causes the ligament to grow shorter and tighter.

Proprioception: The sense (perception) of the movement and position of the body, independent of visual input. This sense helps the child identify his location in space and his relationship to the external world. Proprioception is formed primarily from information coming from sensory nerve fibers in soft tissues and the vestibular apparatus. For example, information from the tendons tells position, length, and to what degree the fibers are being stretched; information from the fibrous capsules of joints gives feedback on joint activity and position.

Pyloristenosis: A malformation of the stomach muscle that blocks the passage of food from the stomach to the small intestine. Pyloristenosis must be treated surgically.

Quadriplegia: Paralysis of both arms and both legs.

Reflex sympathetic dystrophy: Diffuse persistent pain, usually in an extremity, and frequently following some local injury. Reflex sympathetic dystrophy is often associated with limitation or immobility of joints and vasomotor instability. In extreme cases, it leads to joint contractures and osteoporosis.

Retinopathy of prematurity: Damage to the retina caused by the administration of oxygen to premature infants. The child may develop cataracts, glaucoma, nearsightedness, or strabismus.

Spica cast: A cast made up of layers that overlap in a V pattern. It covers two body parts of greatly different size, such as the waist and the hip.

Synapse: A space between two neurons. Nerve impulses are transmitted from one neuron to another by chemicals called neurotransmitters.

Synostosis: When two bones, not normally united, grow together.

Swedish massage: Developed by Per Henrik Ling of Sweden in the nineteenth century, Swedish massage is a combination of five techniques (effleurage, petrissage, friction, tapotement and vibration), combined with passive joint movement.

Strabismus: The turning of an eye, either to the side or up or down, so that both eyes are unable to simultaneously look at the same thing. Also known as *crossed eyes*.

Therapeutic touch: A healing method in which the practitioner does not touch the body; the hands are held above the body in the person's energy field. The goal of therapeutic touch is to release any blockages in the person's energy field, contributing to release of tension, strengthening the person's own healing powers, and improving health.

Torticollis: Twisted neck; the head is persistently flexed and rotated. Commonly caused by fibrous shortening of the sternocleidomastoid muscle as a result of abnormal uterine position; birth trauma; cervical trauma; head tilt caused by vertical strabismus; malformations of the occipital or cervical bones; and inflammatory conditions of the neck tissue, such as pharyngitis or cellulitis. Congenital torticollis resolves spontaneously in 90% of cases, assuming the child does not have vertebral anomalies. Therapy may be prescribed that can be done by parents, with gentle stretches of the tightened sternocleidomastoid muscle. If physical therapy is not successful, children with torticollis may require surgery to release the sternocleidomastoid muscle, with postoperative physical therapy and splinting.

Trigger point: A hyperirritable area in a muscle that, when stimulated, can cause spasm and pain. Trigger points usually manifest as palpable nodules in taut bands of muscle. In contrast to tender points, which hurt only where they are touched, trigger points are tender where they are touched, but pain is also referred to an adjacent area of the body. Trigger points may result from sudden trauma, chronic repetitive strain, or prolonged chilling. Acute and chronic infections and fatigue may also predispose a muscle to develop a trigger point.

Trigger point therapy: Application of concentrated finger pressure to trigger points to break cycles of spasm and pain, as well as for relaxation.

Vestibular stimulation: Stimulation of the inner ear, often by techniques such as rocking or swinging a child.

Watsu: A form of Shiatsu massage performed in a pool of warm water. The therapist cradles the child, who floats in the water as the therapist performs a sequence of movements and Shiatsu pressure.

INDEX

Page numbers followed by t indicate table. Page numbers in *italics* indicate figure or box.

Rice Sensorimotor Stimulation Technique, *159*
Rice, Ruth, 159
Ritalin, 16, 166
Rolfing, 2, *3, 4, 172*, 172

S

Safe environment, for massage, 48–49
Salt glow, *93*, 93–94, 140, 193
Scalp, petrissage, 78–79, *80*
Scar tissue, 109–111
    hydrotherapy for, 110
    massage for, 110–111
    problems related to, 110
School-age children
    adapting massage for, 45
    body image development in, 24
    depression symptoms in, 125
    typical vital signs in, *31*
Scoliosis, 187–189, *188*
    approach and goals, 188–189
    causes of, 187–188
    massage for, 189
Seizure disorder, 176
Self-touching, 26
Sensorimotor Stimulation Technique, Rice, *159*
Sensory stimulation, 67–68, *70* (See also Skin stimulation; Tactile stimulation)
    for developmental delay, 181–182
    effects of massage on, *9, 9*
Sexual abuse, 12, 24, 157–160
    adult health problems related to, 158
    approach and goals, 158–159
    defined, 157
    of disabled children, 155
    massage guidelines, 159–160
Sexual activity, increased, effects on children, 15
Shoulder
    massage for, *78–79*, 144
    muscle tension in, 143–144
    passive range of motion for, 65–66, *68*
Shunting, for hydrocephalus, 184, *184*
Sinus congestion, 120–121, 137
Sinus headache, 137–138
Sinus irrigation, 121
Skin, *38*
Skin stimulation, 67–68, *70*
    arm, 85
    back, 74
    chest and abdomen, 84
    face, 79
    leg (back), 77
    leg (Front), 90
Skull, development of, *37*
Social development
    infant, 33–34
    preschool children, 36
    school-age children, 36–37
    teenagers, 41–42
Social isolation, in disabled children, 153–154
Soft-tissue end-feel, *66*
Sore throat, 144–145
    approach and goals, 144
    hydrotherapy for, 144–145

massage for, 145
Spastic cerebral palsy, 171
Spasticity, 172
Spinal cord injury (SCI), 7, 111–114
    case study, 113
    hydrotherapy for, 112
    massage for, 112–113
    problems related to, 111
Sports
    effect on children, 13
    injuries from, *98*
Sprains, 114–116
    approach and goals, 114–115
    classifications of, 114
    hydrotherapy for, 115–116
    massage for, 116
    treatment of, 114
Steam inhalation, 121, 164
Sternocleidomastoid muscle
    massage of, 128, *128*
    torticollis and, 147–148
Stomach, massage for, 79–84, *82–83*, 124, *125*, 146
Stomachache, 145–146
Stress(es), 156
    asthma and, 162–163
    back pain and, 139
    behavioral effects of, 13, 15–16
    bodily response to, 16–18
    bone response to, *106*
    child stress scale, 14t
    of children, 11–13
    common cold and, *120*
    effects on health, *18*, 18–20
    emotional signs of, 203
    eye fatigue and, 129–130
    headache and, 136–137
    long-term effects, 20–21
    massage therapy for, 21
    mind-body approaches to, 18, *19*
    muscle tension and, 144
    physical signs of, 203
    prenatal, *17*
    screening for, 203
Stretching program
    for contractures, 179
    for growing pains, 133, *133*
Stroke
    selection of, 72
    sequence of, 72
Substance abuse (See also Fetal alcohol syndrome; Fetal drug exposure)
    effects on children, 15
Suicide issues, effects on children, 15
Swallowing problems, 20
Swedish massage, 7 (See also Massage; specific body part; specific disorder)
    adapting for children, 71–72
    advantages for children, 57–59
    components of, 57
        effleurage, 58–59, *59*
        friction, 60, *61*
        passive range of motion (See Passive range of motion)
        passive touch, 58, *58*
        petrissage, 59–60, *60*
        tapotement, 60–62, *61–62*

sequence for full body, 72–90
Synapses, 9

T

Tactile defensiveness, 189–191
    abuse and, 158
    approach and goals, 190
    case study, 52
    defined, 189
    examples of, 189
    hydrotherapy for, 190
    massage for, 190–191
    treatment of, 183
Tactile deprivation, *9*, 9–11
    causes of, 23–24
Tactile stimulation (See also Skin stimulation)
    in disabled children, 152–153
    for tactile defensiveness, 190
Tapotement, 60–62, *61–62*
    cupping, 62, *62*
    pincement, 62, *62*
    tapping, 61, *61*
Tapping, 61, *61*
Teenagers
    adapting massage for, 45, 47–48
    body image development in, 24–25
    depression symptoms in, 125
    typical vital signs in, *31*
Television, 12, 158
Tension stomachache, 145–146
Terminal illness, 170
Therapeutic touch, 163 (See also Touch)
Thumbstroking, 59–60, *60*
    arm, 84, *85*
    back, 73–74, *74*
    foot, 89, *90*
    hand, 84–85, *86–87*
    leg (back), 76, 77
    stomach, 124, *125*
    teaching parents, 201
Thyroxin, 17
Ticklish, 202
Toddlers (See Preschool children)
Toe massage, 89, *90*
Torticollis, *40*, 147, 147–148
Touch (See also Skin stimulation)
    for asthma treatment, 163
    fear of, 1 (See also Tactile defensiveness)
    importance of, 2, *3*, 10–11
    between parent and child, 10
    passive, 58, *58*
    tactile deprivation, *9*, 9–11, 23–24
Trauma
    child's response to, 157–158
    depression and, 125
    early, 21, 143
Trauma Touch program, 159, *159*
Traumatic brain injury, 116–117
    approach and goals, 116–117
    incidence of, 116
    massage for, 117
    problems related to, 116
Trigger points, 4, *4–6*, 7, 21
    early causes of, *40–41*
    fractures and, 107–108
    scoliosis and, 187–188
Type A behavior, in children, 15, *16*